INTRODUCTION TO
HEALTH BEHAVIORS

A GUIDE FOR MANAGERS, PRACTITIONERS & EDUCATORS

MARIETTA ORLOWSKI

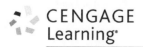

CENGAGE
Learning®

Australia • Brazil • Mexico • Singapore • United Kingdom • United States

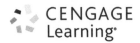
CENGAGE
Learning®

**Introduction to Health Behaviors:
A Guide for Managers, Practitioners &
Educators**
Marietta Orlowski

SVP, GM Skills & Global Product
Management: Dawn Gerrain

Product Manager: Jadin Kavanaugh

Senior Director, Development: Marah
Bellegarde

Product Development Manager: Juliet
Steiner

Content Developer: Lauren Whalen

Product Assistant: Mark Turner

Marketing Director: Michele McTighe

Marketing Manager: Erica Glisson

Senior Director, Production: Wendy Troeger

Production Director: Andrew Crouth

Content Project Management and Art
Direction: Lumina Datamatics, Inc.

Cover Image: Galyna Andrushko/
Shutterstock

Library of Congress Control Number: 2014947842

ISBN-13: 978-1-285-17262-0

Cengage Learning
20 Channel Center Street
Boston, MA 02210
USA

Cengage Learning is a leading provider of customized learning solutions
with office locations around the globe, including Singapore, the United
Kingdom, Australia, Mexico, Brazil, and Japan. Locate your local office at
www.cengage.com/global.

Cengage Learning products are represented in Canada by
Nelson Education, Ltd.

To learn more about Cengage Learning, visit **www.cengage.com**

Purchase any of our products at your local college store or at our
preferred online store **www.cengagebrain.com**.

Notice to the Reader

Publisher does not warrant or guarantee any of the products described herein or perform any independent analysis in connection with any of
the product information contained herein. Publisher does not assume, and expressly disclaims, any obligation to obtain and include information other than that provided to it by the manufacturer. The reader is expressly warned to consider and adopt all safety precautions that might
be indicated by the activities described herein and to avoid all potential hazards. By following the instructions contained herein, the reader
willingly assumes all risks in connection with such instructions. The publisher makes no representations or warranties of any kind, including
but not limited to, the warranties of fitness for particular purpose or merchantability, nor are any such representations implied with respect to
the material set forth herein, and the publisher takes no responsibility with respect to such material. The publisher shall not be liable for any
special, consequential, or exemplary damages resulting, in whole or part, from the readers' use of, or reliance upon, this material.

Printed in the United States of America
Print Number: 01   Print Year: 2022

TABLE OF CONTENTS

SECTION 1	INTRODUCTION TO HEALTH BEHAVIORS & DISEASE PREVENTION	

Learning Objectives

1. Describe a broad multidimensional definition of health.
2. Explain the role of risk and protective factors in disease and injury reduction.
3. Give examples of biological, social, behavioral, and environmental risk and protective factors.
4. Compare the targets of primary, secondary, and tertiary prevention.
5. Classify information into correct levels of the disease prevention model.
6. Discuss current population-level disease, death, and injury targets.

In the News ...

CHAPTER 2	**WHAT IS A HEALTH BEHAVIOR?**	**27**

Learning Objectives

1. Define a health behavior.
2. Distinguish between a behavior and the factors that influence a behavior.
3. Discuss behaviors that have significant impact on population health status.
4. State health behaviors in measurable forms for select target audiences.
5. Recognize the presence and related outcomes of health behaviors in communities.
6. Use existing data sets to prepare a summary of health behavior rates for a defined community.

In the News ...

CHAPTER 3	**SOCIAL DETERMINANTS OF HEALTH**	**54**

Learning Objectives

1. Give examples of social determinants of health.
2. Describe situations in which health behaviors are linked with social conditions of living.
3. Describe components of socioeconomic position and three pathways linking socioeconomic status (SES) components to health outcomes.
4. Identify neighborhood factors that influence a person's ability to perform health behaviors.
5. Discuss the role of early life experiences and the trajectories established with health and behaviors later in life.
6. Assess barriers to health care and health promotion participation across different types of disability.

SECTION 2	HEALTH BEHAVIOR THEORY

CHAPTER 4	SOCIAL ECOLOGICAL MODELS AND HEALTH BEHAVIOR THEORY	80

Learning Objectives
1. Describe the role of health behavior theory in understanding health behaviors.
2. Identify components of health behavior theories.
3. Identify multiple levels of influence within a social ecological model.
4. Describe and classify factors of influence for personal health behaviors.
5. Assess attributes of place-based factors that influence health behavior.
6. Explain why social ecological models are used mainly as a long-term view of health promotion planning and are not often seen in short-term planning.

In the News ...

CHAPTER 7   THEORIES OF NETWORKS AND COMMUNITIES   140

Learning Objectives
1. Describe properties of social networks.
2. Explain how relationship ties influence the spread of information, resources, and health behaviors.
3. Identify properties of groups that influence community action.
4. Categorize stage of community readiness in a population.
5. Classify network members by the extent of innovativeness and explain how membership influences the movement of ideas and behaviors.
6. Compare a system approach to interpersonal approaches to behavioral change.

In the News ...

CHAPTER 8   INTEGRATING HEALTH BEHAVIOR THEORIES AND BUILDING A THEORETICAL MODEL   168

Learning Objectives
1. Determine behavioral constructs common to multiple health behavior theories.
2. Classify health behavior constructs of seven theories by stage of change.
3. Express health behavior constructs in general lay terms.
4. Identify primary and secondary methods for determining behavioral antecedents in populations.
5. Diagram a theory-based logic model, synthesizing constructs from multiple health behavior theories.

SECTION 3 — Applying Theory to Improve Practice

CHAPTER 9   OUTCOME LOGIC MODELS: THE PICTURE OF PROGRAM
PLANNING AND EVALUATION

Learning Objectives
1. Identify the common steps in the process of health promotion programming.
2. Link the process of health assessment, planning, implementation, and evaluation to logic modeling.
3. Identify components of an outcome logic model.
4. Explain a program's assumptions and anticipated outcomes illustrated in an outcome logic model.
5. Construct an outcome logic model, aligning behavioral targets to activities and outcomes.

In the News ...

CHAPTER 10   **EVIDENCE-BASED INTERVENTIONS**   **218**

Learning Objectives

1. Discuss strategies within the five categories of health promotion interventions.
2. Match intervention strategies to type of antecedent and anticipated population health impact.
3. Locate evidence-based health promotion programs.
4. Complete the process for creating evidence-based programs.

In the News ...

CHAPTER 11   **INFANT MORTALITY IN MONTGOMERY COUNTY, OHIO: A CASE STUDY**   **247**

Learning Objectives

1. List five established causes of infant mortality.
2. Discuss behaviors that significantly impact population-level infant mortality.
3. Identify traits and conditions of the social environment associated with birth outcomes.
4. Locate local infant mortality rates and sources of behavioral, social, and geographical factors of influence.
5. Discuss aspects of a life course perspective to improving birth outcomes and how this may differ from traditional health promotion programs.

6. Classify infant death, birth outcomes, and influential factors into correct levels of the disease prevention model.
7. Explain the behavioral assumptions, aligned activities, and anticipated outcomes in an established health promotion program.

PREFACE

Introduction

Introduction to Health Behaviors: A Guide for Managers, Practitioners & Educators is written specifically for professionals who are new to health behavior theory and who feel challenged to shape the health behaviors of others. Health behaviors significantly influence health status and as the country moves toward a population health focus, many more professionals are being called upon to design programs and policies that improve the health status of many. Groups of employees, patients, school-age children, and neighbors are potential audiences for health promotion initiatives. Thus, program managers, health care providers, educators, public health professionals, and community members need to be well versed in evidence-based health behavior strategies.

Successful health promotion initiatives are grounded in health behavior theory, and successful programs often combine concepts from across behavioral theories. The goal of this text is to introduce behavioral science concepts, theories, and planning strategies in a practice-oriented manner.

With its unique applied approach to learning theoretical constructs, *Introduction to Health Behaviors* changes the way learners think and behave in relationship to planning health promotion programs. This text introduces theory as a foundation of deep factual knowledge that is then synthesized and built upon in ways that help students understand the relationships between behaviors and health, antecedents and behaviors, and interventions and antecedents. An innovative chapter on the PER worksheet, a tool that combines the eight most popular health behavior theories into one framework, teaches learners how to organize facts across the different theories as well as incorporate future knowledge. No other textbook includes this or a similar tool for learning. Two additional features, *Model for Understanding* and *Check for Understanding*, also assist readers in synthesizing content and transferring content to practice.

Why I Wrote This Text

I have spent my entire career as a professional health educator, beginning as a health educator working in a multispecialty care medical clinic, progressing to directing community health education for a regional health system, and now in academia serving on teams of both practitioners and fellow academics. This continuum of experience, always grounded in practice, has created a natural tendency to extend content to practical application. An applied approach to health behavior and health behavior theory creates a platform for current as well as future work.

Organization of the Text

Introduction to Health Behaviors is organized into three sections. Section I introduces population health and health behavior basics. The disease prevention model illustrates the importance of the relationship between health behaviors and health status, and serves as a graphic organizer for sorting multiple levels of information across public health. The relationship of social determinants of health (e.g., early life, education, income, place, and stress) is an emerging topic in health promotion and is included in Section I. Section II of the book covers eight health behavior theories commonly used in health promotion programs. Section II concludes with the PER worksheet, a tool that combines the theoretical content into one body of information.

The text concludes in Section III with the mechanisms for building logic models and how theory and models are useful for designing multilevel interventions of change.

Ancillary Package

The complete supplement package for *Introduction to Health Behaviors: A Guide for Managers, Practitioners & Educators* was developed to achieve two goals:

1. To assist students in learning and applying the information presented in the text

2. To assist instructors in planning and implementing their courses in the most efficient manner and provide exceptional resources to enhance their students' experience

Instructor Companion Website

ISBN 13: 978-1-285-17263-7

Spend less time planning and more time teaching with Cengage Learning's Instructor Resources to accompany *Introduction to Health Behaviors: A Guide for Managers, Practitioners & Educators*. The Instructor Companion Website can be accessed by going to http://www.cengage.com/login to create a unique user log-in. The password-protected Instructor Resources include the following:

Instructor's Manual   An electronic Instructor's Manual provides instructors with invaluable tools for preparing class lectures and examinations. Following the text chapter-by-chapter, the Instructor's Manual reiterates objectives, provides a synthesized recap of each chapter's main points and goals, and houses the answers to each chapter's activities.

Online Cognero Test Bank   An electronic test bank generates tests and quizzes in an instant. With a variety of question types, including multiple choice, true or false, and matching exercises, creating challenging exams will be no barrier in your classroom. This test bank includes a rich bank of over 250 questions that test students on retention and application of what they have learned in the course. Answers are provided for all questions so that instructors can focus on teaching, not grading.

Instructor PowerPoint Slides   A comprehensive offering of more than 250 instructor support slides created in Microsoft® PowerPoint outlines concepts and objectives to assist instructors with lectures.

About the Author

Marietta Orlowski, PhD, MCHES, is an associate professor at Wright State University in the Boonshoft School of Medicine and serves as the health promotion and education program advisor in the Master of Public Health Program. Her current work involves health behavior measurement and risk reduction in children and adolescents, and she has developed both undergraduate and graduate courses in the theoretical foundations of health behaviors and program planning. In 2005 she received the Wright State University Presidential Award for Excellence in Early Career Achievement and in 2010 she was honored as Outstanding Faculty Member in the MPH program. In addition to serving as co-principal investigator on multiple federally funded projects to improve the nutrition and activity behaviors of school children, Dr. Orlowski has presented her research on tobacco prevention at the Centers for Disease Control and Prevention as well as served as an evaluator for U.S. Department of Agriculture Team Nutrition projects.

Acknowledgments

I am grateful for and appreciative of colleagues from Wright State University Boonshoft School of Medicine, Public Health-Dayton & Montgomery County, Greene County Combined Health District, and Premier Community Health. I am fortunate to be able to work with skilled professionals across public health disciplines; as a result of these experiences, I have learned much about a variety of topics within this book. Thank you to the graduate students in the public health program—you have challenged me and through your questions and projects, I have refined my own understanding. I also appreciate the willingness of former graduate students Roopsi Narayan, Dustin Ratliff, and Dawn Ebron for sharing their projects.

Early career experiences at the Morehead Clinic and Middletown Regional Hospital were instrumental in forming my career path and allowing me to write this text. Many physicians, nurses, allied health professionals, administrators, and educators took me under their wing and taught me much. They were champions of health promotion long before most. Thank you.

Finally, thank you to my family—Garett, Marilyn, Wendy, Paula, Morgan, Madison, Curt, Ann, Nick, Kristin, Danielle, and Bryan.

Contributors

Kathleen Henschel, MPH

Epidemiologist, Missouri Department of Health and Senior Services

Ms. Kate Henschel contributed the Behavioral Science in Action features in most chapters, completed the research and outline for Chapter 5, and served as a reader and editor of chapter drafts.

Sara Paton, PhD

Associate Professor of Epidemiology, Wright State University

and

Sylvia Ellison, MPH

Instructor of Research and Epidemiology, Wright State University

Project Facilitator, Infant Mortality Reduction, Public Health-Dayton & Montgomery County

Dr. Sara Paton and Ms. Sylvia Ellison co-authored Chapter 11 on infant mortality.

Reviewers

Paul Branscum, PhD, RD

Assistant Professor

The University of Oklahoma

Norman, OK

Crystal Harris, PhD, RN

Associate Professor

Missouri Western State University

St. Joseph, MO

Dr. Amar Kanekar, PhD, MPH, MB, BS, MCHES, CPH

Assistant Professor

University of Arkansas at Little Rock

Little Rock, AR

Marilyn Massey-Stokes, EdD, CHES, FASHA, IC®
Associate Professor
Department of Health Studies, Texas Woman's University
Denton, TX

Lauren Outland, DrPH, MSN, NP, MPH, CNM, BA
Assistant Professor
California State University, Dominguez Hills
Carson, CA

Holly Ann Scheib, PhD, MPH, MSW
Sage Consulting, Inc.
New Orleans, LA

How to Use This Text: A Guided Walk Through

KEY TERMS

antecedents	incidence	prevalence	secondary prevention
chronic disease	injury	primary prevention	tertiary prevention
determinants	lifestyle disease	protective factor	
evidence-based public health	mental health	risk	
health	population health	risk factor	

Key Terms: Key Terms identify important vocabulary for the chapter. Each term appears in bold-face color the first time it is used in the chapter and also appears in the glossary with a definition.

LEARNING OBJECTIVES

1. Describe a broad multidimensional definition of health.
2. Explain the role of risk and protective factors in disease and injury reduction.
3. Give examples of biological, social, behavioral, and environmental risk and protective factors.
4. Compare the targets of primary, secondary, and tertiary prevention.
5. Classify information into correct levels of the disease prevention model.
6. Discuss current population-level disease, death, and injury targets.

Learning Objectives: Chapter Objectives are presented at the beginning of each chapter and introduce the core concepts you should be able to master after reading and studying each chapter. These can be a great review tool as well.

IN THE NEWS ...

Health insurance exchanges filled the news of 2013 and 2014. The Health Insurance Marketplace, one of the key provisions of Affordable Care Act, allows individuals to purchase health insurance in a marketplace at reasonable prices. The exchanges are expected to lower the number of un- and underinsured Americans. The marketplace exchange is the most significant change in health insurance since the creation of Medicaid and Medicare in the 1965. On October 1, 2013, www.healthcare.gov was open for business.

At times, the story of health insurance exchanges read like a soap opera: love, hate, opportunity, disappointment, breakups, and second chances. Far fewer people than expected—just 26,000—were able to sign up for health insurance during the first month of open enrollment. The site crashed, politicians pointed fingers, and many said, "I told you so." New staff was hired, sites were redesigned, outreach workers were dispatched, and enrollment numbers grew. By the end of the open enrollment period on March 31, 2014, a total of 7.4

In the News ...: The In the News ... feature starts each chapter by describing a current event that relates to that chapter's content and ties the text to relevant, real-world events as they relate to health behaviors.

Model for Understanding Tobacco control has been the work of a variety of disciplines: health care, public health, education, law enforcement, substance abuse, media, and business. It has been the work of coalitions, nonprofits, groups of parents, state legislators, lobbyists, researchers, chief executive officers (CEOs), insurers, and many more. Tobacco use has truly been addressed through multilevel interventions that have reached across population segments. Some have called it a model to be applied to other population-level improvements in health behaviors and health status (Brownell & Warner, 2009; Mercer et al., 2003; NCI, 2007).

Tobacco control efforts began with awareness and education interventions, progressed to behavioral and social interventions, and along the way have included numerous policy actions. Individuals learned about the ill effects and the addictive nature of tobacco; individuals were taught methods to quit, including involving the support of others; institutions encouraged and resourced members to quit, adopted policies that restricted tobacco use, and built norms around tobacco; and organizations developed policy statements on use and advocated for change. Governments implemented clean air policies, taxed tobacco, restricted advertising, and regulated retail sales (IOM, 2007; Warner, 2006). This widened system approach to tobacco control has had documented success. The number of adults in this country who smoke cigarettes and use other tobacco products has been cut in half, from over 50% of the adult population in the 1960s to around

Model For Understanding: Models for Understanding use theory and model frameworks from the chapter and then illustrate how they are currently being used to guide practice.

Check for Understanding For the content area of violence, what are possible risk management focus areas at the primary, secondary, and tertiary levels?

Check For Understanding: Checks for Understanding are simple activities placed throughout the chapter that encourage readers to apply the information into a specific content area. They are tools for formative assessment and class discussion.

SUMMARY

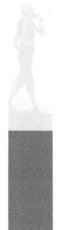

Social ecological models are a way of thinking about the numerous factors that influence health behaviors and health status. The social and built environment has various levels of influence, traditionally labeled intrapersonal, interpersonal, community, organizations, and policy/systems. Social ecological models are most useful in practice when they are behavior specific and when they include specific factors on each level of the model. Health behavior theory is useful for providing details within these broad categories. Health behavior theory consists of factors (called constructs) and hypothesized relationships among the factors. Health behavior theory is a critical part of the process of building evidence-based public health practice.

disciplines addressing multiple levels of influence. Social ecological models have guided the research agendas, strategic plans, and funding offered by national and state organizations. As a result, there will likely continue to be more content-specific models and additional evidence of the impact of outer-level–based interventions. The policy, system, and environment (PSE) agenda of the Centers for Disease Control and Prevention, among others, also has a role in smaller agencies of schools, worksites, and neighborhoods. School wellness committees, employee wellness coalitions, regional health care organizations, and community coalitions are encouraged to adopt a multilevel framework for understanding and impacting change.

Summary: The Chapter Summary is a great place to ensure that you completely understand the information in the chapter and are able to apply it. Look back at the chapter objectives and make sure that you have met those goals by the end of the summary.

BEHAVIORAL SCIENCE IN ACTION

The Ecology of Human Development

Urie Bronfenbrenner, who was born in the Soviet Union in 1917, was a pioneer in the field of child psychology. After serving as a military psychiatrist during World War II, Bronfenbrenner eventually ended up as a professor and researcher at Cornell University. Throughout his tenure, he authored and edited over 300 articles and book chapters and 14 books (Lang, 2005). He was incredibly influential in the fields of

It was widely thought in the 1960s and 1970s that child development was entirely a biological process. Child psychology experiments focused on how children reacted in carefully controlled settings that allowed for the influence of only one particular variable. Bronfenbrenner realized that this was unnatural and hypothesized that children are impacted by the people and environmental influences around them. He theorized that the environment could play a vi-

Behavioral Science in Action: The Behavioral Science in Action feature applies health behavior theory and concepts to the real world and explores their significance when put into action.

IN THE CLASSROOM ACTIVITIES

1) Describe the role of health behavior theory in understanding health behaviors.
2) Compare concepts, constructs, and variables.
3) Take the list of factors that influence one of your health behaviors (see Chapter 2, activity 5). Classify the factors into the corresponding levels of the social ecological model. Knowing the levels of influence, add additional factors to each level.
4) Visit the Pedestrian and Bicycle Information Center and download the Walkability Audit.

Complete a walkability audit of a section of a campus or off-campus location. Take two photos that capture key features of the environment. Compare your walking scores with those of other students. Observe walking for transportation in the area; do perceived walking rates vary? What system- and policy-level factors may be associated with the walking score?

In the Classroom: These activities ask readers to work individually or in groups in the classroom to further explore and discuss health behavior concepts.

WEB LINKS

Active Living Research: http://www.activelivingresearch.org/

Pedestrian and Bicycle Information Center: http://www.pedbikeinfo.org/

World Health Organization: http://www.who.int/en/

Web Links: Utilize the web links section at the end of the chapter for further learning and networking opportunities.

Introduction to Health Behaviors & Disease Prevention

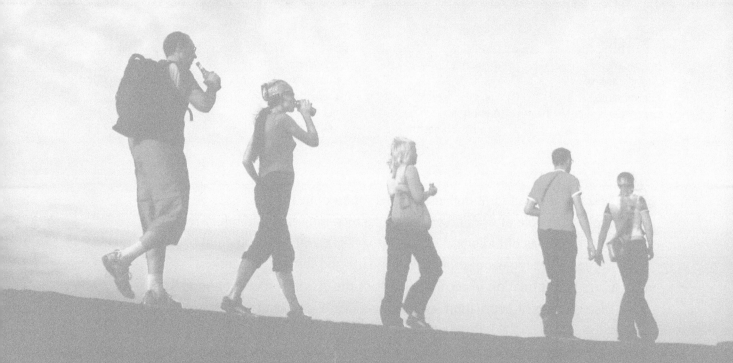

CHAPTER 1

What Is Health?

KEY TERMS

antecedents	incidence	prevalence	secondary prevention
chronic disease	injury	primary prevention	tertiary prevention
determinants	lifestyle disease	protective factor	
evidence-based public health	mental health	risk	
health	population health	risk factor	

LEARNING OBJECTIVES

1. Describe a broad multidimensional definition of health.
2. Explain the role of risk and protective factors in disease and injury reduction.
3. Give examples of biological, social, behavioral, and environmental risk and protective factors.
4. Compare the targets of primary, secondary, and tertiary prevention.
5. Classify information into correct levels of the disease prevention model.
6. Discuss current population-level disease, death, and injury targets.

IN THE NEWS ...

Health insurance exchanges filled the news of 2013 and 2014. The Health Insurance Marketplace, one of the key provisions of Affordable Care Act, allows individuals to purchase health insurance in a marketplace at reasonable prices. The exchanges are expected to lower the number of un- and underinsured Americans. The marketplace exchange is the most significant change in health insurance since the creation of Medicaid and Medicare in the 1965. On October 1, 2013, www.healthcare.gov was open for business.

At times, the story of health insurance exchanges read like a soap opera: love, hate, opportunity, disappointment, breakups, and second chances. Far fewer people than expected—just 26,000—were able to sign up for health insurance during the first month of open enrollment. The site crashed, politicians pointed fingers, and many said, "I told you so." New staff was hired, sites were redesigned, outreach workers were dispatched, and enrollment numbers grew. By the end of the open enrollment period on March 31, 2014, a total of 7.4

million Americans had accessed health exchanges to purchase affordable insurance plans.

States were allowed to start their own exchanges or opt into the federal program. Most states (36) opted into the federal exchange. One of the earliest supporters of health exchanges was the state of Oregon. There, state legislators developed their own marketplace exchange. Like the residents of Maryland, Vermont, and Massachusetts, Oregonians would be able to buy health insurance through a state-organized marketplace. In April 2014, though, another broken heart of the exchange was announced. After spending over $100 million, the state was unsuccessful in launching its own exchange and

announced it would be joining the federal insurance marketplace. Other pieces of this story have included recruitment strategies for younger and healthier Americans, employer-mandated delays, and of course, the breakup letters from insurance companies.

The United States spends more per capita for health care than any other developed country in the world. As a result, health care reform has been an agenda item for three recent presidents: George W. Bush, Bill Clinton, and Barack Obama. Health insurance marketplaces and other provisions of the Affordable Care Act have affectionately (and not so affectionately) become termed Obamacare.

Introduction

The concept of health seems to be ever present. There are daily health articles in the newspaper, and hundreds of websites, blogs, and apps are dedicated to the subject. Products are called healthy or unhealthy. People talk about healthy places to live and work. In the 2012 presidential campaign, health and health care were major issues. Federal agencies dedicate research resources to determining how to achieve health. Communities join walks and buy ribbons to bring awareness to health issues, and the list goes on. The topic of health is everywhere—but what exactly is health?

Health is a multidimensional concept that is a means to end. Individuals seek health because it makes lives easier, more functional, and happier. Society spends considerable resources to assist individuals and populations achieve health. In this chapter, the broad factors that influence health (called determinants) will be discussed, as will the mechanism of disease prevention and health promotion. Before reading on, take a moment to jot down three features of health.

Health Defined

The World Health Organization describes **health** as a state of complete physical, psychological, and social well-being and not simply the absence of disease or infirmity (1948). There are numerous other definitions of health. The wording of definitions differs, but most definitions speak to similar properties of health. Health is *multidimensional*, meaning a person's health is made up of a combination of components. First,

health has a physical component. The strength and condition of the physical body is the common reference for health. Weight, blood pressure, cholesterol levels, and flexibility are often measures taken during a physical examination of health. As reflected in the World Health Organization definition, health is more than physical functions and measures.

Mental health is an equally important dimension of health. **Mental health** refers to a state of well-being in which a person realizes his or her potential, can cope with the normal stresses of life, can work productively and fruitfully, and is able to make a contribution to community (WHO, 2013). Measures of mental health involve emotional, psychological, and social indicators. Emotional and psychological well-being can be indicated by life satisfaction, happiness, and self-acceptance. Social well-being is a reflection of connections to others, social acceptance, and a sense of community (WHO, 2001). It is the combination and reciprocal interactions of these dimensions that define health.

There tends to be a reference to *functionality* in most definitions of health. Health allows individuals to function and complete the activities of daily life. Through health, one is able to work, take care of oneself, interact with others, engage in enjoyable activities, and contribute to meaningful endeavors. In this respect, health is a means to an end.

Health is also *dynamic*. The state of dimensions of health can vary daily and across a lifespan. Health is not a destination; it is not a target with select criteria of physical measures, cognitive abilities and fulfilling social connections. Health is fluid and changes daily, by life circumstance and by lifespan.

Instead of a point on a line, health is a continuum in which the dimensions of health move and slide. This variation in health is normal, given the dynamic interaction of the multiple components. A destination-type definition also implies standardized criteria. Health is much more individualized. Optimal health for someone with an injury-related disability might be different than for a college student—yet both can be equally "healthy."

Leading Causes of Death and Disability

Lifestyle-related diseases top the lists of the leading causes of death and disability in the United States. Heart disease and cancer account for 48% of all deaths in the country (National Center for Health Statistics, 2013). Over 1 million people die each year from heart disease and cancer combined (see Table 1-1). Cancer and heart disease are commonly called **lifestyle diseases** because the greatest amount of risk for developing the disease comes from behaviors and social factors of one's life. Smoking, poor diet, and physical inactivity can significantly increase the likelihood of these diseases. Social factors such as type of employment and lack of connections to others have also been associated with disease rates. Other lifestyle-related diseases include lung disease, diabetes, kidney disease, and liver disease.

Chronic Diseases

A **chronic disease** is a condition that is slow in progression, is long in duration, is void of spontaneous resolution, and often limits the function, productivity, and quality of life of the individual who lives with it (IOM, 2012b). The population reach and magnitude of chronic illnesses is huge. About half of Americans have at least one chronic disease, and medical care of chronic illnesses represents 75% of the dollars spent annually on health care in the United States (USDHHS, 2009; Wu & Green, 2000). In 2012, $2.8 trillion (or $8195 per person) was spent on health care (Martin et al., 2014). With an aging society, the **prevalence**, costs, and productivity losses associated with chronic diseases are only expected to grow.

Many of the leading causes of death are also common chronic diseases. Heart disease, stroke, cancer, lung disease,

TABLE 1-1 Leading Causes of Death in the United States, 2012

Cause of Death	Number of Deaths	Death Rate per 100,000 Population
Disease of the heart	597,689	193.6
Malignant neoplasms (cancer)	574,743	186.2
Chronic lower respiratory diseases	138,080	44.7
Cerebrovascular diseases (stroke)	129,467	41.9
Accidents (unintentional injuries)	120,859	39.1
Alzheimer's disease	83,494	27.0
Diabetes	69,071	20.8
Kidney diseases	50,476	16.3
Influenza and pneumonia	50,097	16.2
Intentional self-harm (suicide)	38,364	12.4
Septicemia (bacteria in the blood)	34,812	11.3
Chronic liver disease and cirrhosis	31,903	10.3

Source: National Center for Health Statistics, 2013

dementia, diabetes, and kidney and liver disease can progressively worsen over years and limit functioning and quality of life. Arthritis, epilepsy, depression, and asthma are other common chronic illnesses that afflict millions of Americans (CDC, 2009). These chronic illnesses may not result in death, but they often detract from overall quality of life through lost days of work, pain, increased hospitalizations, and high medical costs (Ford et al., 2013). For example, asthma is a leading cause of absenteeism from work and school, with nearly 25 million missed days of work and school and a loss of productivity totaling an estimated $3.8 billion (CDC, 2013a). When students are absent, they miss instructional time and, according to some studies, perform worse on standardizes tests (Moonie et al., 2008). Similarly, arthritis and chronic pain, the two most common causes of reported adult disability, can seriously impact the physical, mental, social, and economic health of individuals. Debilitating pain from a chronic disease can cause individuals to miss work and social functions as well as be unable to take care of themselves and family members. This type of pain also often coexists with mental health problems (IOM, 2012b). Arthritis affects 29 million adults, and an estimated 100 million Americans suffer from chronic pain.

Heart Disease and Stroke

Cardiovascular diseases are diseases of the heart and circulatory system. Heart disease and stroke are the two most common cardiovascular diseases. Most often, plaque builds up on the arterial walls and restricts and/or blocks blood flow to various parts of the body. "Heart disease" is a term used to refer to a collection of problems affecting the heart, including atherosclerosis (a build-up of plaque on the arterial walls), heart failure (when the heart is unable to pump enough blood to meet the body's needs), arrhythmia (irregular heartbeat), and heart attack. A heart attack occurs when blood flow to the heart is severely limited or cut off completely. The lack of oxygen can damage the heart muscle. A stroke occurs when a blood vessel in the brain bursts or is blocked. A stroke is similar to a heart attack in that blood flow is impaired, but a stroke occurs in the brain (National Heart, Lung, and Blood Institute, 2013). Heart disease is the leading cause of death, and stroke is the third leading cause of death.

Death from both heart disease and stroke is decreasing; however, the incidence of heart and stroke events and the associated costs remain high. One in three Americans has at least one cardiovascular disease (Go et al., 2014). The American Heart Association estimates that every year, 620,000 Americans will experience a new coronary attack, and about half that number (295,000) will have a recurring event (Go et al., 2014). Similarly, every year 610,000 individuals will experience their first stroke, and an additional 185,000 will experience a recurring stroke. Dollar amounts vary from year to year, but treating cardiovascular diseases accounts for the largest costs in the U.S. health care system. The total costs for cardiovascular diseases are estimated at $315 billion a year, which breaks down to $1 out of every $6 spent on health care in this country (Go et al., 2014; USDHHS, 2011b). Costs include physicians and other health care providers, hospital services, medications, home health care, and lost productivity. The rate of heart disease and stroke does increase with age; it is interesting to note, though, that 32% of adult men under age 65 and 27% of adult women under age 65 report having some form of heart disease. By age 75, 43.5% of males and 31.5% of females report some form of heart disease (National Center for Health Statistics, 2013).

In addition to age, cardiovascular disease prevalence and outcomes vary significantly by race, gender, socioeconomic status, and region (National Center for Health Statistics, 2013). African Americans are two to three times more likely to die from cardiovascular disease than whites, which is due both to differences in vascular risk factors and disparities in treatment (Davis et al., 2007). Risk factors for heart disease and stroke do not appear at the same time in different racial and ethnic groups. For example, hypertension among Black or African Americans tends to manifest at an earlier age, is usually harder to treat and control, and it has a greater prevalence than hypertension in other communities (Davis et al., 2007). Black or African American and Hispanic populations have higher rates of physical inactivity, especially among women, and American Indian and Native Alaskan populations have higher rates of smoking. Treatment disparities are differences in treatment among racial or ethnic groups, particularly among black and Hispanic populations, that are not related to the patients' preferences or differences in underlying health conditions (Davis et al., 2007). Furthermore, place of residence and socioeconomic status can determine the access a patient has to specialists and specialized treatment options, which in turn may influence the quality of care and outcomes (Davis et al., 2007). While race, gender, and socioeconomic status do not account for an individual's entire risk or all outcomes, they are important factors that influence many aspects of disease.

Cancer

Cancer is the second leading cause of death in the United States. According to the National Cancer Institute (2006), cancer is a term used to describe diseases in which abnormal cells divide without control and are able to spread to other tissues. Cancer cells can move to other parts of the body through the blood and lymph systems. There are more than 100 different types of cancer. Skin cancer is the most common, and lung cancer is the most deadly. Most cancer types are named for the place of origin of the cancer cells, for example, breast cancer originates in the breast, and stomach cancer originates in the stomach.

Approximately 574,000 individuals died from cancer in 2012, second only to heart disease (National Center for Health Statistics, 2013). While more than half a million people die from cancer each year, many more are diagnosed with one or more forms of cancer. The American Cancer Society (2014) estimated that 1.67 million Americans were diagnosed with cancer in 2014. Incidence and prognosis vary by cancer type. Excluding skin cancer, breast cancer is the most common cancer in women; currently, one in eight women are likely to receive a breast cancer diagnosis in her lifetime. Breast cancer is also one of the more curable forms of cancer; the 5-year survival rate for early-stage breast cancer can be as high as 90% (American Cancer Society, 2014). Prostate cancer is the most common cancer in men; currently, one in seven men will be diagnosed with prostate cancer in his lifetime. The 5-year survival rate for all prostate cancers is over 99%. By contrast, the lifetime risk of developing colorectal cancer is 1 in 20 (5.1%), with men having a slightly higher lifetime risk (American Cancer Society, 2014).

Like cardiovascular disease, costs to treat cancer represent a significant portion of the money spent on health care. Estimates for the direct costs of cancer care are estimated to be between $86.6 billion and $124.57 billion (American Cancer Society, 2014; Mariotto et al., 2011). The amount climbs to an estimated $216.6 billion when lost productivity is included (American Cancer Society, 2014). Screening tests and protocols for early diagnosis and medical advancements have improved survival rates and have increased incidence/prevalence rates. The incidence rate of diagnosed cases of cancer started increasing in the 1970s; peaked at 510 cases per 100,000 in 1992; and then decreased to 457 cases per 100,000 in 2010 (Howlader et al., 2013). These rates vary by age, sex, and ethnicity, and they will likely continue to change as the population ages. The costs of cancer care are expected to rise with increased cancer incidence in an aging population, along with advances in diagnostic technology and new treatments.

Diabetes

Diabetes is a group of diseases marked by high levels of blood glucose resulting from inadequate insulin production, decreased insulin action, or both (USDHHS, 2011a). Type 1 diabetes develops when the body is unable to produce insulin. People with type 1 diabetes must have insulin delivered by injection or pump. This form of diabetes usually affects children and young adults. Type 2 diabetes is characterized by insulin resistance, that is, the body produces insulin, but the cells do not use it correctly. Type 2 diabetes accounts for 90–95% of diabetes cases and is associated with older age, obesity, family history of diabetes, history of gestational diabetes, impaired glucose metabolism, and physical inactivity. Rates of diabetes are also higher in Black or African Americans, Americans of Mexican origin, and American Indian or Alaska Natives (National Center for Health Statistics, 2013). See Table 1-2 for differences.

Approximately 9.3% of people in the United States have diabetes; 12.3% of adults 20 and older have diabetes, and 25.9% of people 65 and older develop diabetes (CDC, 2014). In addition to being the seventh leading cause of death, diabetes is the leading cause of kidney failure, nontraumatic lower-extremity amputations, and blindness among adults ages 20–74. The direct cost for treating diabetes is approximately $176 billion a year, with an additional $69 million for indirect costs of disability and work loss (American Diabetes Association, 2013).

Injury

Injury is the leading cause of death and disability in young people (ages 1–44) and the fifth leading cause of death for all Americans (National Center for Health Statistics, 2013). Injuries account for 39.1 deaths per 100,000 Americans (see Table 1-1). Falls, motor vehicle crashes, poisoning, fires, and

TABLE 1-2 **Percentage of Adults with Diagnosed Diabetes, 2010–2012**

	Age-Adjusted Rate[a]
White	7.6
Asian American	9.0
Hispanic	12.8
Black or African American	13.2
American Indian or Alaska Native	15.9

a) Age 20 and older

Source: Centers for Disease Control & Prevention, 2014

drowning are the common categories of injuries. When injury tallies include accidents and *violence,* injuries account for 57.9 deaths per 100,000 Americans and become the third leading cause of death (Trust for America's Health, 2012). Violence-related injuries include intimate partner violence, abuse/neglect, murder, and suicide.

Injury is a broad category that includes a variety of actions and outcomes. **Injury** is defined as intentional or unintentional damage or harm to the body resulting in impairment or a diminished level of health (National Research Council, 1999). Injuries are commonly categorized by intent and the mechanism of the injury. Intentional injuries result from an action that was intended to harm; with an unintentional injury, there is no intention to harm self or others. A motor vehicle crash with injuries is likely unintentional, whereas injuries from acts of domestic violence are intentional (CDC, 2011). Injuries are also discussed by the mechanism (or cause) of the injury. The following are mechanisms of injury: motor vehicle crashes, firearms, falls, occupational hazards, poisoning, child maltreatment, and sports. Within each category of causes, numerous specific causes of injury are possible. For example, child maltreatment includes emotional, physical, and sexual acts of maltreatment. In addition to intention and cause, injury data is also tracked by outcome: fatal and nonfatal. Fatal injuries result in death; they can be both intentional and unintentional and from

a variety of mechanisms. Poisoning, motor vehicle crashes, and falls are the leading causes of fatal injury (CDC, 2011).

Prescription drug overdose is a growing, and concerning, trend in the broad category of injury. Prescription drug overdose has surpassed motor vehicle crashes as the leading cause of injury deaths among adults ages 25–64 (see Figure 1-1). *Prescription* drug overdoses represented 60% of all drug overdoses in 2010, with a total of 22,134 deaths attributed to a prescription overdose (Jones, Mack, & Paulozzi, 2013). Painkillers were involved in 75% of prescription overdoses, and one-third of the painkillers involved the drug methadone (CDC, 2012b). Methadone has been used for decades to treat drug addiction, but it is also prescribed for managing pain related to musculoskeletal problems, headaches, cancer, and trauma. Other prescription painkillers involved in overdoses include oxycodone, morphine, and fentanyl (CDC, 2012b).

The current prescription drug overdose epidemic represents a dramatic shift in the source of drugs. Almost all drugs involved in pharmaceutical overdoses are prescribed, not stolen. In a survey of persons who misuse pain relief drugs, more than half (55%) were given the drug for free by a friend (SAMSHA, 2011). Only 17% of the pain relief drugs involved in overdoses were prescribed by a physician for the individual misusing the drugs. Other sources included purchasing from a friend or relative (11.4%), taking without permission from a friend or relative (4.8%), purchasing from a stranger or dealer (4.4%), and other (7.1%) (SAMSHA, 2011).

Injuries result in significant medical and societal costs. Approximately 50 million Americans are treated for injuries each year (Trust for America's Health, 2012). Nearly 12,000 children and teens die from accidental injuries each year, and around 9.2 million are treated in emergency departments. Medical care for injuries costs an estimated $80 billion a year, and the cost of disability and lost productivity is estimated at more than four times that amount—$326 billion (Finkelstein, Corso, & Miller, 2006). Unfortunately, injury as a public health issue tends not to get the attention of the aforementioned chronic diseases, despite its significant cost to society, community, and family (Trust for America's Health, 2012; IOM, 1998). The tendency to discuss injuries as singular and unrelated events or by mechanisms can limit the public's understanding of the magnitude of injuries. Injuries from motor vehicle crashes are discussed as a health concern that is seen

10 Leading Causes of Injury Deaths by Age Group Highlighting Unintentional Injury Deaths; United States, 2010

Rank	<1	1–4	5–9	10–14	15–24	25–34	35–44	45–54	55–64	65+	Total
1	Unintentional Suffocation 905	Unintentional Drowning 436	Unintentional MV Traffic 354	Unintentional MV Traffic 452	Unintentional MV Traffic 7,024	Unintentional Poisoning 6,767	Unintentional Poisoning 7,476	Unintentional Poisoning 9,662	Unintentional Poisoning 4,451	Unintentional Fall 21,649	Unintentional MV Traffic 33,687
2	Homicide Unspecified 154	Unintentional MV Traffic 343	Unintentional Drowning 134	Suicide Suffocation 168	Homicide Firearm 3,889	Unintentional MV Traffic 5,558	Unintentional MV Traffic 4,552	Unintentional MV Traffic 5,154	Unintentional MV Traffic 4,134	Unintentional MV Traffic 6,037	Unintentional Poisoning 33,041
3	Homicide Other Spec., classifiable 82	Homicide Unspecified 163	Unintentional Fire/Burn 89	Unintentional Drowning 117	Unintentional Poisoning 3,183	Homicide Firearm 3,331	Suicide Firearm 2,914	Suicide Firearm 4,092	Suicide Firearm 3,387	Unintentional Unspecified 4,596	Unintentional Fall 26,009
4	Unintentional MV Traffic 76	Unintentional Fire/Burn 151	Homicide Firearm 58	Homicide Firearm 107	Suicide Firearm 2,046	Suicide Firearm 2,594	Suicide Suffocation 1,839	Suicide Poisoning 2,061	Unintentional Fall 2,011	Suicide Firearm 4,276	Suicide Firearm 19,392
5	Undetermined Suffocation 39	Unintentional Suffocation 134	Unintentional Suffocation 31	Suicide Firearm 80	Suicide Suffocation 1,824	Suicide Suffocation 1,910	Homicide Firearm 1,673	Suicide Suffocation 1,965	Suicide Poisoning 1,382	Unintentional Suffocation 3,400	Homicide Firearm 11,078
6	Unintentional Drowning 39	Unintentional Pedestrian, Other 103	Unintentional Other Land Transport 26	Unintentional Suffocation 48	Unintentional Drowning 656	Suicide Poisoning 787	Suicide Poisoning 1,279	Unintentional Fall 1,283	Suicide Suffocation 1,130	Adverse Effects 1,544	Suicide Suffocation 9,493
7	Undetermined Unspecified 35	Homicide Other Spec., classifiable 84	Unintentional Pedestrian, Other 20	Unintentional Fire/Burn 46	Homicide Cut/Pierce 420	Undetermined Poisoning 580	Undetermined Poisoning 712	Homicide Firearm 1,097	Unintentional Suffocation 613	Unintentional Poisoning 1,402	Suicide Poisoning 6,599
8	Adverse Effects 22	Unintentional Natural/Environment 52	Adverse Effects 14	Unintentional Other Land Transport 42	Suicide Poisoning 371	Unintentional Drowning 476	Unintentional Fall 493	Undetermined Poisoning 955	Homicide Firearm 533	Unintentional Fire/Burn 1,088	Unintentional Suffocation 6,165
9	Unintentional Fire/Burn 22	Homicide Firearm 43	Unintentional Natural/Environment 14	Unintentional Poisoning 40	Undetermined Poisoning 282	Homicide Cut/Pierce 438	Unintentional Drowning 409	Unintentional Drowning 578	Undetermined Poisoning 480	Suicide Poisoning 709	Unintentional Unspecified 5,688
10	Unintentional Natural/Environment 22	Unintentional Struck by or Against 37	Unintentional Poisoning 14	Unintentional Firearm 26	Unintentional Other Land Transport 221	Unintentional Fall 299	Homicide Cut/Pierce 349	Unintentional Suffocation 464	Unintentional Fire/Burn 479	Unintentional Suffocation 648	Unintentional Drowning 3,782

Age Groups

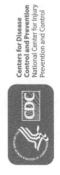

Centers for Disease Control and Prevention
National Center for Injury Prevention and Control

Data Source: National Center for Health Statistics (NCHS), National Vital Statistics System.
Produced by: Office of Statistics and Programming, National Center for Injury Prevention and Control, CDC using WISQARS™.

Figure 1-1 10 Leading Causes of Injury Deaths, United States, 2010

Source: Centers for Disease Control and Prevention, National Center for Injury Prevention and Control

as completely separate from falls or drowning. This singular focus also segments injury prevention issues across different audiences and professional disciplines. Violence, an intentional injury, tends to be associated with law enforcement and mental health professionals, whereas accidental poisonings and choking incidents are often a focus for pediatricians.

Population Health

Health is both an individual and a population measure. Health care tends to be individually focused. A person has his or her individual health assessed, and personalized treatments or preventive measures are prescribed. With population health, the unit of focus is larger than a person. **Population health** is an integrated approach that considers health outcomes *within a population*, the determinants that influence health, and the policies and interventions that impact health determinants (Public Health Accreditation Board, 2011). The goals and challenges of individual- and population-focused health are similar: improve quality of life, increase life expectancy, and effectively utilize resources. Likewise, the challenges are similar: individuals and most population segments die predominantly from lifestyle-related diseases, and both are affected by chronic illness.

Causes of disease, disability, injury, and death are outcome measures for individuals and populations. The methods for assessing the health of a community versus an individual are different, though, as is the threshold for taking action and the strategies employed to achieve change. Population health approaches more often address determinants of health status (tobacco and alcohol use, poor diet, sedentary lifestyles, and environmental factors) as opposed to treating illness.

The well-being of an individual and the well-being of his or her community are important, intertwined, and reciprocal. Individuals who live in a healthy community or environment are more likely themselves to be healthy. The opposite is true as well—unhealthy individuals make for unhealthy communities. A population focus allows for observation of trends in health outcomes and the determinants of health status across segments of the population.

Gaps in Health

A population focus does not imply that outcomes or access by the members of a population will be equal in the end. Segments of the U.S. population can have significantly different levels of chronic diseases and overall life expectancies. Different patterns of disease and disability exist across numerous demographic groups and geographic areas. Age, education level, race, type of insurance, geographic region, and location of residence are categories from which differences are commonly reported (National Center for Health Statistics, 2013). The differences in health are not the result of just one factor. Health differences reflect the influence of a mix of genetic, environmental, and behavioral factors.

Life expectancy and infant mortality, two common health status indicators, illustrate gaps in health by population segments. Life expectancy is the expected number of years of life remaining at a particular age, though most life expectancy figures cited are the expected years of life for a newborn. The current life expectancy in the United States is 78.5 years, which is an average for both sexes and all races (Arias, 2014). When examined by sex and ethnicity, life expectancy ranges from 70.7 for non-Hispanic black males to 83.5 for Hispanic females (Arias, 2014). Recent research has shown that life expectancy is closely correlated to educational attainment and income levels, in addition to sex and ethnicity (Olshansky et al., 2012). As illustrated in Table 1-3, infant mortality races also differ across races. The infant mortality rate (the death of a child before his or her first birthday) is currently 6.05 deaths per 1000 live births (USDHHS, 2013). Racial disparities can be seen in infant mortality rates; the rate for infants born to non-Hispanic white mothers was 5.33 per 1000 live births in 2009, and the rate for infants born to Black or African American mothers was 12.40 (USDHHS, 2013). Of course, race alone cannot explain these gaps in health status indicators. The numerous factors that impact an individual's health status are known as determinants of health.

Determinants of Health

Health is multidimensional, has multiple components (physical, mental, and social) and multiple levels (individual and population), and moves along a continuum. It is no surprise, then, that the factors that create health are diverse. Hundreds of individual factors interact to create health status, including medication use, genetics, air quality, fluoridated water, prenatal care, automobile safety, crime, tobacco use, weight, friend and family support, and much more. These health **determinants** fall into five broad categories: behavior, environment, biology, social conditions, and health care.

TABLE 1-3 Life Expectancy and Infant Mortality by Race/Ethnicity, 2009

Race/Ethnicity	Life Expectancy in Years (both sexes)	Infant Mortality Rate (per 1000 births)
All races	78.5	6.05
White, non-Hispanic	78.9	5.33
Black or African American	74.6	12.40
Hispanic	82.8	5.29
Asian/Pacific Islander	86.5	4.40
American Indian/Alaska Native	76.9	8.47

Sources: Arias, 2014; Kaiser Family Foundation, 2014; USDHHS, 2013.

Behavior

Health behaviors, collectively called lifestyle factors, represent the greatest portion of one's risk for the leading causes of death, disease, and disability. Approximately 40–50% of disease risk comes from health behaviors one chooses to do or not to do (Danaei et al., 2009; Mokdad et al., 2004; National Prevention Council, 2011). Significant population-level changes in disease prevalence and health status must be mediated through the modification of health behaviors.

A health behavior is an activity of an individual or group, regardless of actual or perceived health status, for the purpose of promoting, protecting, or maintaining health (WHO, 2004, 1998). In public health, physical activity, nutrition, sexual behaviors, alcohol and other drug use, tobacco use, and injury prevention are the most commonly discussed categories of behavioral risk factors. Health care utilization, adequate sleep, participating in preventive clinical care, and oral health practices are other types of important health behaviors. Health behaviors are the topic of Chapter 2.

Environment

The environments where people live and work impact their health. The physical environment consists of the conditions of a place that can be seen, touched, heard, smelled, and tasted, as well as other properties, such as radiation and ozone, that are less observable (USDHHS, 2000). Some of these properties may be hazardous to health. Toxic agents, microbial agents, and structural hazards can put individuals at risk for injury, allergies, asthma, pulmonary diseases, cancers, and developmental delays. The physical environment itself may present a risk to health, and the environment can also affect one's exposure to infectious diseases. For example, poor-quality water and food systems may allow pathogens to grow, thus serving as a pathway for pathogens to reach individuals. In general, environmental exposure is associated with 5 to 10% of the risk for premature death (Booke et al., 2010; McGinnis, Williams-Russo, & Knickman, 2002). When social conditions are included with environmental conditions—as a broader concept of environment—McGinnis and colleagues (2002) estimate the percentage of impact to be 20%.

Biology/Genetics

Biology refers to an individual's genetic makeup, family history, and any physical and mental health problem acquired during life (USDHHS, 2000). In addition to an individual's genetic makeup at birth, conditions of living (aging, smoking, stress, drug use, injury, and/or infection) may produce a "newer" biology for the individual. For example, exposure to lead can alter young children's nervous system development, including the brain (Agency for Toxic Substances and Disease Registry, 2007). This compromised nervous system is carried forward as children grow and interact with the environment.

In general, biology is estimated to contribute about 30% to an individual's overall health status (McGinnis et al., 2002). This percentage obviously varies by health condition and by individual. Select health issues have a genetic predisposition, including some cancers, cardiovascular disease, sickle cell disease, and dementia, though genetic predisposition does not guarantee the development of the disease. An individual may have a genetic predisposition to a disease (e.g., cancer), but it is through the interaction of environmental toxins or lifestyle factors that genetic coding signals get triggered, resulting in abnormal cell growth (McGinnis et al., 2002).

Social Conditions

The social conditions of one's life can have a significant impact on health and opportunities for choosing health. Social conditions include income, education level, early life, neighborhood characteristics, and connections to others through work and support networks. These social factors affect health through different pathways, and some of these relationships can be strong. First, social factors operate by creating the conditions through which the individual completes a variety of health behaviors. Where a person lives and works can create tremendous obstacles to completing seemingly simple health behaviors. Taking a walk in the evening is more difficult, and possibly detrimental to safety, in a crime-ridden neighborhood. Similarly, places of work are associated with resources like health and dental insurance, paid sick leave, time to seek preventive care, messages about health behaviors, and stress. Education and income are social factors further upstream to health, but their relationships to health are strong. Income, education, and neighborhood integration influence an individual's opportunities for living and working conditions. The topic of Chapter 3 is the role of social factors (determinants) and their relationships to health status.

Health Care

Access to quality medical care—including health care professionals, facilities, equipment, medications, screenings, and treatments—also influences health status. Some of the largest achievements in population health have been achieved through clinical screenings, primary care, and preventive medical care. Immunizations, prenatal care, and blood pressure and cholesterol screenings have achieved significant improvements in the health of this country (CDC, 1999b). Surprisingly, the impact of access to quality health care on health status is approximately 10% (McGinnis et al., 2002), with individual health behaviors and conditions of living contributing more to overall health status. Being physically active, eating a nutritious and balanced diet, not smoking, getting adequate sleep, and participating in preventive clinical care are foundations for a healthy body.

Technology will continue to advance the practice of medicine. Diagnostic tools, surgical instruments, and pharmacological products evolve and improve the treatment of disease. Clinical preventive care, such as cancer screenings and immunizations, can have significant impact; however, health care budget priorities currently are not geared toward primary and secondary prevention, but on treating illness and disease.

Disease Prevention Model

The fundamental principle of prevention is risk management. Health status is maintained or improved through the minimization of risk for negative outcomes, where risk is defined as an increased probability of a problem or negative event. Specific factors known to increase the likelihood of certain negative health outcomes are called **risk factors**. For example, smoking is a risk factor for heart disease; individuals who smoke are more likely to experience a heart attack. Prevention programs work to maintain health status by altering specific risk factors. **Protective factors** are similar to risk factors but differ in the direction of their relationship to health status. Protective factors are behaviors or traits that decrease the likelihood of disease; physical activity is a protective factor for heart disease.

Each risk factor has a set of antecedents that influence it. In general, certain forms of knowledge, beliefs, skills, resources, and reinforcements facilitate behavior. Collectively, the broad range of factors is called antecedents, and it is the variation of these antecedents that explains variation in behavior. For example, individuals with higher fruit and vegetable intake tend to be able to identify more fruits and vegetables with an appealing taste, report easier access to the foods in home and community environments, and have skills for preparation, storage, and menu planning (Di Noia & Byrd-Breddenner, 2013; Graham et al., 2013; Krolner et al., 2011; Sallis & Glanz, 2009). The disease prevention model (see Figure 1-2) shows the hierarchical relationships of these three facets: health, risk factors, and antecedents.

Level I: Health

Level 1 of the disease prevention model is health, which is the highest level in the hierarchy of population health activities. Surveillance activities, treatments, and programming exist to improve health status. There are numerous examples of health issues that may be relevant to a community, and the opening sections of this chapter have listed numerous examples. Table 1-1 lists the leading causes of death and disability in the United States: heart disease, cancer, respiratory diseases,

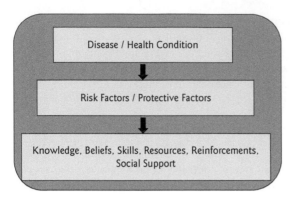

Figure I-2 Disease Prevention Model

and stroke. Health issues deserving of public health attention extend beyond causes of premature death and disability and include unplanned pregnancy, sexually transmitted infections, prescription drug overdose, and foodborne illness. Health issues can also be framed as positive outcomes such as healthy aging, childhood safety, and planned pregnancies.

Level 2: Risk and Protective Factors

Risk factors are behaviors, environmental conditions, or traits that increase the likelihood of a particular disease or injury. The presence of a risk factor increases the likelihood that a particular disease or outcome will occur. Risk factors are specific forms of factors from the broad categories of determinants of health discussed earlier. Specific risks factors include smoking (behavior), air pollution (environment), gender (biology), medication compliance (health care behaviors), and socioeconomic status (social determinants).

Another important categorization within risk factors is modifiable verses nonmodifiable (factors that may increase risk for disease but are not modifiable). Gender, age, race, and family history are nonmodifiable risk factors for a variety of diseases. In Table 1-4, family history is shown as a nonmodifiable risk factor. Children of parents with heart disease are more likely to develop heart disease. Other nonmodifiable coronary heart risk factors include age and gender.

Obviously, interventions cannot be implemented to change nonmodifiable risk factors. However, knowledge of nonmodifiable risk factors may be used to encourage modification of other risk factors. Individuals with increased risk of disease may be encouraged to complete health behaviors at different frequencies because of their risk status. People with nonmodifiable risk factors may begin screenings earlier and follow different dietary

and medication recommendations. For example, the American Cancer Society recommends that all women begin screening mammograms by age 40, but women with a family history of breast cancer are encouraged to discuss with their physicians whether they should start screenings earlier and have them more frequently (ACS, 2014). Similar screening recommendations exist for colorectal cancer; all adults should begin screening by age 50, and individuals with a family history should talk to their physicians about a personalized screening plan (USPSTF, 2012). Thus, this protective behavior—screening—is defined differently for persons with nonmodifiable risk factors.

Environmental Risk Factors

Risk factors can be environmental conditions. The presence of pollutants in the air, water, and general environment can increase the likelihood of disease or injury. For example, if asthma attacks are a health concern (level 1 of the disease prevention model), environmental tobacco smoke (secondhand smoke) could be an important environmental risk factor. Air pollution is a second possible environmental risk factor for asthma attacks (see Figure 1-3). Exposure to either group of airborne pollutants increases the likelihood of an asthma attack. Further examples of environmental risk factors are lead paint exposure, carbon monoxide and air pollution, and contaminated water and food sources (Falk, 2011). Health outcomes with strong relationships to environmental risk factors include birth defects, asthma, cancer, lead poisoning, heart attack, and developmental disabilities (CDC, 2012a).

Level 3: Antecedents

Level 3 of the disease prevention model represents antecedents. **Antecedents** are the factors that drive health behaviors and environmental conditions. For example, antecedents that influence physical activity include positive beliefs about the outcome of physical activity, confidence in completing activities, access to activity opportunities, and a support network (Sallis & Glanz, 2009; Task Force on Community Preventive Services, 2002). When these factors are present, a person is more likely to engage in physical activity. Antecedents fall into the broad categories of knowledge, beliefs, skills, resources, barriers, reminders, and social support (Langlois & Hallam, 2010). If the appropriate antecedents are changed in ample magnitude, then the risk factors change, and thus the likelihood of disease decreases.

Antecedents exist in multiple levels of the environment. Knowledge, beliefs, and skills are individual factors called intrapersonal factors. One's circle of family and friends,

TABLE 1-4 Coronary Heart Disease Risk Factors

Major Risk Factors[a]	
Age	As individuals age, the likelihood of a heart attack increases. About 82% of people who die of coronary heart disease are 65 or older.
Gender	Men have a greater risk of heart attack than women, and men experience attacks at earlier ages. Women's risk for heart disease increases after menopause; however, even after menopause, their risk not as great as men's risk.
Heredity (including race)	Heart disease tends to run in families. Children of parents with heart disease are more likely to develop heart disease. Heart disease risk is also higher among Mexican Americans, American Indians, native Hawaiians, and some Asian Americans. African Americans are more likely to have more severe high blood pressure than whites and a higher risk of heart disease. Most people with a strong family history of heart disease have one or more other risk factors.
Tobacco smoke	Smokers are at a greater risk of developing heart disease than nonsmokers; their risk is between two and four times higher. Smoking one pack of cigarettes a day increases a smoker's risk of a heart attack to twice that of people who have never smoked. Exposure to tobacco smoke promotes plaque buildup in and subsequent narrowing of arteries and thus restricted blood flow. This in turn leads to lower blood oxygen levels and a greater likelihood of clotting.
High blood cholesterol	The risk of heart disease increases as blood cholesterol increases. An individual's cholesterol level is affected by factors such as age, race, sex, and diet. As blood cholesterol rises, so does the risk of coronary heart disease.
High blood pressure	High blood pressure makes the heart work harder, leading to abnormally thickened, stiffer heart muscle. This causes the heart not to work properly. The risk of heart attack or stroke multiplies several times when high blood pressure coexists with obesity, smoking, high blood cholesterol levels, and/or diabetes.
Physical inactivity	Physical inactivity increases an individual's risk for heart disease. It is possible to improve heart and blood vessel health by regular moderate to vigorous exercise.
Obesity and overweight	Carrying excess body fat, especially around the abdominal area, increases one's risk of developing heart disease or having a stroke regardless of whether other risk factors are present. This excess weight forces the heart to work harder and raises blood pressure, cholesterol, and triglycerides. Individuals carrying excess weight are also at an increased risk for diabetes.
Diabetes mellitus	Individuals with diabetes are at a much greater risk for developing heart disease. Heart or blood vessel disease is the cause of death in roughly two-thirds of people with diabetes.

continues

TABLE 1-4 *continued*

Contributing Risk Factors[b]	
Stress	An individual's response to stress may contribute to an increased risk of heart disease. Stress can also influence a person's health behaviors. For instance, people under stress may overeat, start smoking, or smoke more than they normally would. The relationship between stress and heart disease can be challenging to quantify, partly because of the difficulty of measuring stress in populations.
Alcohol	Drinking too much alcohol can raise an individual's blood pressure, cause heart failure, and lead to stroke. It can contribute to high triglycerides and produce irregular heartbeats. The risk of heart disease in people who drink moderate amounts of alcohol is lower than in nondrinkers.
Diet and nutrition	The types and amount of food consumed can affect other controllable risk factors: cholesterol, blood pressure, diabetes, and overweight. A diet rich in vegetables, fruits, whole grains and other high-fiber foods, fish, lean protein, and fat-free or low-fat dairy products is associated with health benefits.

a) Major risk factors are those that research has shown significantly increase the risk of heart and blood vessel (cardiovascular) disease.

b) Contributing risk factors are associated with an increased risk of cardiovascular disease, but their significance and prevalence have not yet been precisely determined.

Source: American Heart Association.

interpersonal factors, also influence behavior via resources, support, and modeling. A third level of behavioral factors includes a person's living and working environments. Environments provide resources, cues, and support that can promote or hinder health behaviors. Program activities are designed and implemented to change antecedents. Thus, a clear understanding of what influences risk factors can determine whether programming is effective or ineffective.

Section 2 of this book uses health behavior theory to explain specific types of antecedents that influence behavioral action. The utility of health behavior theory is to explain, in great detail, possible factors that can influence behaviors. Program activities are designed and implemented to change specific antecedents. Thus, in Chapter 10, interventions will be introduced as a fourth level of the disease prevention model.

Relationships

Relationships within the disease prevention model operate *two levels at a time*. Health is influenced by biological, behavioral, and environmental determinants. Antecedents

influence specific determinants of health, called risk and protective factors. The two-way arrow within the disease prevention model depicts the relationships between the two levels (see Figure 1-2). Measures of obesity (level 1) change when fruit and vegetable consumption or similar behaviors are altered. Fruit and vegetable consumption (level 2) is altered by changing the important antecedents (level 3).

A common mistake in public health practice is skipping a level, or two, in the disease prevention model. Planning strategies of change at a health issue level is common. Community teams identify "obesity" as a community health issue and plan strategies of change, such as health fairs and an awareness walk. Creating a list of activities (level 4) based on the health issue (level 1) lacks focus and is unlikely to produce health status change because it fails to produce behavioral change. A more effective planning approach is to target specific behavioral targets. Common behavioral risk factors for childhood obesity include high caloric intake, low fruit and vegetable consumption, high sugar-sweetened

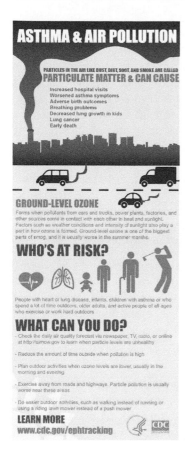

Figure 1-3 Infographic Depicting Air Pollution as an Environmental Risk Factor for Asthma
Source: Centers for Disease Control and Prevention

beverage intake, high fast-food intake, low physical activity levels, and high television viewing and computer gaming time (IOM, 2012a). Multilevel strategies addressing one or two of these behaviors should be implemented. Health fairs and awareness walks may end up as part of an overall program, but the activities are designed to target specific antecedents related to a targeted behavior, for example, knowledge of one's body mass index and amount of social support.

Check for Understanding Draw the disease prevention model for HIV/AIDS. List five risk factors in level 2 of the model.

Levels of Prevention

As noted earlier in this chapter, the fundamental principle of prevention is risk management. **Risk** is defined as an increased probability of a problem or negative event, and prevention programs work to alter risk for disease and injury. Prevention programs can influence disease risk at different stages of the health condition. For example, it is possible to reduce the *incidence* of breast cancer through different activities. Breast cancer **incidence**, the number of new diagnoses of a disease, can be decreased through decreased alcohol consumption, physical activity programs, and radiation exposure programs (Interagency Breast Cancer and Environmental Research Coordinating Committee, 2013). Health professionals can also work to diagnosis early-stage breast cancer. With early diagnosis, positive health outcomes, including survival, are more probable. This type of prevention work promotes early screening via mammography, physician exam, and regular self-exams. Finally, in women who have been diagnosed with breast cancer, health outcomes can be improved through promoting treatment compliance, as well as strength and nutrition programs (Interagency Breast Cancer and Environmental Research Coordinating Committee, 2013). This breast cancer example highlights the three levels of prevention: primary, secondary, and tertiary.

The aim of **primary prevention** is to promote overall health, which limits the number of new cases of a disease or injury. Primary approaches promote health and aim to keep persons healthy, promote good health, and reduce factors that can lead to the onset of disease and disability. This level of health promotion tends to be more holistic and is not typically disease specific (Katz & Ali, 2009). Walking 60 minutes a day promotes overall physical and mental health; it also reduces risk for cardiovascular disease, select cancers, obesity, diabetes, and more. Health promotion also targets larger goals such as entire segments of the population, not individuals (National Public Health Partnership, 2006). It is important to keep in mind that promoting health is more than just avoiding disease. Reflect back to the opening definition of health "... not merely the absence of disease."

Secondary prevention activities seek to identify and treat asymptomatic persons who have developed risk factors but in whom the health condition is not yet evident. Screenings are the primary activities of secondary prevention (Katz & Ali, 2009). Mammography, colorectal, blood sugar, blood

Model for Understanding Disciplines, like health promotion, are organized around big ideas and concepts. As students of the discipline acquire greater competency, they see these schema and use them to organize thoughts and solve problems (National Research Council, 2000). Schemas are patterns of information or behavior. Without linking the big concepts, there is just independent fact. The disease prevention model establishes those relationships. Information for public health and health promotion fits into one of the categories of the disease prevention model. It is *the process of population health*. See this chapter's Behavioral Science in Action feature on the Framingham Heart Study for a description of the process of identifying risk and protective factors for heart disease and how information about behavioral antecedents and interventions were then developed.

The disease prevention model provides a way to organize new facts and information. As new health information emerges, the disease prevention model is a model for organization. It can also help identify gaps in knowledge about a health issue or prevention strategies. Autism spectrum disorder is an example of a common health issue for which professionals are still at the first level of knowing. Autism spectrum disorder is defined and has tools for diagnosis and tracking. To date, though, the risk factors for autism are unclear. Males are more likely to be diagnosed with autism, but other risk factors are still being explored. Some studies have identified maternal and paternal age as possible risk factors (Parner et al., 2012). Others have speculated that exposure to environmental chemicals, maternal stress, and vitamin deficiencies are risk factors (Dietert, Dietert, & DeWitt, 2011). We do not understand autism's risk factors as well as we do those of other health issues such as cardiovascular disease, cancer, obesity, and HIV/AIDS.

Interventions cannot be planned to minimize the risk of autism because it is unclear what influences this risk. Thus, the scientific community must first establish the relationships between autism (level 1) and risk factors (level 2). The next step of knowing and prevention practice will be understanding the antecedents (level 3) that influence the risk factors (level 2).

pressure, vision, and hearing are examples of screenings that can identify early disease onset. Following screenings, subsequent interventions aim to prevent the progression of the disease. Screenings and other awareness activities can be implemented to target both population segments and individuals. The line between primary and secondary prevention activities can at times blur because it is not always possible to differentiate between asymptomatic and unaffected individuals (Katz & Ali, 2009).

Tertiary prevention aims to minimize the negative physical and social effects of disease, prevent future complications and/or progression, and restore function. Treatment, rehabilitation, and self-management programs are the primary activities of tertiary prevention (Katz & Ali, 2009; National Public Health Partnership, 2006). These actions reduce complications and improve the well-being and quality of life of persons with the disease or disability. The target of tertiary prevention is more focused than in the earlier levels, with resources directed toward persons with disease or disability rather than large segments of the population. All three levels of prevention are important in the work of population health improvement; interventions target different behavioral risks factors and/or population segments at differing points in disease progression. Table 1-5 summarizes the three levels.

TABLE 1-5 Three Levels of Prevention

Primary	Approaches that aim to prevent the incidence of disease and disability by promoting determinants of good health and reducing factors that can lead to the onset of disease and disability
Secondary	Approaches that aim to identify and treat asymptomatic persons who have already developed risk factors but in whom the health condition is not evident
Tertiary	Approaches that aim to minimize the negative effects of disease, prevent future complications/progression, and restore function

There are not unique sets of behaviors for each level of prevention. Behaviors that promote health can be important both in the early and later stages of disease. For example, physical activity can be a protective behavior in primary, secondary, and tertiary prevention programs. First, promoting physical activity in healthy children and young adults is primary prevention. Second, offering specialized exercise programs for persons with prediabetes risk factors is secondary prevention. Third, exercise in a supervised cardiac or pulmonary rehabilitation program is an example of tertiary prevention. Nutrition, medication use, and immunizations are other behaviors that also have a role across the continuum of prevention.

> **Check for Understanding** For the content area of violence, what are possible risk management focus areas at the primary, secondary, and tertiary levels?

Evidence-Based Public Health

Evidence-based public health (EBPH) practice is the use of information to identify causes and contributing factors to health and to identify effective health promotion actions to improve health. Simply stated, it is using information (evidence) to make decisions about practice. Evidence-based practice is not a new idea—clinical guidelines in medicine, standards-based education, and total quality improvement are examples of data-driven decision making in other disciplines. Data-driven decision making asks the question "Which method achieves the best outcome?" where outcomes can be patient health, product safety, efficiency, or a combination of outcomes. Evidence-based practice stands in contrast to approaches based on tradition, preference, or anecdotal evidence (AHRQ, 2012b; Rychetnik et al., 2004; SAMSHA, 2011).

In public health, evidence-based practice involves collecting and interpreting information along a continuum of practices. Brownson and colleagues have defined EBPH as "making decisions based upon the best available data and information systems, systematically applying program-planning frameworks, engaging the community in decision making, conducting sound evaluation, and disseminating what is learned" (2009, p. 175). Numerous practices fall within this definition. The first public health practice, surveillance, studies the causes of disease and the magnitude, severity, and preventability of disease. Surveillance information suggests that *something* should be done (Brownson et al., 2009). Table 1-1, which is about the leading causes of death in the United States, lists evidence of this nature. For example, evidence of the leading causes of death indicates that lifestyle-related diseases, not infectious diseases, account for the greatest proportion of deaths and disease.

Surveillance is followed by the second public health practice of programming and treatment. Collecting information through program evaluations can suggest *specifically* what can be done. If certain interventions change behaviors and improve health, then conclusions about their use and efficacy can be drawn. Third is the practice of disseminating information on programs that work. In this stage, programs that have been evaluated are shared with larger audiences. Ideally, information is also collected on this larger scale, and evidence about how and under which conditions interventions work can be generated. This type of evidence suggests *how something should be done*. The collective use of information in the decision-making process along this continuum improves public health outcomes and resource efficacy, which is the goal of evidence-based practice.

Likewise, the Agency for Healthcare Research and Quality (AHRQ) has a similar definition of evidence-based health care. This definition states that evidence-based practice involves applying the best available research results (evidence) when making decisions about health care. Health care professionals who perform evidence-based practice use research evidence along with clinical expertise and patient preferences. Systematic reviews (summaries of health care research results) provide information that aids in the process of evidence-based practice (AHRQ, 2012b). According to this definition, sources of information, from research to medical experience as well as patient context, are all highlighted.

What Is Evidence?

Medicine, health promotion, and other acts of public health should be based on evidence. In all cases, evidence is defined as some form of data used to make judgments and decisions (Brownson et al., 2009). Data exist in various forms. A key to evidence-based practice is to use the *best available data*, recognizing that the most ideal information may not be available. Waiting for the perfect data before acting would be poor practice. Experimental evidence can take years to develop, and often, practitioners must take action earlier. Epidemiologic data about a health issue often exist. As noted in the previous section, the availability of this type of evidence suggests that something should be done. It is this type of information that draws attention to a needed action. As referenced earlier, the understanding of autism spectrum disorder is at this level of evidence. Ideally, information about how and under what conditions interventions work to improve health also is available to guide practice. This best type of data may not be available when working in emerging fields or with specific populations.

Observation and theory are important elements in evidence-based practice. As noted by Brownson and colleagues, "Public health evidence is usually the result of a complex cycle of observation, theory, and experiment" (2009, p. 177). Action begins with the observation of phenomena that is then is further explored. Observation occurs as formal and informal evaluation of relationships and outcomes. A program evaluation or a focus group can be the source of observational information.

Theory plays a critical role in evidence-based practice. Theory organizes observation into hypothesized relationships and outcomes. It becomes a link between observation and experimental evidence. It the absence of content- and audience-specific evidence; theory becomes the road map for understanding behaviors and phenomenon and for designing change. "A theory is a systematic way of understanding events or situations. It is a set of concepts, definitions, and propositions that explain or predict these events or situations by illustrating the relationships between variables" (Glanz & Rimer, 2005). In designing strategies of change, all programs should minimally be based on theory (Brownson et al., 2009; Boyle & Homer, n.d.).

Theories themselves get studied and are generalized so as to apply across content areas. Programs are often designed around a theoretical framework, the theory-based program is evaluated, and then with repeated findings of similar outcomes, the evidence becomes a generalized scientific finding. Theory is particularly useful in new and emerging areas or in areas of practice where there are gaps in the knowledge base. Chapter 4 introduces health behavior theory as a valuable part of the continuum of evidence-based practice.

Other typologies or systems of evidence will be discussed throughout this book. The process and evidence for establishing national behavioral recommendations is the topic of the Behavioral Science in Action feature in Chapter 2. In Chapter 10, a continuum of evidence developed by Puddy & Wilkins (2011) will be introduced as a tool for making informed decisions about interventions. In the continuum, evidence can be well supported, supported, promising, emerging, or undetermined. Evidence-based resources, such as *The Community Guide*, will also be introduced.

Public Health Achievements

Life expectancy and quality of life have changed dramatically in this country. Since the beginning of the 1900s, life expectancy for the average American has increased by more than 30 years (CDC, 1999a). As mentioned previously, the current life expectancy for all Americans is 78.5 years, up from 47.3 years in 1900 (Arias, 2014; National Vital Statistics System, 2012). Approximately 85% of the increase in years is attributed to advances in population-based (public) health initiatives such as safer living and working conditions (CDC, 1999a; McGinnis et al., 2002). The Centers for Disease Control and Prevention identified the following "Ten Great Public Health Achievements" of the twentieth century:

- Vaccinations
- Motor vehicle safety
- Safer workplaces
- Control of infectious diseases
- Decline in deaths from coronary heart disease and stroke
- Safer and healthier foods
- Healthier mothers and babies
- Family planning
- Fluoridation of drinking water
- Recognition of tobacco use as a health hazard

Achievements in public health, both historical and future, have addressed and will address multiple determinants of the health outcomes. They also employ evidence-supported multilevel interventions of change. Through the twentieth century, changes in human factors, vehicle factors, and the driving environment collectively reduced the number of Americans injured or killed while riding in cars (NHTSA, 2014). Individuals increasingly used seat belts, child safety seats, and motorcycle helmets. Vehicles were built with better and additional safety features such as three-point seat belts, headrests, and shatter-resistant windshields. Environmentally, policies for road safety features such as speed, illumination, signage, curves, reflectors, and use of barriers also improved traffic safety (CDC, 1999b). Laws and awareness campaigns changed social norms related to impaired driving and the training of young drivers. No single intervention would have had a drastic impact on the number of vehicle deaths and injuries, but interventions that address multiple determinants resulted in a significant decline. This type of multipronged approach is necessary when tackling complex health issues.

Winnable Battles of the Twenty-First Century

Looking forward, the Centers for Disease Control and Prevention has created a list of health priorities it calls "winnable battles in public health." Winnable battles have a large-scale impact on the health of many, *and* there are evidence-based solutions to address these health issues. Each battle area is a leading cause of illness, injury, disability, or death and/or leads to enormous societal costs. In 2010 and 2011, the agency declared modern-day battles with food safety, health care–associated infections, HIV infections, motor vehicle injuries, obesity/nutrition, unintended pregnancy, and tobacco use.

Readers may notice a few similarities in the lists of twentieth-century achievements and targets for current public health improvements. Immunizations, motor vehicle injuries, food and nutrition, family planning, and tobacco appear on both lists. The topic areas are similar, but the behavioral risk factors and/or the target audiences have changed. For example, with tobacco, early work focused on public awareness and tobacco cessation in nonspecified audiences. As a result, smoking rates were cut in half: from 42% to approximately 21%. Looking forward, desired achievements related to tobacco are to decrease exposure to secondhand smoke in vulnerable populations, increase cessation in "hard-core" smokers, and reduce the proportion of new smokers (see Key Actions in Table 1-6).

Food safety also appears on both lists. The CDC estimates that one in six people get sick each year from foodborne illness and that 3000 Americans will die annually from food illness (CDC, 2013b). Current risks for foodborne illness come from modern farming practices, globalization of the food supply, and more meals being eaten outside the home. No one food group, nor one food practice, is the overarching cause of food illness, though poultry, leafy greens, beef, fruits, and nuts are among the food groups with the largest number of food outbreaks. Foodborne illness can occur in the home or in restaurants due to unsafe preparation habits, including poor hand hygiene, improperly prepared or stored food, or food contaminated during harvest, processing, or transportation. Addressing food safety requires different interventions aimed at the food safety knowledge and handling practices of individuals, food handlers, restaurants, and food manufacturers and processors.

Each battle area has a clear target that can be monitored—either a behavior or an environmental determinant. In 2013, the agency reported progress in motor vehicle deaths, teen births, and some health care–related infections (CDC, 2013b). At this time of reflection, targets and key actions to achieve the targets (evidence-based strategies) were updated, and they are listed in Table 1-6.

TABLE 1-6 Winnable Battles in Public Health: 2015 Targets

Battle Area	Target	Select Key Actions
Food safety	Rate of infections caused by Salmonella and Shiga toxin-producing *Escherichia coli* (STEC)	• Improve knowledge of incidence, trends, burden, and causes of foodborne illness • Improve state and federal epidemiologic, laboratory, and environmental health capacity to quickly detect and respond to foodborne outbreaks
Health care–associated infections	Rates of the following: invasive methicillin-resistant *Staphylococcus aureus* (MRSA), catheter-associated urinary tract infections, surgical site infections, and central line–associated bloodstream infections	• Improve hand washing and other infection prevention guideline behavior • Increase use of the National Healthcare Safety Network (NHSN) to intervene, track, and report infections
HIV infections	The number of new HIV infections	• Increase HIV testing and diagnosis • Improve retention in care and medication adherence for persons with HIV • Increase comprehensive prevention counseling with people who are HIV positive and people who are high-risk negative • Improve data monitoring, data dissemination, and feedback between agencies and states
Motor vehicle injuries	Rate of motor vehicle–related fatalities	• Increase seat belt, child safety seat, and booster seat use • Require all teens to be covered by graduated driving license (GDL) systems with parental monitoring • Employ evidence-based strategies, such as ignition interlock programs, to reduce alcohol-impaired driving
Obesity, nutrition, and physical activity	The prevalence of obesity among U.S. children and adolescents ages 2–19	• Monitor breastfeeding-related maternity care practices • Reduce sodium levels in foods • Reduce trans fats in food supply • Reduce consumption of calories from added sugars • Improve food environments of child care centers, schools, workplaces, and retail outlets • Improve environments and policies of child care centers, schools, workplaces, and communities to support physical activity
Teen pregnancy	The birthrate among adolescent female ages 15–19	• Increase the percentage of youth who delay initiation of sexual intercourse • Promote the use of contraceptive methods among sexually active youth
Tobacco use	Percentage of adults and youth who smoke cigarettes and proportion of the U.S. population covered by smoke-free laws	• Reduce small children's exposure to secondhand smoke • Promote smoking cessation in hard-core smokers • Promote smoking prevention in youth

Source: Centers for Disease Control and Prevention, 2013.

SUMMARY

People seek health because it makes their lives easier, more functional, and more fulfilling. The determinants of health fall into five broad categories: behavior, environment, biology, social conditions, and health care. The disease prevention model and evidence-based public health practice serve as frameworks for population health. Prevention programs work to alter risk for disease among individuals and segments of the population by altering the determinants of a particular health condition and focusing on risk and protective factors. Specific factors known to increase the likelihood of certain diseases are called risk factors, and they include behaviors, environmental conditions, and traits that increase the likelihood of the diseases. Protective factors are behaviors or traits that decrease the likelihood of diseases. Evidence-based public health practice uses the best available information to make decisions about relationships and to make plans for health promotion.

BEHAVIORAL SCIENCE IN ACTION

The Framingham Heart Study

Today, physicians know that eating healthy food, exercising, and not smoking can reduce one's risk of heart disease, but that was not always the case. By the twentieth century, cardiovascular disease (CVD) was the leading cause of death in the United States, killing many seemingly healthy people. Mortality rates steadily increased with each passing year, but scientists and physicians knew little about the disease. The National Heart Institute (now called the National Heart, Lung, and Blood Institute) began the Framingham Heart Study in an attempt to learn more about CVD. Previous research on heart disease included laboratory and clinical research, but these approaches did not lead to answers. Some researchers hypothesized that there might be preexisting and predisposing lifestyle factors present in patients that could be modified to decrease risk or delay the onset of CVD. The Framingham Heart Study set out to solve the mysteries surrounding heart disease.

The Framingham Heart Study, begun in 1948, originally followed over 5000 residents of the town of Framingham, Massachusetts. Scientists chose the town because it was large enough to contain enough volunteer study participants but small enough that it would be possible to monitor all participants. The town was economically stable, so the residents were unlikely to move out due to job loss or other reasons. The town's physicians and health department were committed to the study and provided support throughout the years.

The study was longitudinal, meaning researchers followed the participants before they showed signs of disease and tracked their lifestyles and health status over the course of their lives. Men and women between the ages of 30 and 62 made up the original study group, and they provided information about their lifestyles and completed physical exams and laboratory tests every two years. The study enrolled the children and grandchildren of the original participants into two more cohorts, or distinct groups, to follow new generations using similar longitudinal study techniques.

Over the years, the researchers involved with the Framingham Heart Study have learned much about cardiovascular disease. To learn about the natural course of the disease, they observed how CVD develops over individuals' life spans. With so many participants and such rich details about their lifestyles, physicians recognized trends in the traits and habits that appear in patients who develop CVD that are not present in individuals who do not develop the disease. The researchers coined the term "risk factors" and identified the major risk factors for the disease, including high blood pressure, smoking, high dietary fat intake, diabetes, inactivity, obesity, and high cholesterol. They also learned that only 5–10% of CVD cases are due to genetics, with the vast majority of cases being caused by lifestyle factors.

The original Framingham population was homogenous, as most participants were middle class and white. While the findings of the study apply to most populations, the researchers wanted to expand their pool of participants to include more diverse individuals. A new study cohort, known as the Omni cohort, enrolled in the study in 1994 to add more participants of different racial and ethnic backgrounds from Framingham and surrounding towns. Researchers created a second Omni cohort in 2003 to continue studying how CVD affects people of different backgrounds.

The data obtained through the Framingham Heart Study changed the way cardiovascular disease is viewed. Researchers published over 1200 papers based on the study, and physicians and other health care providers around the world have benefited from knowing about predisposing and risk factors related to heart disease. The study continues to this day, making it the longest longitudinal study ever conducted, and researchers are still learning about the complex relationships between risk factors, lifestyle choices, and CVD.

IN THE CLASSROOM ACTIVITIES

1) List three words that are important elements to a definition of health. Use those terms to create a personalized definition of health.

2) Create a list of at least five unintentional injuries that might be trending on college campuses. Give examples of biological, social, behavioral, and environmental risk and protective factors for each of the injuries.

3) Take the list of injuries and risk and protective factors from activity 2 and place them in the correct category of the disease prevention model.

4) How might interventions differ by the different types of unintentional injuries? Explain the role of risk and protective factors in disease and injury reduction.

5) Read the current edition of a national newspaper and identify health issues that are discussed. Compare the list to the winnable battles in public health discussed in Table 1-6.

WEB LINKS

Agency for Healthcare Research and Quality: http://www.ahrq.gov

American Heart Association: http://www.heart.org/HEARTORG

Centers for Disease Control and Prevention: www.cdc.gov

National Center for Health Statistics: http://www.cdc.gov/nchs

Trust for Americans Health: www.healthyamericans.org

REFERENCES

Agency for Healthcare Research and Quality (AHRQ). (2012a). *The guide to clinical preventive services, 2012.* Rockville, MD: Author.

Agency for Healthcare Research and Quality (AHRQ). (2012b). *What is the Effective Health Care Program.* Retrieved from http://effectivehealthcare.ahrq.gov/index.cfm/what-is-the-effective-health-care-program1

Agency for Toxic Substances and Disease Registry. (2007). *Toxicological profile for lead.* Atlanta: U.S. Department of Health and Human Services.

American Cancer Society (ACS). (2014). *Cancer facts & figures, 2014.* Atlanta: Author.

American Diabetes Association (ADA). (2013). Economic costs of diabetes in the U.S. in 2012. *Diabetes Care, 36*(4), 1033–1046.

American Heart Association (AHA). (2013). *Understanding your risk of heart attack.* Retrieved from http://www.heart.org

Arias, E. (2014). United States life tables, 2009. *National Vital Statistics Reports, 62*(7), 1–63.

Booske, B. C., Athens, J. K., Kindig, D. A., Park, H., & Remington, P. L. (2010). *Different perspectives for assigning weights to determinants of health status* (County Health Rankings working paper). University of Wisconsin Population Health Institute. Retrieved from www.countyhealthrankings.org

Boyle, L., & Homer, A. (n.d.). *Using what works: Adapting evidence-based programs to fit your needs.* U.S. Department of Health and Human Services, National Institutes of Health, National Cancer Institute. Retrieved from http://cancercontrol.cancer.gov

Brownson, R. C., Fielding, J. E., & Maylahn, C. M. (2009). Evidence-based public health: A fundamental concept for public health practice. *Annual Review of Public Health, 30,* 175–201.

Centers for Disease Control and Prevention (CDC). (1999a). Achievements in public health: 1900–1999 motor-vehicle safety; A 20th-century public health achievement. *Morbidity and Mortality Weekly, 48*(18), 369–374.

Centers for Disease Control and Prevention (CDC). (1999b). Ten great public health achievements: United States, 1900–1999. *Morbidity and Mortality Weekly, 48*(12), 241–243.

Centers for Disease Control and Prevention (CDC). (2009). Prevalence and most common causes of disability among adults: United States, 2005. *Morbidity and Mortality Weekly, 58*(16), 421–426.

Centers for Disease Control and Prevention (CDC). (2011). Injury prevention and control: Data and statistics (WISQARS). Retrieved from www.cdc.gov/injury/wisqars/facts.html

Centers for Disease Control and Prevention (CDC). (2012a). *A picture of America: Our health and environment.* Retrieved from http://www.cdc.gov/nceh/tracking

Centers for Disease Control and Prevention (CDC). (2012b). Vital signs: Risk from overdose from methadone used for pain relief; United States, 1999–2010. *Morbidity and Mortality Weekly , 61*(26), 493–497.

Centers for Disease Control and Prevention (CDC). (2013a). *Asthma facts: CDC's National Asthma Control Program grantees.* Atlanta: U.S. Department of Health and Human Services, Centers for Disease Control and Prevention.

Centers for Disease Control and Prevention (CDC). (2013b). *Winnable battles: Progress.* Retrieved from http://www.cdc.gov/winnablebattles

Centers for Disease Control and Prevention (CDC). (2014). *National diabetes statistics report, 2014.* Retrieved from http://www.cdc.gov/diabetes/pubs/estimates14.htm

Danaei, G., Ding, E. L., Mozaffarian, D., Taylor, B., Rehm, J., Murray, C. J. L., & Ezzati, M. (2009). The preventable causes of death in the United States: Comparative risk assessment of dietary, lifestyle, and metabolic risk factors. *PLoS Medicine, 6*(4), e1000058.

Davis, A. M., Vince, L. M., Okwuosa, T. M., Chase, A. R., & Huang, E. S. (2007). Cardiovascular health disparities: A systematic review of health care interventions. *Medical Care Research and Review, 64* (5 Suppl), 29S-100S.

Dietert, R. R., Dietert, J. M., & Dewitt, J. C. (2011). Environmental risk factors for autism. *Emerging Health Threats Journal, 4,* 7111–7118.

Di Noia, J., & Byrd-Bredbenner, C. (2013). Adolescent fruit and vegetable intake: Influence of family support and moderation by home availability of relationships with Afrocentric values and taste preferences. *Journal of the Academy of Nutrition and Dietetics, 113*(6), 803–808.

Falk, H. (2011). Environmental health in *MMWR, 1961–2010. Morbidity and Mortality Weekly, 60*(4), 86–96.

Finkelstein, E. A., Corso, C. S., & Miller, T. R. (2006). *Incidence and economic burden of injuries in the United States.* New York: Oxford University Press.

Ford, E. S., Croft, J. B., Posner, S. F., Goodman, R. A., & Giles, W. H. (2013). Co-occurrence of leading lifestyle-related chronic conditions among adults in the United States, 2002–2009. *Preventing Chronic Disease, 10,* 1–12.

Glanz, N., & Rimer, B. (2005). *Theory at a glance: A guide for health promotion practice* (2nd ed.) (NIH Publication No. 053896). Bethesda, MD: U.S. Department of Health and Human Services, National Cancer Institute.

Go, A. S., Mozaffarian, D., Roger, V. L., Benjamin, E. J., Berry, J. D., Blaha, M. J. …Turner, M. B. (2014). Heart disease and stroke statistics, 2014 update: A report from the American Heart Association. *Circulation, 129*(3), e28–e292.

Graham, D. J., Pelletier, J. E., Neumark-Sztainer, D., Lust, K., & Laska, M. N. (2013). Perceived social-ecological factors associated with fruit and vegetable purchasing, preparation, and consumption among young adults. *Journal of the Academy of Nutrition and Dietetics, 113*(10), 1366–1374.

Howlader, N., Noone, A. M., Krapcho, M., Garshell, J., Neyman, N., Altekruse, S. F., … Cronin, K. A. (Eds.). (2013). *SEER cancer statistics review, 1975–2010.* Bethesda, MD: National Cancer Institute. Retrieved from http://seer.cancer.gov/csr/1975_2010/

Institute of Medicine (IOM). (1998). *Reducing the burden of injury: Advancing prevention and treatment.* Washington, DC: National Academies Press.Institute of Medicine (IOM). (2012a). *Accelerating progress in obesity prevention: Solving the weight of the nation.* Washington, DC: National Academies Press.

Institute of Medicine (IOM). (2012b). *Living well with chronic illness: A call for public health action.* Washington, DC: National Academies Press.

Interagency Breast Cancer and Environmental Research Coordinating Committee. (February 2013). *Breast cancer and the environment: Prioritizing prevention.* National Institutes of Health, National Institute of Environmental Sciences. Retrieved from http://www.niehs.nih.gov/about/boards/ibcercc/

Jones, C. N., Mack, K. A., & Paulozzi, L. J. (2013). Pharmaceutical overdose deaths: United States, 2010. *Journal of the American Medical Association, 309,* 657–659.

Kaiser Family Foundation. (2014). *Life expectancy at birth (in years), by race/ethnicity.* Retrieved from http://kff.org/other/state-indicator/life-expectancy-by-re/

Katz, D. L., & Ali, A. (2009). *Preventive medicine, integrative medicine and the health of the public.* Washington, DC: National Academies Press.

Krolner, R., Rasmussen, M., Brug, J., Klepp, K. I., Wind, M. & Due, P. (2011). Determinants of fruit and vegetable consumption among children and adolescents: A review of the literature. Part II: qualitative studies. *International Journal of Behavioral Nutrition and Physical Activity, 8*(112), 1–38.

Langlois, M., & Hallam, J. (2010) Integrating multiple health behavior theories into program planning: The PER worksheet. *Health Promotion Practice, 11*(2), 282–288.

Mariotto, A. B., Yabroff, K. R., Shao, Y., Feuer E. J., & Brown, M. L. (2011). Projections of the cost of cancer care in the United States, 2010–2020. *Journal of the National Cancer Institute, 103*(2), 117–128.

Martin, A. B., Hartman, M., Whittle, L., Catlin, A., & National Health Expenditure Accounts Team. (2014). National health spending in 2012: Rate of health spending growth remained low for the fourth consecutive year. *Health Affairs, 33*(1), 67–77.

McGinnis, J. M., Williams-Russo, P., & Knickman, J. R. (2002). The case for more active policy attention to health promotion. *Health Affairs, 21*(2), 78–93.

Mokdad, A. H., Marks, J. S., Stroup, D. F., & Gerberding, J. L. (2004). Actual causes of death in the United States, 2000. *Journal of American Medical Association, 291*(10), 1238–1245.

Moonie, S., Sterling, D. A., Figgs, L. W., & Castro, M. (2008). The relationship between school absence, academic performance, and asthma status. *Journal of School Health, 78*(3), 140–148.

National Cancer Institute. (2006). *All you need to know about cancer* (NIH Publication No. 06 1566). Bethesda, MD: U.S. Department of Health and Human Services.

National Center for Health Statistics. (2013). Health: United States, 2012; With special feature on emergency care. Hyattsville, MD: U.S. Department of Health and Human Services, Centers for Disease Control and Prevention.

National Heart, Lung, and Blood Institute. (2013). *Health topics: A–Z index.* Retrieved from http://www.nhlbi.nih.gov/health/health-topics/by-alpha

National Highway Traffic Safety Administration (NHTSA). (2014). Compendium of traffic safety research projects, 1985–2013. Washington, DC: U.S. Department of Transportation.

National Prevention Council. (July 2011). *National prevention strategy.* Washington, DC: U.S. Department of Health and Human Services.

National Public Health Partnership. (2006). *The language of prevention.* Melbourne, Australia: Author.

National Research Council. (1999). *Reducing the burden of injury: Advancing prevention and treatment.* Washington, DC: National Academies Press.

National Research Council. (2000). *How people learn: Brain, mind, experiences and school.* Washington, DC: National Academies Press.

National Vital Statistics System. (2012). Deaths: Preliminary data for 2010. *National Vital Statistics Report, 60*(4), 1–52.

Olshansky, S. J., Antonucci, T., Berkman, L., Binstock, R. H., Boersch-Supan, A., Cacioppo, J. T ... Rowe, J. (2012). Differences in life expectancy due to race and education differences are widening, and many may not catch up. *Health Affairs, 31*(8), 1803–1813.

Parner, E. T., Barton-Cohen, S., Lauritsen, M. B., Jorgensen, M., Schieve, L. A., Yeargin-Allsopp, M., & Obel, C. (2012). Parental age and autism spectrum disorders. *Annals of Epidemiology, 22*(3), 143–150.

Public Health Accreditation Board. (2011). Acronyms and glossary of terms (Version 1.0). Alexandria, VA: Public Health Accreditation Board. Retrieved from www.phaboard.org

Puddy, R. W., & Wilkins, N. (2011). *Understanding evidence part 1: Best available research evidence; A guide to the continuum of evidence of effectiveness*. Atlanta: Centers for Disease Control and Prevention.

Roger, V. L., Go, A. S., Lloyd, D. M., Adams, R. J., Berry, J. D., Brown, T. B. ...Wylie-Rosett, J. (2011). Heart disease and stroke statistics, 2011 update: A report from the American Heart Association. *Circulation, 123*(4), e18–e209.

Rychetnik, L., Hawe, P., Waters, E., Barratt, A., & Frommer, M. (2004). A glossary of evidence-based public health. *Journal of Epidemiology and Community Health 58*, 538–545.

Sallis, J., & Glanz, K. (2009). Physical activity and food environments: Solutions to the obesity epidemic. *Milbank Quarterly, 87*(1), 123–154.

Substance Abuse and Mental Health Services Administration (SAMHSA). (2011). *Results from the 2010 National Survey on Drug Use and Health: Volume 1. Summary of National Findings*. Rockville, MD: SAMHSA, Office of Applied Studies. Retrieved from http://oas.samhsa.gov/NSDUH/2k10NSDUH/2k10Results.htm#2.16

Task Force on Community Preventive Services. (2002). Recommendations to increase physical activity in communities. *American Journal of Preventive Medicine, 22*(4S), 67–72.

Trust for America's Health. (2012). *The facts hurt: Fat; A state-by-state injury prevention policy report*. Washington, DC: Robert Wood Johnson Foundation.

U.S. Department of Health and Human Services (USDHHS). (2000). *Healthy People 2010: Understanding and improving health* (2nd ed.). Washington, DC: U.S. Government Printing Office.

U.S. Department of Health and Human Services (USDHHS), Centers for Disease Control and Prevention (CDC). (2009). *Chronic diseases: The power to prevent, the call to control, at a glance 2009*. Atlanta: U.S. Department of Health and Human Services.

U.S. Department of Health and Human Services (USDHHS), Centers for Disease Control and Prevention (CDC). (2011a). *National diabetes fact sheet, 2011*. Atlanta: U.S. Department of Health and Human Services. Retrieved from http://www.cdc.gov/Diabetes/

U.S. Department of Health and Human Services (USDHHS), Centers for Disease Control and Prevention (CDC), National Center for Chronic Disease Prevention & Health Promotion. (2011b). *Heart disease and stroke prevention: Addressing the nation's leading killers, at a glance*. Atlanta: U.S. Department of Health and Human Services.

U.S. Department of Health and Human Services (USDHHS), Health Resources and Services Administration, Maternal and Child Health Bureau. (2013). *Child health USA, 2013*. Rockville, MD: U.S. Department of Health and Human Services.

U.S. Preventive Services Task Force (USPSTF). (2012). *Guide to clinical preventive services, 2012: Recommendations of the U.S. Preventive Services Task Force*. Rockville, MD: Agency for Healthcare Research and Quality.

World Health Organization (WHO). (1948). Preamble to the Constitution of the World Health Organization as adopted by the International Health Conference, New York, 19–22 June, 1946; signed on 22 July 1946 by the representatives of 61 States (Official Records of the World Health Organization, no. 2, p. 100) and entered into force on 7 April 1948.

World Health Organization (WHO). (1998). Health promotion glossary. Geneva, Switzerland: Division of Health Promotion, Education and Communications. Retrieved from http://www.who.int/healthpromotion/about/HPG/en

World Health Organization (WHO). (2001). *Strengthening mental health promotion* (Fact sheet No. 220). Geneva, Switzerland: Author.

World Health Organization (WHO). (2004). A glossary of terms for community health care and services for older persons. Geneva, Switzerland: WHO Centre for Health Development.

World Health Organization (WHO). (2013). *Mental health: A state of well-being*. Retrieved from http://www.who.int/features/factfiles/mental_health/en

Wu, S. Y., & Green, A. (2000). *Projection of chronic illness prevalence and cost inflation*. Santa Monica, CA: RAND Health.

CHAPTER 2

What Is a Health Behavior?

KEY TERMS

attributed	lifestyle behavior	observable	relative risk
habit	measurable	operationalize	shapeable
health behavior	mortality		

LEARNING OBJECTIVES

1. Define a health behavior.
2. Distinguish between a behavior and the factors that influence a behavior.
3. Discuss behaviors that have significant impact on population health status.
4. State health behaviors in measurable forms for select target audiences.
5. Recognize the presence and related outcomes of health behaviors in communities.
6. Use existing data sets to prepare a summary of health behavior rates for a defined community.

IN THE NEWS ...

January 11, 2014, marked the 50th anniversary of the landmark document *Smoking and Health: Report of the Advisory Committee of the Surgeon General of the Public Health Service*. The 387 pages can be summarized in four words: smoking causes lung cancer. The report has been called one of the most important documents in U.S. public health history. It began the shift in the public's attitude toward tobacco. Per capita tobacco consumption in the United States has dropped every single year since 1964. The Surgeon General's Office on Health and Safety has since issued 33 additional reports drawing attention to additional tobacco–attributable diseases, environmental tobacco smoke, smokeless tobacco, smoking and pregnancy, the physiology of tobacco-attributed disease, youth prevention, and tobacco use among racial/ethnic minorities. In the 2014 report, U.S. surgeon general Boris D. Lushniak added type 2 diabetes, rheumatoid arthritis, and erectile dysfunction to the list of poor health outcomes associated with tobacco.

Introduction

Health behaviors, collectively called lifestyle factors, represent the greatest portion of risk for the leading causes of death, disease, and disability. Approximately half of disease risk comes from health behaviors one chooses to do or not to do (Mokdad, Marks, Stroup, & Gerberding, 2004; National Prevention Council, 2011; U.S. Burden of Disease Collaborators, 2013). Thus, significant population level changes in disease prevalence and health status improvements must be mediated through the modification of health behaviors.

The examination of health behaviors begins within a content area. Content areas are broad topical areas that involve multiple health behaviors and environmental conditions. Population health content areas most commonly discussed are physical activity, nutrition, sexual behaviors, alcohol and other drugs, tobacco, and injury prevention. Less recognized, but also important to the health status of millions of Americans are mental health, oral health, sleep, and food systems. This chapter describes health behaviors in a progression of three phases:

- Within a content area
- As a specific behavioral form
- Framed for a specific target audience

Woven throughout these three phases of behavioral study is the principle that relevant and alterable health behaviors vary by setting and population. While content areas are typically similar, the specific behaviors related to health status can take different forms of relevancy in different settings and communities. Health promotion settings include worksites, health care, schools, and community-based organizations (see Figure 2-1). Settings are a mechanism to reach groups of gathered individuals. Within each setting, various communities, or groups of individuals with a similar trait, exist. Unifying community traits can be demographic characteristics such as age, gender, race, and socioeconomic status. The numbers of communities within a setting, however, extend well beyond these demographic characteristics. Any number of commonalities can identify communities. In health care, clinical staff, administrators, patients, and family are distinct subgroups. At a worksite, communities can be organized by job type, shift, or years of experience. In a university setting, student communities can include traditional and nontraditional students; Greek, club, and nonaffiliated students; part-time and full-time students; and those living on campus, those living in off-campus housing, and those that commute from home. Within settings, a variety of different communities exist, and health promotion interventions should be tailored to the behaviors and interpersonal and contextual factors of each community.

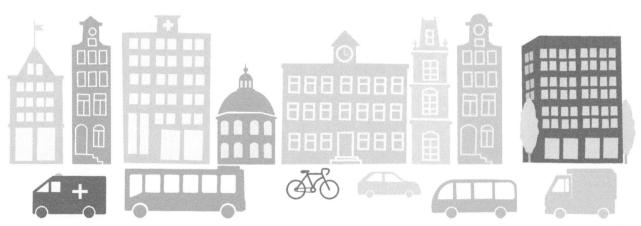

Figure 2-1 Settings for Health Promotion.

What Is a Health Behavior?

The World Health Organization (WHO) defines **health behavior** as any activity undertaken by an individual (or group), regardless of actual or perceived health status, for the purpose of promoting, protecting, or maintaining health, whether or not such behavior is objectively effective toward that end (2004, 1998). Simply stated, a health behavior is an action—regardless of intention, health status, or outcomes—that has a relationship with health.

In specific contexts, a health behavior may be labeled and defined in a more descriptive manner. One set of descriptive definitions published by Kasl and Cobb in 1966 (and since referenced close to 1,000 times, according to Google Scholar) provides health behaviors in which the health status of the actor is described. Kasl and Cobb (1966a, 1966b) differentiate preventive health behavior, illness behavior, and sick role behavior in the following manner:

- Preventive health behavior: Any activity undertaken by an individual who believes himself to be healthy, for the purpose of preventing or detecting illness in an asymptomatic state.

- Illness behavior: Any activity undertaken by an individual who perceives himself to be ill, to define the state of health and to discover a suitable remedy.

- Sick role behavior: Any activity undertaken by an individual who considers himself to be ill, for the purpose of getting well. It includes receiving treatment from health care providers and generally involves a range of dependent behaviors and leads to some degree of exemption from one's usual responsibilities.

Behaviors of Family, Care Providers, and Organizations

The preceding WHO definition specifies individual actions; more current thinking includes actions both of the individual and of others. People influence and are influenced by one another. Actions of family, caregivers, and organizations can have a significant, proximal relationship to another's health. By contrast, *personal health behaviors* are one's own actions that influence an individual's health (Simons-Morton, McLeroy, & Wendel, 2012).

The health-related behaviors of a family member or caregiver can easily impact the health of a child. For example, from conception, the self-care behaviors of a woman during pregnancy can significantly impact the health of the unborn child. Cigarette smoking, alcohol consumption, and inappropriate medication use negatively impact healthy fetal development (CDC, 2013a). Vitamin, mineral, and appropriate caloric intake; physical activity; and rest are associated with healthy development and birth outcomes (Abu-Saad & Fraser, 2010). The infant health–maternal behavior relationship extends beyond the womb. Breastfeeding, immunizations, and automobile driving behaviors influence children's health and safety. These actions are carried out by a parent or caregiver and have a direct, proximal influence on a child's health and development.

Health-related behaviors occur in settings and relationships outside families. Physicians who follow clinical guidelines tend to have patients with better health outcomes (U.S. Preventive Services Task Force, 2012). The health of communities is improved when health care providers report to work in an emergency. The actions of a sexual partner, specifically in disclosing HIV status or wearing a condom, can influence another individual's likelihood of developing a sexually transmitted infection (STI).

Lifestyle Behaviors

Motivation, frequency, and outcomes are additional aspects of behavior that may be reflected in a behavioral definition. Health behaviors can vary in how often they are completed. Some, like immunizations and cancer prevention screenings, are performed infrequently. Ideally, adults receive a flu shot annually, a colorectal exam every 10 years (after age 50), and a Tdap (tetanus, diphtheria, and pertussis) vaccine in adulthood. By contrast, behaviors that are performed more frequently and are integrated into a way of living are called **lifestyle behaviors** (WHO, 1998). Lifestyle behaviors are more complex in execution and reflect a pattern of actions such as those observed in diet, alcohol use, sexual activity, and driving patterns. The term "lifestyle" can also speak to a series of related actions across content areas. A healthy lifestyle may imply regular actions within activity, diet, substance use, and sleep. Further, lifestyle can reflect a series of simple actions that collectively create a pattern, for example, self-care, personal hygiene, and immunizations. Within these categories are simple infrequent acts that collectively describe more repetitive actions.

"Habit" is another term used to describe behaviors that are integrated into patterns of living. **Habit** is defined as an established behavior pattern marked by increasing automaticity, decreasing awareness, and partial independence from reinforcement (Hunt et al., 1979). As with lifestyle behaviors, persons perform habits in a regular and predictable manner. Habits, though, are often void of purposeful intention or motivation to act; a cue or a trigger sparks the habit (Bandura, 1977; Duhigg, 2012; Hunt et al., 1979; Verplanken, 2006). Given the trigger, individuals act in an automatic, almost involuntary, way.

Given one's situation, distinctions in health status, actor, intention, and/or frequency may be helpful. Fundamentally, though, all health behaviors are an individual's or other people's actions when those actions have a relationship to health outcomes.

The Health–Behavior Relationship

The relationship between health and behavior is the fundamental principle of disease prevention and health promotion. If one quits smoking, she is less likely to be diagnosed with lung cancer. If a behavior does not have a relationship with one's health or the health of others, it is not a health behavior. Health-minded individuals care about dietary fat intake because diets high in fat are associated with cardiovascular disease, diabetes, obesity, and select cancers (U.S. Department of Agriculture (USDA) & USDHHS, 2010). Seat belt use is associated with lower automobile fatality rates. Breastfeeding is associated with a lower risk of asthma, childhood obesity, diabetes, and sudden infant death syndrome (SIDS), as well as lower rates of adult breast and ovarian cancer (USDHHS, 2011b).

Health behaviors can have relationships with multiple health outcomes. A behavior can be associated with an increased risk of numerous health outcomes, and conversely, a healthy—or protective—behavior can improve health and lower risk for a number of diseases and disabilities. The relationship of behavior to outcome is not exclusive. Physical activity improves circulation, respiratory function, and insulin sensitivity; lowers blood pressure as well as lipid and carbohydrate metabolism; increases the production of endorphins; burns calories; and may link people socially (Fletcher et al., 1996; USDHHS, 1996). Thus, the protective nature of moderate daily physical activity extends across a number of health issues: cardiovascular disease, stroke, select cancers, diabetes, obesity, arthritis, and mental health issues (e.g., depression). As a result, it is not uncommon to see a small number of health behaviors linked to a large number of health statuses. Table 2-1 presents common health behavior content areas with associated health outcomes.

TABLE 2-1 Select Health Outcomes by Behavioral Content Area

Content Area	Health Outcomes
Accessing health care	Fetal and perinatal health problems Disease progression Chronic disease development
Alcohol and other drugs	Unintended pregnancy Human immunodeficiency virus/acquired immunodeficiency syndrome (HIV/AIDS) Other sexually transmitted infections (STIs) Domestic violence Child abuse Motor vehicle crashes Physical fights Crime Homicide Suicide

continues

TABLE 2-1 *continued*

Content Area	Health Outcomes
Nutrition	Overweight and obesity Malnutrition Iron deficiency anemia Heart disease High blood pressure Dyslipidemia (poor lipid profiles) Type 2 diabetes Osteoporosis Oral disease Constipation Diverticular disease Some cancers
Immunizations	Childhood disease (diphtheria, measles, mumps, whooping cough, polio, chicken pox, tetanus) Childhood development Respiratory infections Hepatitis and tuberculosis Shingles Cancer
Injury prevention (e.g., falls, motor vehicle crashes, and intentional violence)	Premature death Disability (including traumatic brain injury) Poor mental health High medical costs Lost productivity
Oral hygiene	Dental caries (tooth decay) Periodontal (gum) diseases Cleft lip and palate Oral and facial pain Oral and pharyngeal (mouth and throat) cancers
Physical activity	Coronary heart disease Stroke High blood pressure Type 2 diabetes Breast and colon cancer Falls Depression

continues

TABLE 2-1 *continued*

Content Area	Health Outcomes
Responsible sexual behavior	Unintended pregnancy Reproductive health problems (e.g., infertility) Fetal and perinatal health problems Cancer HIV/AIDS Other STIs Violence
Secondhand smoke	Severe asthma attacks Respiratory infections Ear infections Sudden infant death syndrome (SIDS)
Sleep	Fight off infection Support the metabolism of sugar to prevent diabetes Perform well in school and work Injury Heart disease High blood pressure Obesity Diabetes
Tobacco	Cancer Heart disease Lung diseases Premature birth, low birth weight, and infant death

Source: Healthy People 2020.

Check for Understanding Binge drinking, which is common among college students, is a health behavior associated with numerous negative health outcomes. Unlike some other behavioral examples such as smoking, these health outcomes are often realized more quickly. List three negative health outcomes associated with binge drinking.

The Big Four: Tobacco, Diet, Activity, and Alcohol

Four health behaviors contribute disproportionately to the leading causes of death, disease, and injury in the United States. Tobacco, poor diet, physical inactivity, and alcohol use are associated with approximately 37% of all deaths (Mokdad et al., 2004). Of the deaths recorded in a given year, researchers estimate the percentage attributed to behavioral, environmental, and metabolic risk factors. Death certificates list diseases such as heart attack or pneumonia (not smoking or cupcakes), so attributing deaths to risk factors requires advanced statistical analysis with large data sets. The term "actual causes of death" has been adopted to describe the calculated relationships between risk factors and death (Danaei et al., 2009; McGinnis & Foege, 1993; Mokdad et al., 2004). Others call these factors attributed deaths (IOM, 2005; U.S. Burden of Disease Collaborators, 2013). Precise estimates of the deaths **attributed** to particular behaviors can vary because of variations in behavior measurement, data analysis techniques, and population sets. Table 2-2 depicts the number and percentage of deaths, both recent and historical, due to the most common behavioral risk factors.

The unhealthy versions of these four behaviors are bad for health; the opposite is also true. The healthy versions of these behaviors can improve health and life expectancy. The individual and combined impact of behaviors can be significant (Ford, Greenlund, & Hong, 2012; Loef & Walach, 2012; Rasmussen-Torvik et al., 2013). The impact of healthy behaviors on health status appears greatest in combination. The number of healthy behaviors people adopt is positively related to life expectancy and quality of life. Nonsmokers and adults who consume alcohol in moderate amounts, engage in physical activity, and consume fruits and vegetables are three times more likely to age in a healthy manner (Sabia et al., 2012). Healthy aging implies good cognitive, respiratory, and cardiovascular functions as well as the absence of functional disability, mental health issues, and chronic disease. Likewise, adults ages 60 and older are 75% less likely to develop

a functional disability if they have never smoked, drink no more than moderate alcohol, sleep 6 to 8 hours a night, and engage in regular exercise (Liao et al., 2011). The powerful relationship between these behaviors and **mortality** are discussed next.

Tobacco Use

Tobacco use was declared public health enemy number one by former surgeon general C. Everett Koop, who in 1982 declared tobacco use as the leading cause of death and disability in this country. Three decades ago, this was a pretty significant statement. Analysis published by McGinnis and Foege (1993) quantified the numbers of deaths attributed to tobacco use as 400,000 a year; 10 years later, the number of per annum deaths had risen to 435,000 (18.1% of preventable deaths) (Mokdad et al., 2004). The current estimate of tobacco-attributed deaths is 465,000 per year; one in five deaths is attributed to tobacco (USDHHS, 2014; U.S. Disease Collaborators 2013; CDC, 2008).

TABLE 2-2 Tobacco-, Diet-, Inactivity-, and Alcohol-Attributed Causes of Death, 1990, 2000, and 2010

	No. (%) in 1990[a]	No. (%) in 2000[b]	No. in 2010[c]
Smoking	400,000 (19)	435,000 (18.1)	465,651
Dietary Patterns	300,000 (14)	365,000 (15.2)	678,282
Physical Inactivity			234,022
Alcohol Use	85,000 (5)	100,000 (3)	88,587
Microbial Agents	90,000 (4)	75,000 (3.1)	See Figure 2-2
Toxic Agents	60,000 (3)	55,000 (2.3)	
Motor Vehicle Crashes	25,000 (1)	43,000 (1.8)	
Firearms	35,000 (2)	29,000 (1.2)	
Sexual Behaviors	30,000 (1)	20,000 (0.8)	
Illicit Drug Use	20,000 (< 1)	17,000 (0.7)	
TOTAL	1,060,000 (50)	1,159,000 (48.2)	

Sources: [a]McGinnis & Foege, 1993; [b]Mokdad et al., 2004; [c]U.S. Burden of Disease Collaborators, 2013

One-third of all cancers are tobacco related (CDC, 2008). For certain diseases, the percentage of deaths attributed to tobacco use is much higher. Deaths attributed to tobacco use are highest for lung cancer (87%), chronic obstructive pulmonary disease (79%), and heart disease (32%). In addition, 8% of infant deaths are attributed to tobacco—either sudden infant death syndrome or low birth weight and respiratory problems (CDC, 2008). On an individual level, the life expectancy of a smoker is approximately 11 years short than that for a nonsmoker (Jha et al., 2013). Quitting smoking, before age 40, though and with time for the body to repair, can return life expectancy to that near a nonsmoker (Jha et al., 2013; USDHHS, 2014).

Tobacco use is also an expensive health behavior. Few smokers die of a sudden event; it is more likely for smokers experience chronic conditions and symptoms that are medically treated and/or result in disability (CDC, 2003). Damaged blood vessels, plague build up, reduced blood flow, inflamed airways and linings, and toxin exposure create conditions that require medical treatment (USDHHS, 2010). As a nation, 7% to 9% of health care expenditures are tobacco related. In 2013, direct medical care costs were $175 billion, up from $132 million in 2009 (USDHHS, 2014).

Looking at employer health care costs by behaviors is another method to calculate economic costs of health behaviors. Calculations can vary by the structure of the health care plan, age of employees, and calculation methods. In any case, costs for individual smoker are high. On average, the health care costs for a smoker are approximately $2056 higher, ranging from a low of $899 to a high of $3598 (Berman et al., 2013). In reviewing records for self-insured companies, Goetzel and colleagues (2012) found a smaller difference, $587 per year, which comes out to 16% higher costs than for nontobacco users. In a separate analysis, researchers found health care spending highest for recent quitters; spending was about $2500 higher ($7650) for a recent quitter versus a nonsmoker ($5040) or a current smoker ($5540). To explain the recent quitter versus current smoker gap, researchers hypothesize that recent quitters may have experienced illness that triggered both quitting and entering the medical care system (Baumgardner et al., 2012; CBO, 2012; USDHHS, 2014).

Today, tobacco retains its spot as public health enemy number one. In a recent report from the surgeon general, director of the CDC Dr. Thomas Frieden reflected that despite the dramatic progress the nation has made reducing tobacco use, there is a significant continuing burden of disease and death caused by smoking (USDHHS, 2014). Its reign as king killer is being challenged, though. A recent analysis by the U.S. Burden of Disease Collaborators (2013) found that dietary patterns contribute to more death and disability than tobacco (Figure 2-2).

Eating Patterns

Diet is a risk factor for four of the leading causes of death; heart disease, select cancers, stroke, and diabetes have associations with various food and nutrient intakes (USDA, 2010). Further, the likelihood of obesity, hypertension, and osteoporosis is also associated with one's eating patterns. In 1993, McGinnis and Foege quantified the numbers of deaths attributed to diet and inactivity as 300,000 a year; 10 years later, the number of deaths had risen to 365,000 (15.2% of preventable deaths) (Mokdad et al., 2004). These two calculations combined the impact of diet and physical activity. The most recent estimates, with diet contributions calculated alone, are 678,000 deaths, which represents one in four preventable deaths (U.S. Burden of Disease Collaborators, 2013).

Calculations and discussions of health outcomes and the economic impact of diet are a bit trickier than tobacco due to the large number of behaviors and the complexity of behaviors involved with diet. Caloric balance, sodium intake, saturated and trans fat intake, cholesterol intake, added sugar, and fruit and vegetable consumption are specific behaviors given attention within the Dietary Guidelines for Americans 2010 (USDA and USDHHS, 2010). Further, in one of the most recent calculations of diet's impact on health status, a team of researchers included 14 specific measures of diet (U.S. Burden of Disease Collaborators, 2013). Fruits, vegetables, sodium, and fat intakes were components of the calculations, but the researchers also considered intake of nuts and seeds, omega-3 fatty acids, whole grains, fiber, sugar-sweetened beverages, calcium, milk, and red and processed meats.

In addition, diet behaviors are co-mingled because one specific form of a behavior can be associated with other forms of

Risk factors and related deaths

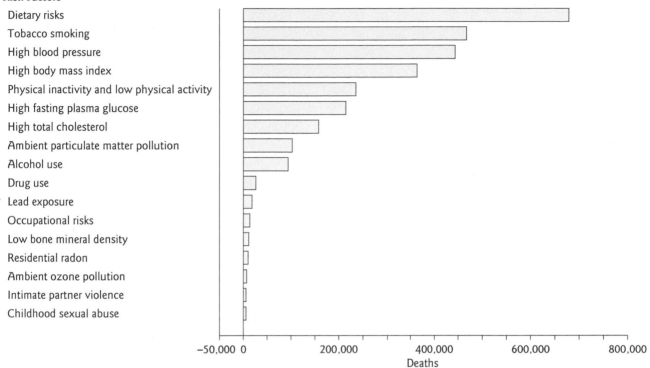

Figure 2-2 Attributed Causes of Death by Risk Factors, 2010.
Source: Adapted from U.S. Burden of Disease Collaborators (2013)

diet behaviors. One's overall diet intake is a pattern of these different behaviors. Eating foods high in sodium, for example, has a strong relationship with caloric intake. The more calories a person consumes, the higher his or her sodium intake tends to be (Hoy et al., 2011). Eating foods high in calories may also be associated with eating foods high in sugar, as well as lower fruit and vegetable consumption. These types of patterns and co-mingling exist across all content areas. Co-mingling relationships may lead researchers to overestimate the precise number of deaths attributed to certain behaviors or risk factors.

Discussing the economic costs associated with dietary behaviors is easiest when examining specific forms of behavior. Dietary sodium intake is a significant contributor to

health outcomes, in particular high blood pressure and stroke (Danaei et al., 2009; Ford et al., 2012; Go et al., 2013; U.S. Burden of Disease Collaborators, 2013). Most adults (90%) consume more than the recommended amount of sodium, with the majority of the intake coming from processed and/or combination foods (like casseroles and mixed dishes)—not from a table shaker (CDC, 2012a). A wide variety of foods contribute to total sodium intake; however, 10 food categories account for 40% of sodium consumption in the United States: cold cuts/cured meats, breads, pizza, poultry, soups, sandwiches, cheese, pasta dishes, meat dishes, and salty snacks (CDC, 2012a; Hoy et al., 2011).

The pharmaceutical and medical care costs to treat high blood pressure are high. Approximately $50 billion was spent in 2013 to treat high blood pressure (Go et al., 2013). One-third of adults have high blood pressure (Go et al., 2013; Roger, et al., 2012). Age, ethnicity, family history, weight, tobacco, stress, sleep, and excessive alcohol use all contribute to an individual's blood pressure measurement (Ford et al., 2012; Go et al., 2013). There is also strong, consistent evidence that a diet low in sodium can lower blood pressure. A DASH diet (Dietary Approaches to Stop Hypertension) can reduce blood pressure and blood cholesterol levels (Chen, Maruther, & Appel, 2010).

That dietary patterns are increasingly implicated in cause of death is not surprising, and some people even predicted this shift. As rates of obesity—of which diet is a strong behavioral correlate—increased to epidemic proportions, researchers predicted the rise of deaths attributed to dietary intake and physical inactivity (McGinnis & Foege, 2004). Diet's movement up the list could represent the beginning of a shift in causes of attributed deaths; this will be important to monitor for replicated findings by other researchers.

Physical Activity

Physical activity is associated with 5 of the 10 leading causes of death and disability. Rates of cardiovascular disease, stroke, select cancers, diabetes, and chronic respiratory diseases are higher in individuals who are not physically active (Murphy, Xu, & Kochanek, 2012). The latest estimates, using 2010 data, are that 234,022 deaths in the United States are attributed to physical inactivity (see Table 2-2) (U.S. Burden of Disease Collaborators, 2013). In a focused analysis using 2008 data and examining only inactivity as a risk factor, a group of researchers estimated that physical inactivity was the cause of approximately 6% of the coronary heart disease, 8% of type 2 diabetes, 12% of breast cancer, and 10% of colon cancer in the United States (Lee et al., 2012).

In 1992, physical inactivity was classified as a "major cardiovascular risk factor." (USDHHS, 1996). Following scientific recognition of the strength of the health–behavior relationship, promotion of physical activity has garnered widespread public and private efforts (Bouchard, Blair, & Haskell, 2007; Fletcher et al., 1996; USDHHS, 1996). The impact of inactivity is often discussed specifically in terms of health conditions, obesity, and diabetes. In studies of specific health care costs to employers, obesity was shown to be the fourth most expensive modifiable factor, with only depression, high glucose (related to diabetes), and high blood pressure higher. Overall, just examining behavioral differences by health care costs, physically inactive employees incurred about $600 (or 15%) higher annual health care claims than physically active employees (Goetzel et al., 2012).

As a health promotion behavior, physical activity has numerous benefits. Moderate amounts of activity increase cardiovascular and muscle fitness, promote bone health, increase cognitive function, and promote a healthy body mass and composition (Lee et al., 2012; USDHHS, 1996). Physically active adults are more likely to age in a healthier manner; they may maintain greater independence and live an addition 0.5 to 7 years (Reimers, Knapp, & Reimers, 2012).

Alcohol Use

The relationship of alcohol use to death and disability has been described as "j shaped." Light to moderate amounts of alcohol can be healthy and are associated with a lower risk of mortality, particular from cardiovascular disease, but heavy drinking is related to a greater risk of mortality and poor health outcomes (Kloner & Rezkalla, 2007; Plunk et al., 2013). The low hook part of the *j* signifies the low risk of mortality that then increases with increased consumption. An analysis published by McGinnis and Foege (1993) quantified the numbers of deaths attributed to alcohol use as 100,000 a year and decreasing to 85,000 deaths (3.5%) in 2000 (Mokdad et al., 2004). Current estimates are similar ranging between 87,798 and 88,587 deaths per year (U.S. Burden of Disease Collaborators 2013; Stahre et al., 2014).

Alcohol use is expensive, with excessive alcohol use costing states about $2.9 billion a year. These excessive drinking costs are largely due to losses in workplace productivity, medical expenses, and other costs related to the criminal justice system, motor vehicle crashes, and property damage (Sacks et al., 2013). Surprisingly, medical expenses represents 11.6% of the total cost associated with excessive drinking. A much larger part of the total costs associated with excessive alcohol consumption (70.5%) are nonmedical costs: productivity losses, lost wages due to premature death, injury, incarceration, and absenteeism. The combined medical care and productivity losses cost each state about $1.91 per drink (Bouchery et al., 2011; Sacks et al., 2013).

Fetal alcohol spectrum disorders (FASD) are groups of conditions that result from alcohol use during pregnancy. Alcohol use can impair physical development, intellectual capabilities, and emotional disposition. The effects on the person range from mild to severe. Fetal alcohol syndrome (FAS) represents the severe end of the FASD spectrum. Outcomes include fetal death and developmental disabilities. People with FAS can also have problems with learning, memory, attention span, communication, vision, or hearing. Behaviorally, people with fetal alcohol syndrome often struggle in school and in getting along with others (CDC, NCBDDD, 2014). "Alcohol-related neurodevelopmental disorder (ARND)" is a second term used to describe FASD conditions. Persons with ARND may have intellectual disabilities and/or behavioral and learning problems. The third category of conditions within FASD is alcohol-related birth defects (ARBD). People with ARBD may have heart, kidney, or bone abnormalities as well as hearing and/or vision impairments (CDC, NCBDDD, 2014). Because of the range of outcomes associated with FASD, the estimated direct (medical-related care) and indirect (lost productivity) costs also vary. Lupton and colleagues (2004) reviewed previously published costs estimates and then calculated 2002 per person and population costs. They predicted a lifetime cost for one individual with FAS to be $2 million (with $1.6 million being direct care, i.e., medical, residential, and support care). Persons with severe problems, such as profound intellectual disability, have much higher costs. Collectively the cost to the United States for FAS alone was over $4 billion annually (Lupton, Burd, & Harwood, 2004).

Binge drinking, a specific behavior within alcohol use, is both prevalent and costly. Binge drinking, defined as four or more drinks on one occasion for women, and five or more drinks on one occasion for men, is a risk factor for adverse health and social outcomes, including unintentional injuries (e.g., motor vehicle crashes), violence, suicide, hypertension, acute myocardial infarction, sexually transmitted infections, unintended pregnancy, fetal alcohol syndrome, and sudden infant death syndrome (National Institute of Alcohol Abuse and Alcoholism, 2000). Binge drinking is responsible for half of alcohol-related deaths and three-fourths of the economic costs (Bouchery, et al., 2011; Sacks et al., 2013). About 18% of adults report at least one episode of binge drinking in the past 30 days (Kanny et al., 2013). The average number of drinks in an episode was 7.7 (8.7 for men and 5.7 for women).

By contrast, heavy drinking is defined as on average consuming more than two drinks per day (men) or one drink per day (women).

Three Phases of Operationalizing a Behavior

Tobacco use, dietary patterns, physical activity, and alcohol use are significant, fundamental determinants of health status. A number of specific behaviors are found within these broad categories. In the previous section, the discussion of the content area of alcohol use presented three versions of a behavior: total amount, binge drinking, and drinking during pregnancy. Other forms of behavior not yet mentioned are underage drinking and driving under the influence. The specific forms of the behaviors within these categories are the versions that are actually studied, linked to health status, and shaped via interventions. All three forms—by content area, in a specific form, and then framed for an audience—are important in health promotion and discussed in the following sections.

Phase 1: Behaviors by Content Area

Health behaviors are often presented in terms of content areas. Content areas are broad, topical areas that can involve multiple health behaviors. One might easily confuse a topic area with a health behavior, and though these two are related, they are not interchangeable. Content areas are broad topic areas that may or may not describe an action. Access to care and nutrition are two such content areas that were presented in Table 2-1. Health behaviors are specific, measurable actions within content areas. Fruit and vegetable consumption is a health behavior within the content area of nutrition. Using a specific and ongoing source of primary health care is a behavioral target within the access to care content area. Behaviors that contribute to the leading causes of death and disabilities for defined populations are typically communicated to the general public by content areas. The specific actions within each content area influence health status.

Interventions that target content areas are limited in effectiveness and are difficult to evaluate. Content area–directed interventions tend to employ change strategies that are overly broad and lack a behavioral focus. As will be addressed in upcoming chapters, knowledge, beliefs, skills, resources, and support mechanisms drive behaviors and environments. Interventions that include clearly defined behaviors and intervention strategies are more likely to change and maintain changes to health behaviors. Designing interventions will be discussed in Chapter 10.

In any case, broad topic areas are helpful for discussion and when communicating information to the public. Human brains like to group information together by patterns; these "chunks" of information help with absorption of new information as well as information retention (National Research Council, 2000). Talking to others about "healthy eating" and "responsible sexual behaviors" can help individuals make sense of the information as well as link it to previous knowledge. Thus, communicating information about health behaviors by content areas is helpful; yet designing of strategies to change behaviors is best completed within a specific behavioral form.

Phase 2: Health Behavior Form

The second part of defining a health behavior is describing a specific form of that behavior. Within content areas, there are numerous forms of a behavior that can vary by the action and by the occurrence/frequency of the behavior. Figure 2-3 illustrates a few examples of physical activity.

How many forms of physical activity can you list?

Specific forms of physical activity include number of steps per day, minutes of physical activity per day, number of weekly sessions of moderate to vigorous activity, number of times per week of engaging in recreational activities, minutes per week of stretching and flexibility, number of sessions of strength training, and sessions of walking to and from school.

Clearly defined behavioral targets increase the likelihood of action. Eating fruits and vegetables, limiting sodium intake, and limiting solid fats define the target more clearly than "healthy eating." Being active 150 minutes a week or 10,000 steps a day again are clearly defined behavioral targets. Behaviors also need to be performed at certain intensity or frequency levels to realize health benefits. To clearly define a behavior for an intended audience, health behaviors should be observable, measureable, should have a relationship to a health issue, and be shapeable for target audience. Table 2-3 lists specific forms of health behaviors by content areas and setting.

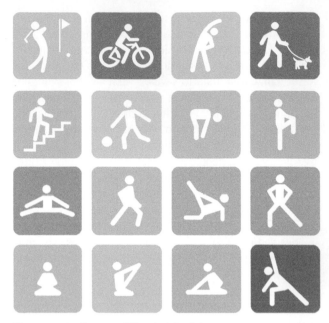

Figure 2-3 Forms of Physical Activity

Observable

Health behaviors are actions that one can see. Being **observable** captures the verb part of the behavior. As the behavior is described to others, *what* is it that one intends to see? If the behavior is not an observable action, it is not a behavior. Some forms may be small and difficult to observe, but they are observable nonetheless. Similarly, persons may not engage in a particular action (e.g., smoking), but that behavior sill does have an observable form.

Personal attributes, consequences, and outcomes of behavior are incredibly important to the execution of behaviors and receive substantial attention in this book. However, determinants and outcomes of behavior are not the behavior. According to Merriam-Webster's dictionary (2014), behaviors are the way a person acts or behaves. In other words, attributes like beliefs do not lower one's risk of a heart attack. Rather, it is the actions of activity, diet, medication, and so on that lower the risk of disease. The belief of self-efficacy is often confused with a behavior. Self-efficacy, one's confidence in completing forms of activity, is a strong predictor of behavior (Bauman et al., 2012). Confidence in one's ability to be physically active in specific situations facilitates physical activity,

TABLE 2-3 Health Behaviors by Content Area and Setting

	Nutrition	Physical Activity	Sexual Behaviors	Alcohol and Other Drugs	Tobacco	Injury Prevention	Other
GENERAL	Fruit and vegetable consumption	60 minutes a day	Sexual intercourse before marriage	Drinking alcohol underage	Smoking cessation	Gun violence	Hand washing
	Calorie intake	Sessions of moderate/vigorous each week	Consistent and correct condom use	Driving under influence of alcohol	Smoking initiation	Protective eyewear and gear compliance by farm workers	Exposure to environmental asthma triggers
	Low-fat milk consumption	10,000 steps a day	Monogamy: one sexual partner	Using prescription drugs as prescribed	Smokeless tobacco cessation	Falls	Use of pesticides by local farmers
SCHOOL HEALTH AND PHYSICAL EDUCATION	Fast-food and sugar-sweetened beverage intake	Active commuting to school three days a week	Age of sexual initiation	Binge drinking: drinking five or more drinks in one session		Bystander behavior during harassment (bullying) by peers	7 hours of sleep a day
	Dark green and red/orange vegetable consumption	Minutes of daily activity in the classroom	"Healthy Relationship"	Inhalant use		Head, eye, mouth equipment during physical activity	Indoor/outdoor tanning
	Adoption of nutrition policy for competitive foods	Minutes of activity time in PE class				Suicide attempts	Connectedness via school community

continues

TABLE 2-3 *continued*

	Nutrition	Physical Activity	Sexual Behaviors	Alcohol and Other Drugs	Tobacco	Injury Prevention	Other
PUBLIC	Breastfeeding for 12 months	Organized recreation four times per week	HIV testing and returning for results	Alcohol use by pregnant women	Smoking cessation: pregnant women	Emergency preparedness kit and plan	Childhood immunizations
	Buying local foods		Intravenous drug needle sharing	Riding in a car with a driver under influence of alcohol	Retailer compliance with smoking ban	Health care providers report to work in an emergency	Staying home when sick
		Asthma management plan	Disclosure of HIV status to partner		Children's exposure to secondhand smoke	Seat belt use	Adoption of a community mosquito control program
ALLIED HEALTH	Dietary compliance in type I diabetics	Asthma management plan compliance by athletes	Natural family planning	Medication compliance: antibiotics, hypertension medicine		Screening and referral by HCP for posttraumatic stress disorder (or depression)	Male and female cancer screenings: breast, cervical, testicular, prostate, colon
	Weight screening and counseling by primary care physician	Organized physical activity by individuals with a disability	HPV vaccination	Steroid and other performance enhancing drug use		Screening by HCP for intimate partner violence	Infant safe sleeping
	Sodium intake	Moderate to vigorous activity in those with chronic disease				Distracted driving: texting and cellular phone use	Prenatal care initiated in first trimester

but belief—along with other antecedents—is not itself a health behavior. Numerous other behavior mediators will be discussed in Chapters 4 through 8.

Measurable

Observable actions are countable, and **measurement** of the action occurs on a continuum. At one end of the continuum, behaviors are measured in a simple binary scale to count whether the action occurred. Preventive health screenings and immunizations are behaviors that might be assessed with a binary yes/no count. Behaviors can also be measured on continuous scales from zero upward to indicate how frequently an action occurs. Alcohol consumption and dietary behaviors might be measured as frequencies.

In addition to frequency, time is also important element in measuring behavior. All behaviors have an element of time, that is, *how often* and over what period of *time* a behavior occurs. Time frames can be daily, weekly, or yearly. It may also be of interest to know how often a behavior occurs when paired with another action, like bicycle riding and helmet use. Repetitiveness of an action may also be a desired element of health behaviors. Condom use, seat belt use, medication compliance, and breast cancer screenings are examples of behaviors that have a desired element of consistency. The protective and disease detection benefits of breast cancer screenings are rarely realized through one screening; rather, they are realized through monthly, annual, and/or semiannual screenings. Consistency of behavior is determined through the combination of frequency and time elements. This step of describing a behavior in a measurable form is referred to as **operationalizing** a behavior.

Relationship to Health

At the beginning of this chapter, a health behavior was defined as an action that has a relationship to some type of health outcome. As health behaviors become clearly defined for an intended audience, the health–behavior relationship is revisited. Planners need to consider both the presence of the behavior in a community as well as the strength of the health–behavior relationship. Not all health–behavior relationships are equal in strength or importance. The strength of the relationship between the health outcome and the health behaviors needs to be explored. Some behaviors can have a greater impact on health status than others. Altering behaviors that have stronger relationships with a health outcome will have a greater impact on the health of the population.

For example, caloric intake is the most reliable predictor of weight status, and the obesity-caloric intake relationship is strong (IOM, 2012; Kumanyika et al., 2008). If someone's caloric intake is altered, his body weight is likely to change. Sodium intake, fat intake, and sugary beverage intake also relate to weight status, but the relationships are not as strong. Thus, successful population-level interventions to alter sodium or fat intake will likely alter weight status but not to the degree produced by altering caloric intake. This strength of relationship issue is often at the center of debates concerning national dietary recommendations. See the Behavioral Science in Action feature later in this chapter for information on the development of national behavior recommendations.

The health–behavior relationship can be expressed quantitatively as a relative risk. **Relative risk** is an estimated measure of the strength of the relationship between risk factors and a particular disease. Relative risk compares the likelihood of developing a disease in persons with a certain trait or behavior to the risk in persons who do not have that trait or behavior. A relative risk of one indicates that an individual exhibiting the behavior or trait has the same likelihood of developing the disease as someone without. The higher the relative risk value, the greater the risk associated with that trait or behavior, though there is no specific relative risk value that signals a dangerous health behavior. For example, male smokers have a relative risk of 23 for developing lung cancer, meaning they are about 23 times more likely to develop lung cancer than nonsmokers (ACS, 2014). It is important to note, however, that relative risk does not indicate cause and effect. Many factors—such as behavior, genetics, and environment—play into an individual's ultimate health outcomes.

Shapeable for Target Audience

Finally, when defining health behaviors, the behavior form should be alterable in the intended audience. **Shapeability** implies that given intervention, people will be able to change the desired behavior. Programs should target behaviors that are both relevant to health status and changeable. The concept of changeability is different from behavior relevance. Relevance means that a behavior is prevalent in a community and is linked to the community's health status.

Changeability involves issues of abilities and resources. If a health behavior requires specific skills and resources, it can be completed only to the extent that individuals can perform the necessary skills and acquire the needed resources. In the previous section, caloric intake was identified as a strong predictor of weight status. Given the strength and reliability of the obesity-caloric intake relationship, and that caloric intake can also be stated in an observable, measurable and specific form, why do all weight status interventions not target caloric intake?

The answer to this question has to do with the complexity of the behavior. Caloric intake is a difficult behavior to shape. To monitor and shape calorie intake, one needs to know the calorie count of all foods eaten, be able to estimate portion size, calculate calories of "combination foods," and keep a food diary. Few people are able to successfully calculate and track their intake. The introduction of electronic food diaries for smartphones and tablets has lessened the required skill level, but individuals still struggle with estimating portion size and menu planning. As a result of the difficulty in tracking caloric intake, less complicated versions of the behavior have been introduced. These substitute health behaviors capture the spirit of caloric intake but are framed in more shapeable forms. In children, caloric intake–related behaviors include (1) sugar-sweetened beverage intake, (2) fruit and vegetable intake, (3) number of weekly fast-food meals, and (4) processed snacks intake. Sugar-sweetened beverage intake, fast-food meals, and consumption of processed snacks are associated with higher caloric intakes in children (IOM, 2012). Thus, shaping versions of these less complicated behaviors will in turn lower caloric intake. Weight Watchers™ Points Plus is a similar substitute behavior. Instead of counting calories, individuals count food points. Food groups are designated to be worth a certain number of points. Higher-calorie foods are worth more points than low-calorie foods. Using these methods, individuals may be able to more easily manage caloric intake.

Check for Understanding Take the following broad behaviors and modify them to be observable, measurable, in a specific form, and shapeable for an intended audience (behavioral forms can be primary, secondary or tertiary targets):

- Excessive alcohol intake
- Oral health
- Intimate partner violence
- Distracted driving
- Responsible sexual behaviors

Nontraditional Health Behaviors

The health–behavior relationship can exist between health and a "nontraditional" behavior. Behaviors that may not be typically thought of as health related can have strong relationships to the health of specific communities. For instance, high school graduation is a health behavior identified in Healthy People 2020. The adolescent health objective 5.1 (AH 5.1) states that the goal is to "increase the proportion of students who graduate with a regular diploma 4 years after starting 9th grade" (USDHHS, 2011a). A related objective for a specific population of high school students is to improve graduation rates for students with disabilities (AH 5.2). Acculturation of recent immigrants and social connectedness are two other behaviors that have a relationship to health status. The relationship of education level, income, and early life experiences to health status are discussed as social determinants of health in Chapter 3.

Phase 3: Framing a Behavior for a Specific Audience

The final phase of defining a health behavior is to frame or position that behavior for the intended audience. Framing a behavior refers to the manner in which it is communicated to the intended audience. How a behavior is presented influences community understanding, receptivity, and likelihood of adoption. Framing a behavior is based on the behavioral objective of a program but also targets possible attitudes, perceived barriers, or behavioral milestones.

Framing a behavior largely occurs when the actual health promotion intervention is being planned. Program planners consider the communication goal, health literacy, language, and patterns when developing community-specific communication tools and mediums. Tailored messages that appeal to, educate, and resonate with intended audiences are developed. Table 2-4 shows the progression of a health behavior from content area to a tailored message for specific audiences. Health communications and interventions will be discussed more in Chapter 10.

Community Variations in Health Behaviors

Identifying community-specific risk factors is important for improving population health and maximizing return on allocated resources. Positive health status and disease risk can

TABLE 2-4 Progression of a Health Behavior by Content Area

Content Area	Health Behavior	Tailored Message
Healthy eating	Consume five servings of fruits and vegetables a day	Make half your plate fruits and vegetables.[a]
Physical activity	Engage in a minimum of 60 minutes of activity a day	Play 60[b]
Alcohol use	Zero alcohol consumption during pregnancy	Not a single drop.[c]

Sources: [a]USDA and USDHHS, 2010; [b]National Football League, n.d.; [c]Ohio Department of Health, n.d.

come from different behaviors in different populations. The prevalence of risk factors varies by community, and it is necessary to identify specific risk factors for subgroups within a community in order to deliver tailored interventions to those in need.

Analysis of state-level cigarette use demonstrates how risk behaviors vary throughout communities. Healthy People 2020 Tobacco Use Objective 1.1 (TU-1.1) is to reduce the percentage of U.S. adult smokers from 20% to no greater than 12%. However, both between and within states, there are significant differences in tobacco use. Smoking rates vary across states from a low of 10.6% in Utah to a high of 28.3% in Kentucky. Cigarette use rates also vary across communities by gender, race/ethnicity, geography, socio-economic status, and job type. In Ohio, 23% of the adult population smokes, but this rate varies by several socio-demographic characteristics (see Table 2-5). Males have higher smoking rates, and tobacco use is inversely related to education level. Further, there are community trends. Approximately half (53%) of people across the country who receive Medicaid smoke, a percentage that is significantly higher than the rate in the general population (Armour, Finkelstein, & Fiebelkorn, 2009). To be most effective, efforts to reduce state-level smoking should target communities where risk is most prevalent.

Check for Understanding What are the tobacco rates in your state? How have they varied across years? List three populations with rates higher than the state average.

Health Behaviors Data Sources

The primary federal agency that collects, analyzes, and disseminates information on health and health determinants is the National Center for Health Statistics (NCHS). Working with partners throughout the health community, the NCHS uses a variety of approaches to collect information from the sources most able to provide information. NCHS collects data from birth and death records, medical records, interview surveys, and direct physical exams and laboratory testing. Federal reports on a wide range of topics are produced through this collection: birth trends, leading causes of death and disease, health behavior rates, nutrition and growth trends, use of preventive services, reproductive health indicators, health insurance coverage, health care use and services, and health care services environment (National Center for Health Statistics, n.d.). *Health, United States* is an annual report on the health status of the nation that the secretary of health and human services submits to the president and Congress. The large (more than 400 pages) report contains tables showing national trends related to health status and its determinants as well as health care resources and their use. Each year, the report presents a special feature on a topic of importance to current public health discussions. Emergency care (2012), socioeconomic status (2011), and death and dying (2010) have been featured topics. The NCHS also releases national vital statistic reports and numerous data briefs. In addition, researchers and practitioners can access data sets.

TABLE 2-5 Cigarette Use by Socio-Demographic Characteristics, 2012

	United States	Ohio
Gender		
Male	20.5%	25.4%
Female	15.8%	21.3%
Race		
American Indian/Alaska Native	21.8%	38.5%
Asian	10.7%	15.0%
Black/African American	18.1%	28.1%
Hispanic	12.5%	20.5%
White	19.7%	23.5%
Education		
Adults with less than 12 years of school	24.7%	45.6%
Adults with high school diploma	23.1%	27.7%
Adults with at least some college	9.1%[a]	16.5%
Geographic regions		
Low	10.6% Utah	14.8% Delaware County
	12.6% California	19.0% Warren County
High	28.3% Kentucky	30.2% Highland County
	28.2% West Virginia	30.7% Noble County

a) with an undergraduate degree

Sources: Centers for Disease Control & Prevention; Dwyer-Lindgren et al., 2014

Table 2-6 provides a partial list of national data sources and the data's content area. Three specific data sets collected under the umbrella of the NCHS are the Behavioral Risk Factor Surveillance Survey, the National Health and Nutrition Examination Survey, and the National Health Interview Survey.

Behavioral Risk Factor Surveillance Survey

As the name implies, the Behavioral Risk Factor Surveillance Survey (BRFSS) assesses behaviors, preventive health practices and health care access related to chronic disease and injury. State health departments in collaboration with the Centers for Disease Control and Prevention to operate the state-based surveillance system. This survey is unique in that it generates state-level data; most state behavioral comparisons use data from the BRFSS. Comparisons can also be made between metropolitan areas within the states. Piloted in 1984 and nationally adopted in 1993, the BRFSS is the largest telephone survey in the world (CDC, 2011). Data are collected monthly in all 50 states, the District of Columbia, American Samoa, Palau, Puerto Rico, the U.S. Virgin Islands, and Guam. In 2011, more than half a million (506,000) interviews were conducted (CDC, 2011).

The questionnaire has three parts: the core components with rotating and emerging questions, optional modules, and

TABLE 2-6 Health Behavior Data Sources at the National Level

Data Source (Acronym)	Website	Content Area
National Center for Health Statistics (NCHS)	http://www.cdc.gov/nchs	Principal health statistics agency
Behavioral Risk Factor Surveillance Survey (BRFSS)	http://www.cdc.gov/brfss	Risk factors in adults
Youth Risk Behavior Surveillance Survey (YRBSS)	http://www.cdc.gov/HealthyYouth/yrbs/index.htm	Risk factors in youth
National Health and Nutrition Examination Survey (NHANES)	http://www.cdc.gov/nchs/nhanes.htm	Nutrition and health
Surveillance Epidemiology and End Results (SEER)	http://seer.cancer.gov	Cancer
National Hospital Care Surveys (NHCS)	http://www.cdc.gov/nchs/nhcs.htm	National patterns of health care delivery
National Health Interview Survey (NHIS)	http://www.cdc.gov/nchs/nhis/about_nhis.htm	Broad range of topics
National Vital Statistics System (NVSS)	http://www.cdc.gov/nchs/nvss.htm	Birth, death, marriage, and divorce certificates
Pregnancy Risk Assessment Monitoring System (PRAMS)	http://www.cdc.gov/prams	Pregnancy and women's health
Injury Prevention	http://www.cdc.gov/injury/wisqars/index.html	Injury
Child & Adolescent Health Measurement Institute	http://www.childhealthdata.org	Broad range of topics related to children and children with special needs
Monitoring the Future	http://www.monitoringthefuture.org	Behaviors, attitudes, and values of U.S. secondary school students, college students, and young adults
U.S. Department of Transportation (USDOT)	http://www.dot.gov	Transportation
Agency for Healthcare Research and Quality (AHRQ)	http://www.ahrq.gov/data/dataresources.htm	Health care–related behaviors and outcomes
National Survey of Family and Growth (NSFG)	http://www.cdc.gov/nchs/nsfg.htm	Family life, marriage and divorce, pregnancy, infertility, use of contraception, and men's and women's health
National Immunization Survey (NIS)	http://www.cdc.gov/nchs/nis.htm	Estimates of vaccination coverage rates for all childhood vaccinations

continues

TABLE 2-6 *continued*

Data Source (Acronym)	Website	Content Area
The Longitudinal Studies of Aging (LSOA)	http://www.cdc.gov/nchs/lsoa.htm	Multicohort study of persons 70 years of age and over designed primarily to measure changes in health, functional status, living arrangements, and health services utilization
Institute for Health Metrics and Evaluation (IHME)	http://www.healthmetricsandevaluation.org	Independent research center that measures health and health determinants in the United States and worldwide
Robert Wood Johnson Foundation (RWJF)	http://www.rwjf.org	Children, obesity, other topics

state-added questions. The core consists of a series of set questions across 16 to 18 content areas. There is a core set of questions on demographics, health status, and select health behaviors (tobacco, alcohol, exercise, seat belt use, and HIV/AIDS). There are also two sets of questions that alternate each year. The 2013 survey asked about fruits and vegetables, immunizations, and arthritis; the 2012 survey included questions on various cancer screenings, drinking and driving, and falls. Within the core, up to five questions related to emerging issues can be added. H1N1 immunization was a recent emerging topic. Optional modules are additional sets of questions that states may choose to ask their residents. Topics include diabetes, sugary beverages, asthma, sodium intake, human papillomavirus (HPV), and mental illness. Finally, states may add their own questions. Again, the data sets are available online (see Table 2-6). Numerous reports by the CDC as well as health departments and researchers are created with BRFFS data.

The Youth Risk Behavioral Factor Surveillance Survey (YRBFSS) provides data on health behaviors among high school students. There are six areas of interest: behaviors that contribute to unintentional injury, sexual behaviors, alcohol and other drug use, tobacco use, diet, and physical activity (CDC, 2013b).

National Health and Nutrition Examination Survey (NHANES)

The NHANES is designed to assess the health and nutritional status of adults and children in the United States. The survey is unique in that it combines interviews and physical examinations. The NHANES program began in the early 1960s and has been conducted as a series of surveys focusing on different population groups or health topics. In 1999, the survey became a continuous program under the NCHS that has a changing focus on a variety of health and nutrition measurements. The survey examines a nationally representative sample of about 5,000 persons each year who are located in counties across the country, 15 of which are visited each year (National Center for Health Statistics, n.d.).

The NHANES interview includes demographic, socioeconomic, dietary, and health-related questions. The examination component consists of medical, laboratory, dental, and physiological measurements. Key diet variables that are examined include energy intake, fruit and vegetable intake, and intake of carbohydrates, protein, fat, and mineral/vitamins. Body weight, body fat, blood pressure, and cholesterol levels are related physiological measures. This data set is also publically available to practitioners and researchers and appears as a data source in many publications.

National Health Interview Survey

The National Health Interview Survey (NHIS) is another survey of the nation's health and its determinants. Established in 1957, data on a broad range of health topics are collected through personal household interviews. The U.S. Census Bureau has been the data collection agent for the National Health Interview Survey (National Center for Health Statistics, n.d.). As with the BRFSS, there is a core set of questions as well as rotating supplemental items. The core contains four major components: household, family, sample adult, and sample child. Data collected through the NHIS can be grouped, analyzed, and compared on a variety of demographic characteristics: age, gender, education level, income, household properties, type of heath insurance, and more. The NHIS is a primary source for information about health insurance enrollment and trends by demographics and health conditions. The survey also is a source of information on children's health (Bloom, Cohen, & Freeman, 2012).

The Early Release Program of the National Health Interview Survey aims to provide data and summaries on a timely schedule. Quarterly reports are released on 15 key indicators. Indicators related to health insurance, accessing medical care, vaccinations, obesity, physical activity, smoking, alcohol use, HIV testing, health status, personal care and psychological distress, diabetes, and episodes of asthma were reported on during 2013. Two related specialized reports are the National Health Interview Survey-Disability Survey (NHIS-D) and the National Immunization Provider Record Checks Survey.

Foundations and Community Agencies

Foundations and community agencies are valuable sources of national, state, and local behavioral data. Hospital systems, physician groups, health insurance companies, community groups, worksites, school districts, local nongovernmental organizations (NGOs), local funding agencies, and universities are examples of sources that are available in most communities. Nonprofit hospitals are required to complete community health assessments, and school districts receiving federal school meal funds are required to have written wellness policies that include goals and evaluated outcomes. Community assessment and program evaluation data help the United Way and similar nonprofits make decisions about funding needed and effective programs.

SUMMARY

A health behavior is an action of an individual or a group that influences health status. Health behaviors can be performed consciously, under great motivation—or not. Health behaviors can be performed rarely or frequently. Health behaviors are often discussed in terms in content areas, such as healthy eating and driving patterns, but interventions target specific forms of the behavior that are measurable and shapeable for a target audience. Health behaviors are driven by a great number of individual- and community-level factors.

BEHAVIORAL SCIENCE IN ACTION

National behavior guidelines—where do they come from?

It often seems as if recommendations for healthy living are everywhere. The ones listed here are just a few common examples:

- Sleep 7 to 8 hours a night.
- Eat 5 to 10 servings of fruits and vegetables a day.
- Exercise 30 to 60 minutes a day most days of the week.
- Drink alcohol in moderation—no more than one drink a day for women and two drinks for men.
- Infants should be breastfed exclusively for at least six months.

- Get an annual flu shot.
- After the age of 50, get an annual colonoscopy.

National guidelines come from both federal agencies and professional organizations. Experts meticulously review scientific research to identify the benefits and potential risks of select health-related actions. It is based on this scientific evidence that guidelines and recommendations related to dietary intake, physical activity, cancer screenings, immunizations, and other health behaviors are developed. In addition to the efficacy and/or benefits of the action, population-level recommendations must also consider the cost effectiveness of said recommendations.

The U.S. Preventive Services Task Force (USPSTF), made up of experts in prevention and evidence-based medicine, develops national cancer screening guidelines. The results of the organization's scientific evidence-based reviews covering a wide range of clinical preventive health care services are developed into recommendations for health care professionals that are then accepted and promoted by the CDC. The USPSTF will make recommendations or create guidelines only when the benefits of the service outweigh any associated harms and risks. Other groups, such as the National Heart, Lung, and Blood Institute (NHLBI), use expert panels to systematically review medical research and literature to develop recommendations that are then released to the general public.

Just as individuals have differing opinions, so do various groups working in preventive health. For example, the American Cancer Society and the American College of Obstetricians and Gynecologists are in agreement that *women age 40 and older should have a mammogram every year and should continue to do so for as long as they are in good health.* In contrast, the USPSTF recommends that *women should have mammograms every two years from age 50 to 74.* These recommendations both deal with the same health behavior, but the experts reviewing the evidence-based studies may have interpreted the data differently or weighed the costs and benefits in a different manner. In cases such as this, individuals should discuss their own personal medical and family histories with a health care provider to determine which clinical guidelines are most appropriate for their care.

Variation in recommendations is possible for non-clinical behaviors, too. For example, the American College of Sports Medicine, the American Heart Association, the U.S. surgeon general, and the Institute of Medicine all have guidelines regarding physical activity. Due to the many variables related to the health behavior, including the frequency, intensity, and duration of the physical activity, and the intended outcome of the behavior, such as weight loss or improved cardiovascular health, the guidelines differ among the organizations. Health professionals need to be familiar with the various guidelines and promote the recommendations that best meet the needs of their patients.

The USPSTF has a useful website that can help one begin to understand health behavior and medical screening recommendations (http://www.uspreventiveservicestaskforce.org/). This site provides resources such as an A-Z Topic Guide, Recommendations for Adults, Recommendations for Children and Adolescents, and Topics in Progress. Many national not-for-profit nongovernmental organizations (NGOs) and some professional organizations develop and promote guidelines for specific preventive measures. These organizations include the American Heart Association (www.heart.org), American Cancer Society (www.cancer.org), American Diabetes Association (www.diabetes.org), American Academy of Pediatrics (www.aap.org), the American College of Sports Medicine (www.acsm.org), and the U.S. Department of Agriculture (www.dietaryguidelines.gov).

IN THE CLASSROOM ACTIVITIES

1) Read a current edition of a national newspaper and list up to 10 health behaviors that are discussed. Are the health behaviors discussed by a content area, in a specific form, framed for a specific audience? Can you locate a nontraditional health behavior?

2) Select a behavioral content area from Table 2-4. Applying concepts from Chapter 1, create a primary, secondary, and tertiary version of the behavior.

3) Several new topic areas have been added to Healthy People 2020. A number of these new

topic areas represent subgroups of the population. Go to the Healthy People 2020 website (http://www.healthypeople.gov/2020/) and explore one of the following new topic areas: adolescent health; early and middle childhood; lesbian, gay, bisexual, and transgender health; and older adults. Create a list of the health behaviors of particular relevance in one of the subgroups.

4) Contact an organization from one health promotion setting (community-based organization, health care, public health, school, and/or worksite). Explore behavioral data that the organization collects. What are the content areas, methods, and tools, and what is the frequency of collection?

5) Identify two personal health behaviors: one that has a positive impact on health (protective factor) and one that may increase the likelihood of negative health outcomes (risk factor). List five factors that influence each action, in order of possible influence from most to least. After sharing the list with others, save it for future reference. Chapters 4 through 8 discuss factors that influence health behaviors.

6) Create a trend report on tobacco use in a defined population. Visit the State Tobacco Activities Tracking & Evaluation (STATE) System (http://www.cdc.gov/tobacco). Select a specific behavioral measure and include trends by at least three variables: states, years, gender, or age.

WEB LINKS

Healthy People 2020: http://www.healthypeople.gov/2020/

Centers for Disease Control and Prevention, Smoking and Tobacco Use: http://www.cdc.gov/tobacco

Office of the Surgeon General: http://www.surgeongeneral.gov/

REFERENCES

Abu-Saad, K., & Fraser, D. (2010). Maternal nutrition and birth outcomes. *Epidemiology Reviews, 32*(1), 5–25.

American Cancer Society (ACS). (2014). *Cancer facts & figures, 2014.* Atlanta: Author.

Armour B. S., Finkelstein E. A., & Fiebelkorn I. C. (2009). State-level Medicaid expenditures attributable to smoking. *Preventing Chronic Disease, 6*(3), 1–10.

Bandura, A. (1977). Self-efficacy: Toward a unifying theory of behavior change. *Psychological Review, 84*(2), 191–215.

Bauman, A. E., Reis, R. S., Sallis, J. F. Wells, J. C., Loos R. J. & Martin, B.W. (2012). Correlates of physical activity: Why are some people physically active and others not? *Lancet, 38,* 258–271.

Baumgardner, J. R., Bilheimer, L. T., Booth, M. B., Carrington, W. J., Duchovny, N. J., & Werble, E. C. (2012). Cigarette taxes and the federal budget: Report from the CBO. *New England Journal of Medicine, 367,* 2068–2070.

Berman, M., Crane, R., Seiber, R., & Munur, M. (2013). Estimating the cost of a smoking employee. *Tobacco Control* (published online first: June 3, 2013).

Bloom, B., Cohen, R. A., & Freeman G. (2012). Summary health statistics for U.S. children: National Health Interview Survey, 2011. *Vital and Health Statistics 10*(254). Washington DC: U.S. Department of Health and Human Services, Centers for disease Control and Prevention, National Center for Health Statistics.

Bouchard, C., Blair, S. N., & Haskell, W. L. (2007). *Physical activity and health*. Champaign, IL: Human Kinetics.

Bouchery E. E., Harwood H. J., Sacks J. J., Simon C. J., & Brewer R. D. (2011). Economic costs of excessive alcohol consumption in the United States, 2006. *American Journal of Preventive Medicine, 41*, 516–524.

Centers for Disease Control and Prevention (CDC). (2003). Cigarette smoking: Attributable morbidity; United States, 2000. *Morbidity and Mortality Weekly, 52*(35), 842–844.

Centers for Disease Control and Prevention (CDC). (2008). Smoking: Attributable mortality, years of potential life lost, and productivity losses; United States, 2000–2004. *Morbidity and Mortality Weekly, 57*(45), 1226–1228.

Centers for Disease Control and Prevention (CDC), Office of Surveillance, Epidemiology and Laboratory Services, (2011). *At a glance: Conducting the 2011 Behavioral Risk Factor Surveillance System*. Retrieved from http://www.cdc.gov/brfss/pdf/238974_BRFSS-AAG.pdf

Centers for Disease Control and Prevention (CDC). (2012a). Vital Signs: Food categories contributing the most sodium consumption; United States, 2007–2008. *Morbidity and Mortality Weekly, 61*(05), 92–98.

Centers for Disease Control and Prevention (CDC). (2012b). *State Tobacco Activities Tracking and Evaluation (STATE) System*. Retrieved from http://www.cdc.gov/tobacco/data_statistics

Centers for Disease Control and Prevention (CDC). (2013a). *Maternal and infant health*. Retrieved from http://www.cdc.gov/reproductivehealth/MaternalInfantHealth/index.htm

Centers for Disease Control and Prevention (CDC). (2013b). Methodology of the Youth Risk Behavior Risk Factor Surveillance System. *Morbidity and Mortality Weekly, 62*(1), 1–25.

Centers for Disease Control and Prevention (CDC), National Center for Birth Defects and Developmental Disabilities (NCBDDD). (2014). *Facts about FASD*. Retrieved from http://www.cdc.gov/ncbddd/fasd/facts.html

Chen, S. T., Maruthur N. M., & Appel, L. J. (2010). The effects of dietary patterns on estimated coronary heart disease risk: Results from the Dietary Approaches to Stop Hypertension (DASH) trial. *Circulation: Cardiovascular Quality and Outcomes, 3*(5), 484–480.

Congressional Budget Office (CBO). (2012). *Raising the excise tax on cigarettes: Effects on health and the federal budget*. Washington DC: U.S. Congress.

Danaei, G., Ding, E. L., Mozaffarian, D., Taylor, B., Rehm, J., Murray, C. L., & Ezzati, M. (2009). The preventable causes of death in the United States: Comparative risk assessment of dietary, lifestyle and metabolic risk factors. *PloS Medicine, 6*(4), 1–23.

Duhigg, C. (2012). *The power of habit: Why we do what we do in life and business*. New York: Random House.

Dwyer-Lindgren, L., Mokdad, A. H., Srebotnjak, T., Flaxman, A. D., Hansen, G. M. & Murray, C. L. (2014). Cigarette smoking prevalence in US counties: 1996–2012. *Population Health Metrics, 12*(5), 1–13.

Fletcher, G. F, Balady, G., Blair, S. N., Blumenthal, J., Caspersen, C., Chaitman, B., ... Pollock, M. L. (1996). Statement on exercise: Benefits and recommendations for physical activity programs for all Americans. *Circulation, 94*, 857–862.

Ford E. S., & Dietz W. H. (2013). Trends in energy intake among adults in the United States: Findings from NHANES. *American Journal of Clinical Nutrition, 97*(4), 848–853.

Ford, E. S., Greenlund, K. J., & Hong, Y. (2012). Ideal cardiovascular health and mortality from all causes and diseases of the circulatory system among adults in the United States. *Circulation, 125*(8), 987–995.

Go, A. S., Mozaffarian, D., Veronique, R. L., et al. (2013). Heart disease and stroke statistics, 2013 update: A report from the American Heart Association. *Circulation, 125*, e2–243.

Goetzel, R. Z., Pei, X., Tabrizi, M. J., Henke, R. M., Kowlessar, N., Nelso, C. F., & Metz, R. D. (2012). Ten modifiable health risk factors are linked to more than one-fifth of employer-employee health care spending. *Health Affairs, 31*(11), 2474–2484.

Hoy, M. K., Goldman, J. D., Murayi, T., Rhodes, D. G., & Moshfegh, A. J. (2011). Sodium intake of the U.S. population: What we eat in America, NHANES 2007–2008 (Food Surveys Research Group Dietary Data Brief No. 8, October 2011). Retrieved from http://www.ars.usda.gov/services/docs.htm?docid=19476

Hunt, W. A., Matarazzo, J. D., Weiss, S. M. & Gentry, W. D. (1979). Associative learning, habit and health behavior. *Journal of Behavioral Medicine, 2*(2), 111–124.

Institute of Medicine (IOM). (2005). *Estimating the contributions of lifestyle-related factors to preventable death: A workshop summary.* Washington, DC: National Academies Press.

Institute of Medicine (IOM). (2012). *Accelerating progress in obesity: Solving the weight of the nation.* Washington DC: National Academies Press.

Jha, P., Ramasundarahettige, C., Landsman, V., Rostron, B., Thun, M., Anderson, R. N., McAfee, T., & Peto, R. (2013). 21st-Century hazards of smoking and benefits of cessation in the United States. *New England Journal of Medicine, 368*(4), 341–350.

Kanny, D., Liu, Y., Brewer, R. D., & Lu, H. (2013). Binge drinking, United States, 2011. *Morbidity and Mortality Weekly, 62*(03), 77–80.

Kasl, S.V., & Cobb, S. (1966a). Health behavior, illness behavior, and sick role behavior: I. Health and illness behavior. *Archives of Environmental Health, 12*(2), 246–266.

Kasl, S. V., & Cobb, S. (1966b). Health behavior, illness behavior, and sick role behavior: II. Sick role behavior. *Archives of Environmental Health, 12*(4), 531–541.

Kloner, R. A., & Rezkalla S. H. (2007). To drink or not to drink? That is the question. *Circulation, 116*(11), 1306–1317.

Kumanyika, S. K., Obarzanek, E., Stettler, N ... Hong, Y. (2008). Population-based prevention of obesity: The need for comprehensive promotion of healthful eating, physical activity, and energy balance; A scientific statement from American Heart Association Council on Epidemiology and Prevention, Interdisciplinary Committee for Prevention. *Circulation, 118*, 428–464.

Lee, I. M., Shiroma, E. J., Lobelo, F., Puska, P., Blair, S. N., & Katzmarzyk, P. T. (2012). Effect of physical inactivity on major non-communicable diseases worldwide: An analysis of burden of disease and life expectancy. *Lancet, 380*(9638), 219–229.

Liao W. C., Li, C. R., Lin, Y. C., Wang, C. C., Chen, Y. J., Yen, C. H., et al. (2011). Healthy behaviors and onset of functional disability in older adults: results of a national longitudinal study. *Journal of the American Geriatrics Society, 59*(2), 200–206.

Loef, M., & Walach, H. (2012). The combined effects of healthy lifestyle behaviors on all cause mortality: A systematic review and meta-analysis. *Preventive Medicine, 55*(3), 163–170.

Lupton, C., Burd, L., & Harwood, R. (2004). Cost of fetal alcohol spectrum disorders. *American Journal of Medical Genetics, 127c*(1), 42–50.

McGinnis J. M., & Foege, W. H. (1993). Actual causes of death in the United States. *Journal of the American Medical Association, 270*(18), 2207–2212.

McGinnis J. M., & Foege, W. H. (2004). The immediate vs the important. *Journal of the American Medical Association, 291*(10), 1263–1264.

Merriam-Webster. (2014). *Merriam-Webster online: Dictionary and thesaurus.* Retrieved from http://www .merriam-webster.com

Mokdad, A. H., Marks, J. S., Stroup, D. F., & Gerberding, J. L. (2004). Actual causes of death in the United States, 2000. *Journal of the American Medical Association, 291*(10), 1238–1245.

Murphy, S. L., Xu, J. Q., & Kochanek, K. D. (2012). Deaths: Preliminary data for 2010. *National Vital Statistics Reports, 6*(4), 1–52.

National Center for Health Statistics. (n.d.). Surveys and data collection systems. Retrieved from http://www.cdc.gov/ nchs/surveys.htm

National Football League. (n.d.). *About the NFL Play 60.* Retrieved from http://www.nfl.com/play60

National Institute of Alcohol Abuse and Alcoholism (NIAAA). (2000). *Tenth special report to the US Congress on alcohol and health.* Bethesda, MD: National Institutes of Health.

National Prevention Council. (2011). *National prevention strategy.* Washington, DC: U.S. Department of Health and Human Services, Office of the Surgeon General.

National Research Council. (2000). *How people learn: Brain, mind, experiences and school.* Washington, DC: National Academy Press.

Ohio Department of Health (n.d.). Ohio FASD Initiative. Retrieved from https://notasingledrop.mh.state.oh.us/

Plunk, A. D., Syed-Mohammed, H., Cavazos-Rehg, P., Bierut, L. J., & Grucza, R. A. (2013). Alcohol consumption, heavy drinking, and mortality: Rethinking the J-shaped curve. *Alcoholism: Clinical and Experimental Research, 38*(2), 471–478.

Rasmussen-Torvik, L. J., Shay, C. M., Abramson, J. G., Friedrich C. A., Nettleton, J. A., Prizment, A. E., & Folsom, A. R. (2013). Ideal cardiovascular health is inversely associated with incident cancer: The atherosclerosis risk in communities study. *Circulation, 127*(12), 1270–1275.

Reimers C. D., Knapp, G., & Reimers A. K. (2012). Does physical activity increase life expectancy? A review of the literature. *Journal of Aging Research,* 1–9.

Roger, V. L., Go, A. S., Lloyd-Jones, D. M., et al. (2012). Heart disease and stroke statistics, 2012 update: A report from the American Heart Association. *Circulation, 125*(1), e2–220.

Sabia S., Singh-Manoux, A., Hagger-Johnson, G., Cambois, E., Brunner, E. J., & Kivimali, M. (2012). Influence of individual and combined healthy behaviors on successful aging. *Canadian Medical Association Journal, 184*(18), 1985–1992.

Sacks, J. J., Roeber, J., Bouchery, E. E., Gonzales K., Chaloupka, F. J., & Brewer, R. D. (2013). State costs of excessive alcohol consumption, 2006. *American Journal of Preventive Medicine, 45*(4), 474–485.

Simons-Morton, B., McLeroy, K. R., & Wendel, M. L. (2012). *Behavior theory in health promotion practice and research.* Burlington, MA: Jones and Bartlett.

Stahre, M., Roeber, J., Kanny, D., Brewer, R. D., & Zhang, X. (2014). Contribution of excessive alcohol consumption to deaths and years of potential life lost in the United States. *Preventing Chronic Disease 11,* 1–11.

U.S. Burden of Disease Collaborators. (2013). The state of US health, 1990–2010: Burden of diseases, injuries, and risk factors. *Journal of the American Medical Association, 310*(6), e1–118.

U.S. Department of Agriculture (USDA) & U.S. Department of Health and Human Services (USDHHS). (2010). *Dietary guidelines for Americans, 2010* (7th ed.). Washington, DC: U.S. Government Printing Office.

U.S. Department of Health and Human Services (USDHHS). (2010). *A report of the surgeon general: How tobacco smoke causes disease; The biology and behavioral basis for smoking-attributed disease.* Atlanta, GA: U.S. Department of Health and Human Services, Centers for Disease Control and Prevention, National Center for Chronic Disease Prevention and Health Promotion, Office of the Surgeon General.

U.S. Department of Health and Human Services (USDHHS). (2011a). *Healthy people 2020.* Retrieved from http://www.healthypeople.gov/2020/

U.S. Department of Health and Human Services (USDHHS). (2011b). *The surgeon general's call to action to support breastfeeding.* Washington, DC: U.S. Department of Health and Human Services, Office of the Surgeon General.

U.S. Department of Health and Human Services (USDHHS). (1996). *Physical activity and health: A report of the surgeon general.* Atlanta, GA: U.S. Department of Health and Human Services, Centers for Disease Control and Prevention, National Center for Chronic Disease Prevention and Health Promotion, Office of the Surgeon General.

U.S. Department of Health and Human Services (USDHHS) (2014). *The health consequences of smoking: 50 years of progress; A report of the surgeon general.* Atlanta, GA: U.S. Department of Health and Human Services, Centers for Disease Control and Prevention, National Center for Chronic Disease Prevention and Health Promotion, Office of Smoking and Health, Office of the Surgeon General.

U.S. Preventive Services Task Force (USPSTF). (2012). *Guide to clinical preventive services, 2012: Recommendations of the U.S. Preventive Services Task Force.* Rockville, MD: Agency for Healthcare Research and Quality.

Verplanken, B. (2006). Beyond frequency: Habit as a mental construct. *British Journal of Social Psychology, 45*(3), 639–656.

World Health Organization (WHO). (1998). *Health promotion glossary.* Geneva, Switzerland: Division of Health Promotion, Education and Communications. Retrieved from http://www.who.int/healthpromotion/about/HPG/en/

World Health Organization (WHO). (2004). *A glossary of terms for community health care and services for older persons.* Geneva, Switzerland: WHO Centre for Health Development.

CHAPTER 3

Social Determinants of Health

KEY TERMS

activities of daily living	early life	mediate	toxic stress
adverse childhood	gradient	mobility	trajectories
experience (ACE)	instrumental activities	social determinant of health	upstream factor
downstream factor	of daily living	socioeconomic position	
		socioeconomic position	

LEARNING OBJECTIVES

1. Give examples of social determinants of health.
2. Describe situations in which health behaviors are linked with social conditions of living.
3. Describe components of socioeconomic position and three pathways linking socioeconomic status (SES) components to health outcomes.
4. Identify neighborhood factors that influence a person's ability to perform health behaviors.
5. Discuss the role of early life experiences and the trajectories established with health and behaviors later in life.
6. Assess barriers to health care and health promotion participation across different types of disability.

IN THE NEWS ...

"Blue-collar workers top charts for worst employee health" was the headline in an August 2012 article in *USA Today*. Based on a survey by Gallup and Healthways, blue-collar workers reported higher rates of select risk behaviors and poorer health outcomes. On average, blue-collar workers reported higher rates of smoking, high blood pressure, and obesity, and half had not visited a dentist in a year.

Introduction

Persons reading this chapter have likely heard a factoid about health status and income, such as the *USA Today* story about blue-collar workers and health outcomes. In general, as income increases, health status improves (Adler & Stewart, 2010b). Few in the general public, though, stop to ask why this relationship between income and health remains so consistent. Income can influence a person's ability to provide resources for oneself and one's family. The home in which a person lives, the neighborhood environment, and social opportunities are also made available through income. Furthermore, income can increase a person's sense of control and sense of identity. Income is an example of a social determinant of health. **Social determinants of health** are social factors that have important direct and indirect relationships with health outcomes (Braveman, Egerter, & Williams, 2011; WHO, 2008). Social determinants influence immediate opportunity, such as having the money to purchase healthy food, but also influence health behaviors indirectly by influencing the neighborhood where one lives, which influences access to stores that may or may not have healthy foods available for purchase.

Attention to the social determinants of health has increased as the health status of the country has stagnated, health disparities have continued, health care costs have increased, and documentation of the association of social factors with health outcomes has improved. Health disparities are differences in health status between segments of a population (Carter-Pokras & Baquet, 2002). In the United States, population segments are typically defined by demographic, environmental, and geographic attributes (Carter-Pokras & Baquet, 2002). Table 1-3 in the opening chapter shows disparities in U.S. life expectancies and infant mortality across racial and ethnic groups. Over the past two decades, the understanding about differences in health status and determinants has deepened beyond racial differences. The impact of social factors on one's ability to be healthy and make healthy choices has been repeatedly documented. In addition to differences by income, education, and ethnicity, variations in early life experiences, living and work environments, and the chronic stress associated with disadvantage can have profound influences on health (Adler & Stewart, 2010a; Braveman et al., 2011; RWJF, 2008 and 2013; WHO, 2008).

Upstream Factors

Social determinants of health are often called upstream factors. Upstream factors are issues or conditions located "up river," or away from the person or object of interest. They may be out of immediate eyesight but can represent root causes of a problem or circumstance. In studying the health of populations, **upstream factors** are "fundamental causes that set in motion causal pathways leading to (often temporally and spatially distant) health effects downstream" (Braveman et al., 2011). General examples of upstream factors that relate to health are income, housing, employment, addiction, and social support. By contrast, **downstream factors** are actions more closely linked to health outcomes and are often seen as the cause but may in fact be only a symptom.

In a classic example of upstream versus downstream factors, Braveman and colleagues (2011) describe a scenario of a community exposed to contaminated drinking water. Drinking contaminated water can cause individuals to get sick. The downstream factor, the health behavior, is drinking the contaminated water, and people should not be drinking the contaminated water. Upstream thinking, though, would lead one to explore factors that cause the water to become contaminated. In this scenario, the community was located on a river where upstream industrial dumping was occurring. The upstream approach would lead the community to improve living conditions within the neighborhood, in this instance the water quality supply, by changing industrial dumping practices. The traditional downstream intervention would be to teach individuals to test and filter the water in their homes. Both solutions, filtering water and eliminating industrial dumping, would clean the water that community members are drinking. The upstream solution, while more difficult to implement, is more likely to produce a sustainable improvement in the health practices and health status of this community.

Table 3-1 compares specific social factors as listed in various national and international reports. Other social factors exist, but the factors listed in these reports represent the most significant opportunities for improving the health of communities and reducing health disparities. Later in the chapter, specific factors of neighborhood, family (including early life), income, employment, and disability will be discussed.

TABLE 3-1 Social Factors That Influence Health

Report	Healthy People 2010	Healthy People 2020[a]	Commission to Build a Healthier America	The Solid Facts (2nd ed.)
Organization	U.S. Department of Health and Human Services	U.S. Department of Health and Human Services	Robert Wood Johnson Foundation	World Health Organization
Factors	• Gender • Race and ethnicity • Income and education • Disability • Geographic location • Sexual orientation	• Resources to meet daily needs • Education, economic and job opportunities • Health care services • Recreational opportunities • Transportation • Public safety • Social support • Social norms and attitudes • Exposure to crime, violence, and social disorder • Socioeconomic conditions • Residential segregation • Language/literacy • Access to mass media and emerging technologies • Culture	• Early life experiences • Education • Income • Work • Housing • Community • Race and ethnicity • The economy	• Social gradient • Stress • Early life • Social exclusion • Work • Unemployment • Social support • Addiction • Food • Transport

a) Social determinants of health are a new and emerging focus area in Healthy People 2020. Actual indicators are being developed.

Personal health behaviors are important determinants of health status. Being physically active, eating a nutritious and balanced diet, not smoking, receiving adequate sleep, and participating in preventive clinical care are all foundations for a healthy body. In some segments of the population, completing those actions can be more difficult. Even with knowledge and motivation to act, the conditions of a particular place can make completing health behaviors more difficult. The infrastructure of a system and policies that direct funding create a context that influences individual action. For example, a neighborhood's retail and recreational facilities can promote or deter physical activity. Similarly, places of employment are associated with resources such as health and dental insurance, paid sick leave, time to seek preventive care, messages about health behaviors, and stress.

Addressing health behaviors in both upstream and downstream fashion is important to improve the health of communities. The critical distinction in the work is that downstream solutions do not fix upstream problems. For behavioral interventions to produce sustainable population improvements, root causes need to be addressed, and appropriate strategies need to be put in place.

Pathways to Health

Before considering specific social factors, it is important to recognize the different ways in which social factors affect personal behavior and population health. Understanding the different pathways deepens comprehension and therefore the ability of persons designing effective interventions. In using the river example, social factors are located at different places along the riverbank; some may be midstream while others are significantly further upstream. First, neighborhood, community, and workplace environments create an environmental context from which individual health behaviors are completed (see Figure 3-1). Health-promoting neighborhoods and larger communities offer safe streets, sidewalks, clean and toxin-free housing, accessible transportation, and recreation spaces (RWJF, 2013). Similarly, healthy communities include nutritious food choices in schools and retail outlets, include

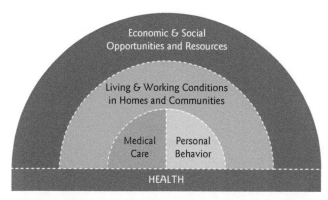

Figure 3-1 Robert Wood Johnson Foundation Commission to Build a Healthier America Model for Understanding the Social Determinants of Health.

Source: Copyright 2013 Robert Wood Johnson Foundation Commission to Build a Healthier America

opportunities for members to participate in community life and offer affordable, high-quality health care. The very access to these factors creates opportunity to take action. Lack of access and the presence of obstacles can create tremendous challenges to performing seemingly simple health behaviors. For example, completing immunizations can be difficult for someone who works an hourly job and lacks transportation. Taking time off from work can mean a decrease in income, and without transportation, the time to get to the appointment may create an additional obstacle. Providing immunizations to populations will absolutely improve health status. The provision of the medical services alone, though, may not be adequate to improve long-term health status. A person's living and working conditions surround medical and personal care and thus **mediate** the healthy action. Mediating factors act as a source of influence between two other factors. In this example, living or working conditions influence actions between intention and health behavior.

Further upstream, social factors shape economic and education opportunities that then influence living and working conditions. Economic opportunities are the possibilities to work a job associated with a living wage in a physically and emotionally safe environment (RWJF, 2013; Wilkinson & Marmot, 2003). Educational opportunities are realized through the completion of high-quality education at the primary, secondary, college, and/or vocational levels (RWJF, 2013; Wilkinson & Marmot, 2003). Further, access to education and employment opportunities creates **mobility**, that is, the ability of individuals to move upward in a manner that improves the conditions of living and social position. Finally, community social factors such as race relations and integration also create pathways to an individual's living and employment opportunities. Exclusion prevents individuals from participating in educational activities and gaining access to timely services, civic activities, and social relationships (Brondolo et al., 2011; USDHHS, n.d.; Wilkinson & Marmot, 2003). Poor community relations can also increase community members' stress levels (Bravemen et al., 2011). In the river metaphor, economic and societal factors can be the "really" upstream factors in many health disparities. They create a platform from which all other opportunities and struggles originate. In the model of social determinants and health developed by the Commission to Build a Healthier America, the broad economic conditions of a population surround all other factors within the model (see Figure 3-1).

Neighborhood and Families

It may seem an obvious statement, but people are products of their environment. As a result, different environments often lead to differences in health status (LaVeist et al., 2011). Health status differences exist by geographical regions of the county, by state, and by neighborhood. Across the country, states with the longest life expectancies and lowest rates of chronic diseases are located in the Northeast and West. Hawaii, California, and Connecticut have the lowest age-adjusted death rates per 100,000 people (NCHS, 2012). By contrast, the most "unhealthy" states are in the South. Louisiana, Mississippi, Arkansas, and West Virginia have the highest age-adjusted death rates per 100,000 people. Differences in health status can be significant. State percentages of adult obesity range from a low of 20.5% (Colorado) to a high of 34.7% (Louisiana). Similarly, the prevalence of hypertension in Alabama (40%) is almost double that of Utah (22.9%) (Trust for America's Health, 2013). Health status differences at the state level represent a collection of upstream factors at work—economic, social, living, working, normative health behaviors, and medical care. It should be no surprise, though, that two of the least healthy states (Mississippi and Louisiana) also have lower median household incomes and education levels than the national average (U.S. Department of Commerce, U.S. Census Bureau, 2012). The broad economic conditions of the overall population surround all other factors on the pathway to health behavior and health outcomes.

A neighborhood is a place of physical and social health. Neighborhoods influence health through their physical characteristics, such as air and water quality, noise, exposure to environmental toxins, and structures of safety (Braveman et al., 2011; LaVeist et al., 2011). Service-based organizations such as grocery stores, health care facilities, transportation, social and/or spiritual support, and recreation also vary by neighborhood and affect one's ability to take positive actions toward a healthier lifestyle.

Two health behaviors that have been studied in terms of neighborhood correlates are physical activity and healthy eating. Research has found that environments that are functional, safe, and aesthetically pleasing promote physical activity (McCann, 2005). Functional environments have well-connected streets, sidewalks, mixed land use, and lighting. Furthermore, when adults and children have access to quality and safe places of recreation, they are more active and have lower body mass indexes (Frank, Anderson, & Schmid, 2004). Neighborhood access to supermarkets combined with limited convenient store retail also appear to be environmental factors associated with higher rates of healthy eating (e.g., high consumption of fruits and vegetables, appropriate amount of calories from fat, and overall high diet quality). Supermarkets offer a greater variety of fresh affordable produce; residents with this access have improved food choice and tend to have lower levels of obesity (Larson, Story, & Nelson, 2009). By contrast, food at convenient stores has more calories, and these stores offer limited fresh produce. The study of relationships between health behaviors/outcomes and environmental factors is increasing and in Chapter 11, methods used by a community coalition to assess rates of infant mortality by neighborhood factors will be discussed.

> **Check for Understanding** Before reading further, jot down a list of the 10 healthiest states and the 10 least healthy states. List at least five factors considered in your rankings. After finishing the chapter, access County Health Rankings or the Center for Health Statistics to locate a list of state-level health outcomes.

Early Life

Early life is particularly important to the health status of individuals and population segments. Early life is a life stage (childhood) and includes the developmental, economic, and social experiences during that life stage. Economic resources, neighborhood and home conditions, early education, stress and trauma, nurturing, and health care utilization influence the health of children through the direct and indirect pathways introduced earlier. Early childhood is a time of significant physical, emotional, and intellectual development. Therefore, early childhood is a period in one's life span in which health can be particularly influenced, positively and negatively, by one's physical and social environments (Adler & Stewart, 2010b; Cohen et al., 2010; RWJF, 2013; Wilkinson & Marmot, 2003).

Parents' income and education levels can create opportunities and resources for establishing healthy and nurturing environments for children. Despite motivation and hard work, lack of income and/or education can create obstacles for establishing health-enhancing neighborhood environments and family behaviors. From the beginning of life, being born into poverty has detrimental effects on children's health (Adler & Stewart, 2010b; Cohen et al., 2010). Children born into poverty have a child mortality rate that is two to three times higher than children born into more affluent families (Singh, 2010). Some of the differences in birth outcomes are explained through combinations of maternal health and prenatal behaviors such as smoking, nutrition, vitamin and mineral intake, and environmental exposures (Braveman, Sadegh-Nobari, & Egerter, 2011). However, numerous social factors can also lead to poor birth outcomes. These factors include access to healthy foods, racial equity, good air and water quality, safe areas designated for physical activity, and programs designed to increase a community's financial literacy and social capital (Lu et al., 2010).

Children who live in poverty continue to experience postnatal differences in health status. Asthma is the most common chronic disease experienced by children; approximately 9% of children have asthma. As family income decreases, rates of childhood asthma increase; 12.1% of children living below the federal poverty level have asthma. By contrast, 10.2% of children within 100% to 199% of the poverty level have asthma (Federal Interagency Forum on Child and Family Statistics, 2013).

Family income provides some of the most basic resources for development—food, child care, and safe housing. Food consumption and the early establishment of eating habits are mediated through the food that is in the home environment. Children living around or below the federal poverty level are less likely to eat fruits and vegetables (Federal Interagency Forum, 2013). Where a child lives can also determine exposure to environmental pollutants, violence, air quality, and lead paint—factors that are disproportionately experienced by certain segments of the population.

The home and neighborhood climate also affect current and future health. Living in disadvantaged circumstances often creates chronic stress and a sense of anxiety. Research has found that difficult home lives can affect children's brain development, which in turn affects emotional development and ability to learn. When someone is stressed, the body releases adrenaline (which increases blood pressure and heart rate and redirects blood flow) and cortisol (which can age the immune system and damage the cardiovascular system) (AAP, 2012; Egerter, Braveman, & Barclay, 2011). A chronic state of

stress can cause serious damage to the body, and damage due to childhood stress can influence how an adult's body responds to stress (AAP, 2012; Egerter et al., 2011). Chronic stress can also negatively impact a child's ability to concentrate, and it interferes with one's ability to self-regulate and pay attention. Similarly, social factors such as negative school climate, poor quality of education, and racism can disrupt cognitive and emotional development (Cohen et al., 2010; National Scientific Council on the Developing Child, 2014).

Pediatricians have called chronic early life stress **toxic stress** because of the harm it can cause. Specifically, toxic stress is "severe, chronic stress that becomes toxic to developing brains and biological systems when a child suffers significant adversity, such as poverty, abuse, neglect, neighborhood violence, or the substance abuse or mental illness of a caregiver" (AAP, 2012). Toxic stress differs from positive and tolerable stress in its duration and social support mechanisms. Positive stress refers to moderate, short-lived stress responses. Positive stress is normal and an essential part of healthy development, and it is characterized by brief increases in heart rate and mild elevations in hormone levels. Positive stress and learning to cope with short-term adverse events generally occurs in safe, nurturing relationships. When an individual experiences more severe, longer-lasting difficulties, tolerable stress activates the body's alert systems to a greater degree. This activation is time limited and buffered by relationships with adults who help the child adapt, so the brain and other organs can recover from what might otherwise be damaging effects (National Scientific Council on the Developing Child, 2014).

Negative early childhood experiences are also associated with poor health outcomes later in life. The Adverse Childhood Experiences Study is one of the largest studies measuring the impact of occurrences of maltreatment during childhood with adult rates of health behaviors, chronic diseases, and emotional health. Initiated in 1995 by Kaiser Permanente and still active today in collaboration with the Centers for Disease Control and Prevention, the study's researchers have found numerous examples of a dose/response relationship between the number of childhood occurrences of traumas, household dysfunction, and neglect with adult health (Felitti et al., 1998), collectively called **adverse childhood experiences (ACEs).** ACEs included childhood physical, emotional, or sexual abuse; witnessing domestic violence; and growing up with household substance abuse, mental illness, parental divorce, and/or an incarcerated household member. ACEs are associated with higher rates of heart disease, cancer, chronic bronchitis or emphysema, hepatitis or jaundice, skeletal fractures, and poor self-rated health (Felitti et al., 1998). More recently, others have documented relationships between ACEs and autoimmune hospitalizations (Dube et al., 2009), headaches (Anda et al., 2010), alcoholism (Dube et al., 2002), homelessness (Patterson, Moniruzzaman, & Somers, 2014), and self-reported quality of life (Corso et al., 2008). In 2009, a subset of 11 ACE-related questions was developed for addition to the Behavioral Risk Factor Surveillance System. Five states that adopted the subset found that 59.4% of respondents reported having at least one ACE, and 8.7% reported five or more ACEs. The highest prevalence rate was for substance abuse (25.9%), followed by verbal abuse (25.9%) and physical abuse (14.8%). When considering family dysfunction, 26.6% reported separated or divorced parents; 19.4% reported that they had lived with someone who was depressed, mentally ill, or suicidal; and 16.3% reported witnessing domestic violence (CDC, 2010).

Not all children living in stressful neighborhoods experience poor health. Studies have documented that early parental nurturing can prepare children to navigate these pathways. Secure attachments, coping skills, resilience, and optimism can all be shaped in children. A supportive family or community can also help a child or adult deal with the stressors in life, which can reduce the damaging physical effects of stress (Egerter et al., 2011; National Scientific Council on the Developing Child, 2014).

What happens during the early years of life places children on life trajectories. **Trajectories** are paths that are determined by one's previous experiences; current and future opportunities and resources available to a person on his or her path are based upon prior experiences (Berkman, 2009). Similarly, obstacles such as lack of resources and feelings of helplessness and isolation are carried forward on the path. The power of early childhood development is in the cumulative effect of early health and behavioral/cognitive development. An obese child is likely to be an obese adult. A child with diabetes is likely to be an adult with diabetes *and* with secondary health conditions related to the diabetes. A child with poor cognitive development is likely to be an adolescent with poor cognitive achievement. The cumulative effects of carcinogens, poor air quality, and social isolation are apparent in individuals who

seek treatment in the emergency department, but the roots of the problem appear much earlier in life. Early experiences influence health at the time those experiences are lived, but the effects of those early experiences and outcomes are also carried forward (Adler & Stewart, 2010a). Much like genetic makeup, childhood experiences are carried forward to alter the likelihood of future outcomes.

> **Check for Understanding**   Babies born to mothers who have not finished high school are nearly twice as likely to die in infancy compared to babies born to mothers with a college degree. List three possible health-related behaviors (downstream factors) that might be associated with high infant mortality. Then list three upstream factors that may be associated with the health-related behaviors.

Socioeconomic Position

Economic opportunities are the furthest upstream factors impacting the health of a community. Economic achievements are fundamental platforms from which people develop a sense of purpose and worth, accumulate and trade resources, and are able to pursue upward mobility. **Socioeconomic position** is a composition of many individual concepts, the three foundations being education, income, and occupation (Adler & Newman, 2002; Herd, Goesling, & House, 2007; Krieger, 2001). Education, income, and occupation are intertwined, much like a rope. They twist around one another, and it can be difficult to tell where one strand begins and the other ends. Income is the primary benefit of a high-quality education; generally, income increases as levels of education increase. Yet, income is required to attain education and the ability to live in certain neighborhoods and school districts as well as afford tuition. The presence of one factor influences the opportunities of the others.

Socioeconomic position also includes a prestige- or position-based component. Prestige-based measures refer to individuals' rank or status in a social hierarchy (Krieger, 2001). A person's rank may be evaluated within the context of type of employment, level of education completed, or amount of wealth or resource type accrued. In any case, persons further down a social ladder have fewer resources, and they lack power to influence resource decisions and trajectories. The

gradient relationship between socioeconomic position and educational outcome has significant implications for subsequent employment, income, living standards, behaviors, and mental and physical health (RWJF, 2013; Wilkinson & Marmot, 2003).

Individual concepts within socioeconomic position may take on more active roles with health status at different points of time in the life span. Educational attainment is largely established earlier in one's life and has a stronger relationship with the onset of health problems. Education may act as a protective factor. In an analysis of the chronic diseases and functional limitations of over 3100 adults across a 16-year period, persons with higher education levels had fewer and later onsets of chronic diseases and reported fewer physical limitations (Herd et al., 2007). By contrast, income may have a more active role in the progression of health issues (Herd et al., 2007). Income seems to slow the progression of health problems, whereas education does not. Income allows persons to access health care and coping resources, as well as make modifications to home and work situations, thus slowing the progression of chronic disease and illness.

Education

There is a very strong correlation between education and health, as education is a significant upstream factor for health. Higher education levels are associated with increased life expectancy and quality of life, and lower levels of chronic disease and stress (NCHS, 2014, 2012). A 25-year-old college graduate can expect to live 8 to 9 years longer than similar persons without a high school diploma, and 2 to 4 years more than those who graduated high school and completed some college (NCHS, 2012). Figure 3-2 illustrates a growing gap in life expectancy by education level. Between 1996 and 2006, life expectancy increased for persons with a bachelor's degree or higher and remained unchanged for persons with less than a bachelor's degree. Further, persons with at least some college education are less likely to report their health as fair or poor (NCHS, 2012).

Success in education brings many advantages. Most notably, education is associated with higher incomes. In 2013, college graduates earned 70% more than high school graduates; $1108 per week compared with $651 per week, respectively (USDL Bureau of Labor Statistics 2014). For every milestone in

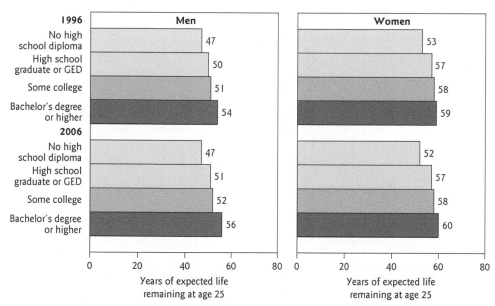

NOTE: GED is General Educational Development high school equivalency diploma.

Figure 3-2 Life Expectancy by Level of Educational Attainment

Source: Courtesy of Centers for Disease Control and Prevention, National Center for Health Statistics

educational attainment completed (high school to associate; associate to bachelor; bachelor to master; master to doctorate), weekly income increases by at least 20% (see Figure 3-3). College graduates also experience lower unemployment rates: 4.0% for college graduates versus 7.5% for high school graduates and 11.0% for high school dropouts (USDL Bureau of Labor Statistics 2014). Through income, individuals are able to purchase resources associated with health and have expanded choice in living, working, education, and recreational options (Herd et al., 2007). Higher levels of education also are associated with "safer" jobs and involvement in social, civic, and political life (Southern Education Foundation, 2008).

Figure 3-4 summarizes three interrelated pathways in which educational attainment is linked with health status: health knowledge and behaviors, employment and income, and social and psychological factors (Braveman et al., 2011; RWJF, 2013). The first path, at the top of the chart, reflects the link between education and health behaviors. Broadly, individuals with increasing educational completion tend to have knowledge and skills (most notably health literacy) that are associated with health behaviors. For example, rates for cigarette smoking, physical activity, and breastfeeding vary across levels of education. Smoking rates decrease as education increases, with 17% of high school graduates smoking cigarettes versus

7% of college graduates (NCHS, 2014). Approximately one-fourth (26%) of persons with only a high school diploma or GED smoke cigarettes. Leisure-time physical activity increases as educational levels increase: 7.6% (no high school diploma or GED), 12.4% (high school diploma or GED), and 25% (some college or more) (NCHS, 2014). Likewise, mothers with a college degree are much more likely to breastfeed up to the baby's first birthday: 65.8% compared with varying rates between 37% and 49%, respectively (NCHS, 2014).

Education influences adult occupation, work conditions, resources, and income. In the second pathway, education is linked to income, and income is the means to numerous material, service, and social resources. Those resources then provide means for seeking and improving health (Herd et al., 2007; RWJF, 2013). Job type and work conditions impact exposure to work hazards and stress. Jobs that require higher levels of training and education tend to have fewer environmental hazards (USDL Bureau of Labor Statistics, 2013a). Further, work generates resources associated with health behavior, namely health insurance, sick leave, wellness benefits, and messages about health. Work and health will be discussed in more detail in the upcoming section. Work and income may be the most important pathway through which education affects health (RWJF, 2014).

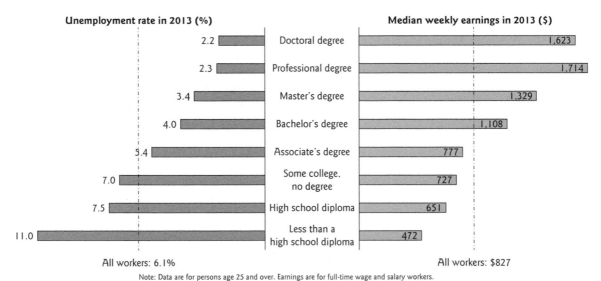

Note: Data are for persons age 25 and over. Earnings are for full-time wage and salary workers.

Figure 3-3 Earnings and Unemployment Rate by Level of Educational Attainment.
Source: Courtesy of U.S. Bureau of Labor Statistics

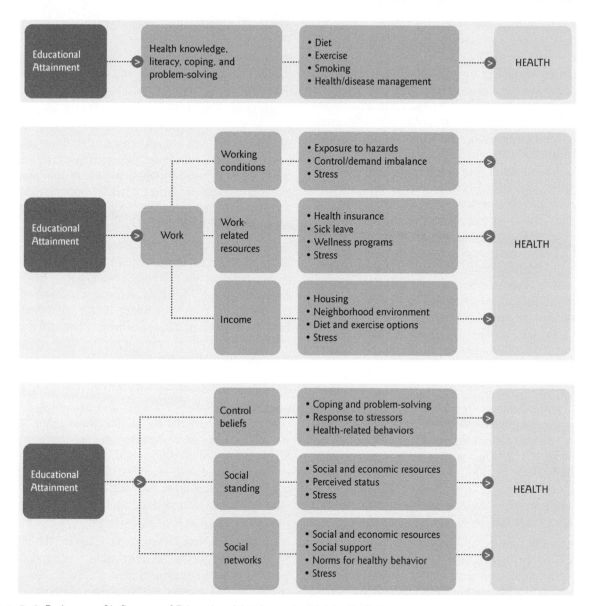

Figure 3-4 Pathways of Influence of Educational Attainment with Health Status.

Source: Copyright 2013 Robert Wood Johnson Foundation Commission to Build a Healthier America

The third path is an indirect means through social and psychological factors of control, standing, and support. Educational attainment can improve a person's sense of control, social standing, and social support (Braveman et al., 2011). These factors can then improve health through reducing stress, supporting health behaviors, and providing informational and emotional support (Herd et al., 2007; RWJF, 2013). Social support, buffering, and social networks will be discussed in Chapters 6 and 7.

For the aforementioned reasons, a number of Healthy People 2020 objectives include increasing educational attainment. Adolescent Health Objective 5.1 (AH-5.1) is to increase the proportion of students that graduate with a regular high school diploma within 4 years after starting ninth grade. The national target graduation rate is 82.4%, approximately 10% above the baseline rate (2007–2008) of 74.7%. High school graduation rates are increasing; the 2009–2010 rate was up to 78.2% (USDHHS, 2014). AH-5.1 is a leading health indicator (LHI), that is, a subset of objectives that are considered high-priority objectives. Of the 1200 objectives within Healthy People 2020, there are 26 designated as LHIs. Further, high school graduation is *the* leading health indictor measure for the topic area of social determinants of health. Other related adolescent health education objectives include increasing the proportion of students with a disability who graduate (AH-5.2), increasing grade-level reading skills (AH-5.3) and mathematic skills (AH-5.4), increasing the proportion of schools with a breakfast program (AH-6), and increasing school environment safety (AH-8, AH-9, AH-10, AH-11). Objectives can be accessed at http://www.healthypeople.gov.

Employment

There is a preponderance of evidence that health status and behaviors vary by job type. As described in the opening In the News case study, blue-collar workers report lower health status and are less likely to engage in preventive clinical care. Further, individuals from tougher economic environments with lower educational attainment are more likely to occupy lower-wage, stressful, blue-collar jobs (Clougherty, Souza, & Cullen, 2010; USDL Bureau of Labor Statistics, 2013a).

As the middle pathway in Figure 3-4 illustrates, work is associated with health first through the conditions in which work is completed. Some jobs are clearly more dangerous than others. Jobs with repetitive tasks, physically demanding jobs, shift work, and required overtime raise the likelihood of physical injury. Truck and bus drivers; police officers; correctional officers and jailers; firefighters; nursing aides; freight, stock, and material movers; construction laborers; emergency medical technicians; and paramedics have the highest incidence of nonfatal workplace injuries (USDL Bureau of Labor Statistics 2013c). Logging workers, fishermen and related fishing workers, aircraft pilots, flight engineers, roofers, and steel and iron workers are among the workers with highest fatal work injury rates (USDL Bureau of Labor Statistics 2013b). The physical environment of the workplace influences health; exposure to toxins, physical demands, repetitive demands, air quality, and noise can create environments that are hazardous to health.

The associations between work and health are more complicated than just exposure to physical danger, however. Working conditions are also created through organization policy, practices, and climate. Downsizing and restructuring, temporary and part-time labor, and use of lean production practices are examples of recent trends in organizational practices that have been associated with job stress (Caruso et al., 2004; Grosch & Sauter, 2005; USDHHS, CDC, NIOSH, 2002).

Type of work also provides differences in resources. Work-accrued resources associated with health status include income (amount and reliability), health and/or dental insurance, paid time off, sick leave, retirement benefits, education reimbursements, and workplace health promotion activities (Braveman et al., 2011; USDHHS & National Prevention Council, 2011). Simply having a job is not enough to secure these benefits of employment. The type and degree of these benefits are disproportionately dispersed. For example, 7.2% of those in the workforce generally do not earn enough in wages to cover basic necessities and are unlikely to receive health-related benefits (USDL Bureau of Labor Statistics 2013a). Type of job can be associated with other important benefits that make managing individual and family health easier. Flexible scheduling, quality child care, and social support are resources sometimes provided through employers that make health, sick, and medical care behaviors easier.

Work environments can also have a hierarchy that creates a real or perceived class system. Certain jobs and the employees who fill them may appear more valuable to an organization. A hierarchy of worth then compromises the contribution, sense of control, and interpersonal connections of workers. This can be psychologically stressful and physically damaging to those at the bottom of the system (Clougherty et al., 2010). Lower wages, contract work (as opposed to full-time employment), and shift work are symptoms of a class system that can make workers feel stressed. The Whitehall Study was a longitudinal study originating in 1967. It looked at British civil employees and documented inverse relationships between employment type or class and mortality. Men in the lowest-status jobs had three times higher rates of coronary artery disease and were more likely to die at a younger age (Marmot et al., 1978). A second study, Whitehall II, conducted 20 years later, found similar differences in health status by employment type (Marmot et al., 1991). Psychologically, being treated unfairly also had an independent relationship with poor health outcomes. The risk of coronary events among workers who strongly or moderately agreed that they were often treated unfairly was 55% higher than for those who reported fair treatment, controlling for age, gender, employment grade, established coronary risk factors, and other work-related psychosocial characteristics (De Vogli et al., 2007).

Workplace stress is a significant factor to consider when examining the relationship of work and health. Most employed Americans report job stress, both physical and psychological. Psychological job strain—a composite of perceived demand, control, and reward—is associated with higher rates of hypertension, cardiovascular disease, and depression. Workers who perceive higher demands, lower sense of control, and/or fewer rewards are more likely to experience chronic disease and injury (Clougherty et al., 2011; De Vogli et al., 2007).

Stress

Stress is the body's response to a demand, whether physical or emotional. Moderate amounts of stress can be healthy, particularly when stressors are time limited and persons have emotional and tangible support for coping with the stress (Thoits, 2010). Chronic exposure to stress, though, can create wear and tear on the body and ultimately be associated with chronic disease and impaired emotional health. Stress has been linked with hypertension, diabetes, depression, obesity, injury, and cardiovascular disease (Egerter et al., 2011). Numerous researchers believe that chronic stress is a central concept when seeking to understand how social disadvantage produces ill health (Adler & Stewart, 2010a; Thoits, 2010).

When presented with a stressor, the body initiates its stress response, preparing to fight the stressor or flee (i.e., the fight-or-flight response). Heart rate and respiration increase; blood flow is redirected from the digestive tract, kidneys, and skin to the brain, heart, and skeletal muscles; and senses become heightened (Egerter et al., 2011). Stress causes the pituitary gland to stimulate the adrenals to release cortisol, the main stress hormone. In acute stress, cortisol helps maintain blood sugar and stimulates the release of adrenalin. Some stress can

be healthy and is associated with productivity, a sense of control, and the ability to deal with future stressors (Egerter et al., 2011). Chronic stressors lead to persistent cortisol elevation, which causes increased insulin resistance, increased belly fat, decreased protein synthesis, a weakened immune system, and decreased DNA repair (Egerter et al., 2011; Salpolsky, 1998). Chronic stress creates wear and tear on the body, including the brain (McEwen & Gianaros, 2010).

Modern life is full of stressors—the commute to work, weather, deadlines, physical challenges, and more. Adults and children who live and work in disadvantaged environments are exposed to a far greater *number* of acute stressors, and they experience higher *chronic* exposure to stressors (Adler & Stewart, 2010b). Living a day-to-day existence that includes noisy and unsafe housing, long work hours, physical demands, and lack of a sense of control can create a chronic state of stress. The impact of the stressors becomes chronic due to repeated exposure and limited resources to manage the stressors (National Scientific Council on the Developing Child, 2014). Given a stressor, persons with higher incomes (and therefore likely a greater sense of control) are better prepared psychologically to deal with it (Adler & Stewart, 2010b).

There is no standardized measure of stress and therefore, the full magnitude of the relationships between stress and disease, disability, and quality of life is not fully understood. To measure the relationship of factor A to disease B, factor A and disease B need reliable and valid measures that are uniformly adopted. Risk factors with strong evidentiary relationships to disease have standardized tools to measure their presence. A blood pressure cuff, a scale, a blood test, and the observation of a behavior such as smoking can measure major risk factors for cardiovascular disease. No such tool for directly measuring stress exists (Thoits, 2010). The strong and growing body of evidence of the relationship between stress and health uses validated questionnaires or life scale tools. These indirect measures are good tools, but their limited adoption by practitioners likely leads to underreporting of the population-level impact of stress and health.

Check for Understanding Hourly workers are less likely than salaried employees to stay home when sick. Why do you think that is?

DISABILITY

Having a disability is associated with poorer health outcomes. A significantly higher number of adults with disabilities report having one or more chronic diseases compared to adults without a disability (40.5% versus 13.7%) (CDC, 2014). One in five individuals with a disability reports diabetes (19%) and heart disease (21%), and almost half of persons with a disability experience obesity (45%) (CDC, 2014). Individuals with disabilities are also more likely to experience psychological distress and to self-report lower levels of health (Altman & Bernstein, 2008; Drum et al., 2011, NCHS, 2014).

Disability can be discussed in a number of ways. First, many health issues are considered to be disabilities, including autism, arthritis, cerebral palsy, Down syndrome, hearing loss, vision loss, Parkinson disease, and spinal cord injury. In addition to referring to a specific health issue or loss, categories of disabilities can also be described by type of functional or activity limitation: communication, mental, and physical. People with disabilities in the *communication* domain report difficulty seeing, hearing, or having their speech understood. A communication-related disability includes blindness and deafness. People with disabilities in the *mental* domain may have a learning disability, intellectual disability, a developmental disability such as dementia, or similar conditions. People with disabilities in the *physical* domain may use assistive equipment such as a wheelchair, crutches or walker; have difficulty walking, carrying objects, or other activities of daily living; or have a chronic disease that limits physical functioning, such as arthritis, back problems, cancer, or diabetes (Brault, 2012).

Level of disability is another category to consider when talking about disability and health. Persons with a disability are able to function at different levels, and the distinction between difficulty with basic actions and complex activity limitation is important (NCHS, 2014; CDC, 2013; Brault, 2012; WHO and World Bank, 2011). Basic action difficulty captures limitations or difficulties in movement and sensory, emotional, or mental functioning associated with a health problem. Complex activity limitation describes limitations or restrictions on a person's ability to participate fully in social role activities such as working or maintaining a household (NCHS, 2014). The U.S. Census Bureau presents information in terms of nonsevere disability versus severe disability. In general, persons with nonsevere disabilities report *difficulty* with communication, mental, or physical tasks. Persons with a severe disability are *unable* to perform select communication, mental, or physical tasks (Brault, 2012).

Figure 3-5 outlines distinctions in disability severity by communication, mental, and physical tasks. Assessing difficulty and the need for assistance with self-care and independent living is a means to measure severity as well as to arrange clinical and social services. **Instrumental activities of daily living** (IADL) are basic self-care activities that include going outside the home, managing money, preparing meals, doing housework, taking prescription medications, and using the phone. **Activities of daily living** (ADL) include getting around inside the home, getting in and out of bed, bathing, dressing, eating, and toileting (Brault, 2012). Disability severity increases as a person's abilities to complete activities of daily living decrease.

Overall, 18.7% of the U.S. population reports having some type of disability, and 12.6% of the population has a severe disability (Brault, 2012). A person can be born with a disability or can develop a disability through injury, illness, or aging (USDHHS, 2005). Therefore, disability rates tend to increase with age. Approximately half of adults 65 and older (49.8%) report difficulty with one or more tasks (nonsevere disability), and approximately one-third (36.6%) report a severe disability.

One may not think about disability as a social factor, but persons with disabilities encounter environmental, social, and service barriers that make completing basic health and health care utilization behaviors difficult. In terms of the paths to health, the environmental platform from which health behaviors are completed may contain numerous barriers for persons with disabilities. For example, persons with disabilities often face obstacles to participating in physical activities that persons without a disability do not face. Space, equipment, or instructions may need to be modified to enable persons with disabilities to participate in a community-based activity. Similarly, persons with disabilities face biases and obstacles to accessing adequate health care (USDHHS, 2005). To participate in preventive cancer screenings (breast, cervical, or colorectal), procedure time, equipment, and space may need to be modified. The accessibility of medical examination and diagnostic equipment is particularly problematic for individuals who use a wheelchair. Navigation around examination tables and mammography machines can be difficult for a person with a mobility disability. In addition, individuals with disabilities may require special arrangements related to transportation and support personnel.

Types of disabilities (applicable age group)	Severity	
	Nonsevere	Severe
Had difficulty seeing words in ordinary newsprint, hearing a normal conversation, or having speech understood (aged 6 and older).	X	
Was deaf, blind, or was unable to see, hear, or have speech understood (aged 6 and older).		X
Had difficulty moving arms or legs (under 3 years).	X	
Had difficulty walking, running, or playing/taking part in sports (aged 3 to 14).	X	
Had difficulty performing one or more functional activities: walking, using stairs, lifting/carrying, or grasping small objects (aged 15 and older).	X	
Unable to perform one or more of the functional activities (aged 15 and older).		X
Used a wheelchair, cane, crutches, or walker (aged 6 and older).		X
Had difficulty with one or more activities of daily living (ADLs): getting around inside the home, getting in or out of bed or a chair, bathing, dressing, eating, or toileting (aged 6 and older).	X	
Needed assistance of another person to perform one or more ADLs (aged 6 and older).		X
Had difficulty with one or more instrumental activities of daily living (IADLs): going outside the home, managing money and bills, preparing meals, doing light housework, taking prescription medicines, or using the telephone (aged 15 and older).	X	
Needed assistance of another person to perform one or more IADLs (aged 15 and older).		X
Had difficulty with schoolwork (aged 6 to 19).	X	
Was limited in the kind or amount of housework (aged 16 and older).	X	
Had difficulty finding a job or remaining employed (aged 16 to 72).		X
Had a learning disability such as dyslexia (aged 6 and older).	X	
Had Attention Deficit Hyperactivity Disorder (aged 6 to 14).	X	
Had Alzheimer's disease, dementia, or senility (aged 15 and older).		X
Had a developmental delay (under 6 years).		X
Had an intellectual disability or a developmental disability, such as autism or cerebral palsy (aged 6 and older).		X
Had some other developmental condition for which received therapy or diagnostic services (aged 6 to 14).		X
Had difficulty getting along with other children of the same age (aged 6 to 14).	X	
Had one or more selected symptoms that interfered with everyday activities: was frequently depressed or anxious, had trouble getting along with others, had trouble concentrating, or had trouble coping with stress (aged 15 and older).		X
Had some other type of mental or emotional condition (aged 15 and older).	X	

Note: The definition of disability shown here is consistent with the definition used in the prior report, "Americans With Disabilities: 2005," (P70-117). The definition of ADLs and IADLs is consistent with other national surveys like the Medicare Current Beneficiary Survey and the National Health Interview Survey.

Figure 3-5 Definition of Disability by Severity.

Source: Courtesy of U.S. Census Bureau

The presence of a disability also limits economic and social opportunities, the very upstream factors associated with health. Employment is a significant upstream factor that influences the health of people with disabilities. Data from the U.S. Census indicate a wide gap in employment status between people with a disability and those without. Less than half of adults ages 21 to 64 with a disability are employed (41%), compared with approximately 79% of adults without a disability. Employment rates are higher (71%) for adults with a nonsevere disability (Brault, 2012). Remember that employment is affiliated with numerous midstream resources such as money, housing, and social connections. Disability and Health Objective15 (DH-15) of Healthy People 2020 is to reduce the unemployment rate of individuals with disabilities by 10%.

Persons with disabilities experience difficulties in securing affordable housing and transportation and integrating themselves into a community. Again, lack of employment opportunities can be associated with living and neighborhood conditions, but even separate from employment, obstacles in living, neighborhood, and social conditions can further remove a person with a disability. Many persons with

disabilities experience difficulty accessing wellness and organized spiritual activities. Churches and other places of worship may be difficult to maneuver with mobility equipment, and sometimes individuals with sensory disabilities report difficulty connecting with the material. Further, despite higher rates of smoking, substance abuse, obesity, and unplanned pregnancies, interventions of change tailored to the needs of persons with specific disabilities (sight, hearing, intellectual, and mobility) are lacking (USDHHS, 2005). A small number of federal, state, and local initiatives tailored for persons with disabilities are quietly emerging. Figure 3-6 shows a poster from a social marketing campaign for improving mammography and Pap screening rates among women with disabilities.

Housing First

Housing First is an approach to ending homelessness that centers on providing people experiencing homelessness with housing as quickly as possible and then providing services as needed (National Alliance to End Homelessness, 2009). Housing First differs from traditional approaches that require sobriety or employment before housing is offered/rewarded. The approach reflects a paradigm shift—put people in safe

Model for Understanding   Discussing social determinants of health can be difficult. At times, statistics can sound preachy, imply finger-pointing, or take on an "us versus them" tone (Adler & Newman, 2002). Neither preaching nor finger-pointing are the intentions of the current discussion or of the cited reports. The goal is a deeper upstream understanding of differences in health outcomes. Health behaviors and health care utilization have direct relationships with health, yet their execution by some segments of the population is impaired by obstacles of place, employment, and/or exclusion. Solutions of a downstream nature alone—directly altering health behaviors and health care utilization—are unlikely to close gaps in health disparities (Docteur & Berenson, 2014). Evidence-based practices for a given segment of the population can be hampered by unseen upstream factors.

Social determinants of health should be added to *our* Model for Understanding. In coaching health behaviors and guiding the use of health care, it is essential to understand that living conditions and larger systems may create obstacles

to personal health. Applying a one-size-fits-all solution to both upstream and downstream health problems will fail to improve health for segments of the population; further, misaligned resources can lead to terrible amounts of waste (IOM, 2014). A broader purpose of the health care system is to address nonmedical factors that affect health and connect community members to resources and services in the community that can improve their ability to pursue better health (RWJF, 2013). For example, medication and behavioral compliance for a person with diabetes can be impaired by food insecurity, housing conditions, and lack of social support. Failing to understand a person's conditions of living (nonmedical factors) is failing to offer the best solution for the individual. Coaching diabetes self-management through evidence-based strategies of building functional knowledge and monitoring skills requires the individual to have access to healthy foods, refrigeration, and opportunities for activity. Looking through a broader lens, asking questions and enriching understanding can lead to better interventions. Housing First is an example of such an intervention.

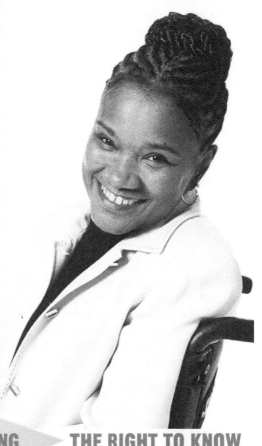

Breast cancer was just another obstacle I had to fight.

—DIANE, SURVIVOR

As a young mother, a spinal cord injury left Diane with a disability. And at 40, she was first in her family to be diagnosed with breast cancer. She calls the cancer her wake-up call, and credits early detection with still being alive today.

Breast cancer is the most common cancer in women. And living with a disability doesn't make you immune. If you are between the ages of 40 to 49, talk to your doctor about when and how often you should have a screening mammogram. If you are between the ages of 50 to 74, be sure to have a screening mammogram every two years.

BREAST CANCER SCREENING   THE RIGHT TO KNOW

For more information, visit
www.cdc.gov/RightToKnow
or call **1–800–CDC–INFO** (232–4636)
1–888–232–6348 (TTY)

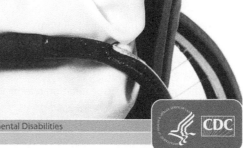

National Center on Birth Defects and Developmental Disabilities
Division of Human Development and Disability

Figure 3-6 Poster to Promote Mammograms by Women with a Disability
Source: Courtesy of Centers for Disease Control and Prevention

housing, provide basic necessities, reduce stress levels, and then approach health and health care behaviors. Housing First initiatives involve a system redesign that requires social, health care, legal, law enforcement, government, and funding agencies to collaborate.

Twelve metropolitan areas that have implemented a housing first model have measured decreased rates of homelessness. Homelessness decreased 12%, from 6715 in 2005 to 5922 in 2007 in Chicago; 25% between 2006 and 2008 in Norfolk, Virginia; and 39% from 2005 to 2007 in Portland, Oregon (National Alliance to End Homelessness, 2009). In Chicago, a 4-year randomized study of homeless people with chronic medical problems also documented that permanent housing and case management reduced hospital days by 29% and emergency department visits by 24% (Sadowski et al., 2009). Researchers estimated an average annual savings of $6307 per person and $9809 for persons who had been chronically homeless (Basu et al., 2011).

Successful initiatives are tailored to local communities, with most providing a combination of prevention efforts and efforts to quickly rehouse individuals when needed. Prevention efforts address underlying causes of homelessness—impaired mental health, substance abuse, and unemployment. In more detailed analyses, researchers have documented that permanent housing is associated with decreased substance use and relapse, as well as maintained housing (Fitzpatrick-Lewis et al., 2011). Housing has also been associated with improved psychiatric outcomes (Patterson et al., 2013; Fitzpatrick-Lewis et al., 2011).

First Things First: Education

As previously discussed, earning a high school diploma has many benefits for both the health and the economic situation of individuals. The public school system in Kansas City, Kansas, decided to completely change the way it approached education by adopting the First Things First education reform model (Gambone et al., 2004). The schools focused on creating stronger relationships between students and teachers, improving student attendance, improving teacher performance, and setting higher standards for student conduct and academic performance (Gambone et al., 2004). The First Things First intervention seeks to improve the education of all students in kindergarten through 12th grade, allowing children of all ages to benefit from the advantages of a stronger

education. It took several years before the results of the intervention could be measured, but the outcomes were significant. In the four high schools in the district, students were 20–27% more likely to graduate from high school. Across all socioeconomic levels and ethnicities, the graduation rates increased from 80% to 85% three years following implementation of the interventions (Gambone et al., 2004). More graduating students, especially in urban areas, can strengthen the health and economic conditions of the entire community.

Moving Upstream

Solutions seeking to address social determinants of health have historically been called social programs, not public health programs. In the shift toward addressing upstream factors, issues such as housing, employment, high school graduation, and neighborhood conditions are being considered in terms of their impact on the health of multigenerational segments of the population (USDHHS, n.d.). National policy initiatives that created Head Start and the Americans with Disabilities Act should be called public health initiatives, as they have the potential to alter places of living and work, as well as environmental and social opportunities that mediate the ability to choose health and health care behaviors. Building places and systems where healthy behaviors are possible requires focusing on neighborhoods, family, inclusion, and economic opportunities across all segments of the population.

In Chapter 1, the idea of winnable battles in public health was introduced. Winnable battles are health issues that have a significant effect on the health of segments of the population *and* have evidence-based, efficacious interventions. The documentation and dissemination of evidence-based solutions is a challenge in the battle to address social determinants of health. Solutions often must involve system and environmental changes achieved through policy and environmental interventions (Alder and Newman, 2002; IOM, 2014; RWJF, 2013; Wilkinson and Marmot, 2008; Woolf & Braveman, 2011). Policy and environmental interventions can be harder to implement, and it may take generations to see measured change, for example, it may take generations following the improvement of neighborhood conditions to see changes in rates of diabetes, obesity, and infant mortality. This length of time between implementation and improvement can hurt the ability to disseminate information on whether the intervention works. Similarly, social issues are complex, with various factors affecting a particular health issue and the implementation of a solution. The appropriate solution to a specific social factor issue in one segment of the population may be different from the right solution in another community.

Pursuing a culture of health for all persons means adopting policies and system changes that support individual action.

Given motivation, all people should have the ability to choose and pursue health. Chapter 4 introduces the social ecological model in which individual action is surrounded by the multiple layers of social, environmental, and policy influence. The model collectively represents upstream and downstream factors that directly and indirectly influence health behavior.

SUMMARY

Social determinants of health are social factors that have direct and indirect impacts on an individual's health status. Social factors include income, education, inclusion, and living and family environment. Social factors influence health at all stages of life. Socioeconomic factors may be upstream, meaning they influence an individual's health at a more distant level. Other upstream factors may include government policies or environmental influences that are out of an individual's control. Disability is another factor that can seriously impact one's health status. Interventions designed to address socioeconomic and other social factors can profoundly affect community's health.

BEHAVIORAL SCIENCE IN ACTION

Can you hear me? Framing messages about social factors that speak to policy makers

The Robert Wood Johnson Foundation Commission to Build a Healthier America funded a study to gain greater understanding of how policymakers and private sector leaders process information about social determinants of health. The goal was to be able to develop messages that would in turn capture attention and raise awareness about social factors. At the time of the commission's work, and despite decades of work documenting health disparities and the influence of social factors, professionals outside public health and related disciplines were unfamiliar with the topic of social determinants. This lack of awareness created a significant barrier to action in that solutions to these upstream factors involve policy and system change. Again, the purpose of the study was not to evaluate evidence about the impact of social factors on health outcomes; rather, it aimed to explore how

policymakers, identified as Republicans or Democrats, processed and reacted to the research.

The first part of the study consisted of one-on-one interviews with legislators and legislative representatives. The goal of the interviews was to identify the pathways or frames through which individuals process information about health disparities. Researchers have documented that all individuals process information through physical pathways in the brain. If we are presented with information that does not fit on one of our pathways, we tend to disregard it (Zaltman & Zaltman, 2008). Metaphors used in speech can reveal one's pathways or ways of seeing the world. In this study, researchers used a specific interviewing technique—Zaltman Metaphor Elicitation Technique (ZMET)—to identify "deep metaphors" for processing messages about differences in health status. By understanding the pathways that both political parties use to process similar information about health differences, the commission believed that more effective messages could be developed. Three metaphors emerged and were translated to social factor messages: journey, connection, and resources.

Journey was a primary deep metaphor for overall life experience. Life is a journey where there may be twists and turns along the path to a destination. Seeing life as a long journey allows for optimism and creates references to starting points. For example, health status (measured via life expectancy) has improved significantly in this country. Despite current population differences, the overall journey toward population health might be viewed as successful. Resources and connections were two additional themes that emerged as possible frames for introducing messages about health status differences. Resources are needed and are essential on life's journey. Yet, some people may not have adequate resources to make healthy choices. Finally, people and conditions are connected. Determinants and resources for health affect all people, not just certain ethnic and socioeconomic groups. Messages of commonalities were more receptive to some people than were messages of exclusion or divide.

In another phase of the study, researchers developed and tested new messages about differences in health status and different social conditions. *Overcoming Obstacles to Health: Stories, Facts and Findings* (2008) is one product of this understanding and discusses translating messages to new audiences. The road on the cover of this report represents the journey. The sole car on the road represents the individual and individual responsibility. Words such as "obstacles to choosing" and "resource-poor" were used instead of "inequality" and "disparity." Wasting resources is also a part of the new messages about health differences. In this report and others, readers are reminded that the United States spends more on health care than any other developed country, yet it experiences poorer aggregate health outcomes.

To find out more about the seven lessons learned from this research, read *A New Way to Talk about Social Determinants* (2010) from the Robert Wood Johnson Foundation. For more information about the study, see *Breaking Through on the Social Determinants of Health and Health Disparities: An Approach to Message Translation* (2009) from the Robert Wood Johnson Foundation.

IN THE CLASSROOM ACTIVITIES

1) Write a definition for social determinants of health. Give specific examples of social conditions that could impact the academic success of fellow college students.

2) Explain three pathways in which social factors are linked to asthma outcomes in young children.

3) From the *Unnatural Causes* series, watch the segment "Bad Sugar" about diabetes and empowerment in two Native American communities. Discuss the impact of water on downstream behaviors and health. Use Figure 3-4 to organize your thoughts and draw the model pathways using the diversion of water as the upstream factor.

4) Visit an on-campus health promotion program. Assess the program for participation by persons with a specific type of communication, mental, or physical impairment.

5) Exclusion is a broad factor on the list of social determinants of health. In what ways can aging members of the population be excluded from the resources of healthy living?

WEB LINKS

ACE Study: http://www.cdc.gov/violenceprevention/acestudy/

American Academy of Pediatrics, Public Health Approach to Toxic Stress: http://www.aap.org/en-us/advocacy-and-policy/aap-health-initiatives/EBCD/Pages/Public-Health-Approach.aspx

California Newsreel Documentary Series, *Unnatural Causes*: http://www.unnaturalcauses.org/

Center for Disease Control and Prevention, National Center for Birth Defects and Developmental Disabilities: http://www.cdc.gov/ncbddd/disabilityandhealth/

Harvard University, Center for the Developing Child: http://developingchild.harvard.edu/

National Alliance to End Homelessness, Housing First: www.endhomelessness.org

Robert Wood Johnson Foundation, Commission to Build a Healthier America: http://www.commissiononhealth.org/

REFERENCES

Adler, N., & Newman, K. (2002). Socioeconomic disparities in health: Pathways and policies. *Health Affairs, 21*(2), 60–76.

Adler, N., & Stewart J. (2010a). Health disparities across the lifespan: Meaning, methods and mechanisms. The biology of disadvantage: Socioeconomic status and health. *Annals of the New York Academy of Science, 1186,* 5–23.

Adler, N., & Stewart J. (2010b). Preface to the biology of disadvantage: Socioeconomic status and health. *Annals of the New York Academy of Science, 1186,* 1–4.

Altman, B., & Bernstein, A. (2008). *Disability and health in the United States, 2001–2005*. Hyattsville, MD: National Center for Health Statistics.

American Academy of Pediatrics (AAP). (2012). Early childhood adversity, toxic stress, and the role of the pediatrician: Translating developmental science into lifelong health. *Pediatrics, 129*(1), e224–e231.

Anda, R., Tietjen, G., Schulman, E., Felitti, V. J., & Croft, J. (2010). Adverse childhood experiences and frequent headaches in adults. *Headache, 50*(9), 1473–1481.

Arkin, E., DeForge, D., & Rosen, A. M. (2009). *Breaking through on the social determinants of health and health disparities: An approach to message translation*. Commission to Build a Healthier America, Robert Wood Johnson Foundation. Retrieved from http://www.commissiononhealth.org

Basu, A., Kee, R., Buchanan, D., & Sadowski, L. (2011). Comparative cost analysis of housing and case management program for chronically ill homeless adults compared to usual care. *Health Services Research, 47*(1), 523–543.

Berkman, L. F. (2009). Social epidemiology: Social determinants of health in the United States; Are we losing ground? *Annual Review of Public Health, 30,* 27–41.

Brault, M. (2012). Americans with disabilities, 2010. In *Current Population Reports* (pp. 70–131). Washington, DC: U.S. Department of Commerce, Census Bureau.

Braveman, P., Egerter, S., & Williams, D. R. (2011). The social determinants of health: Coming of age. *Annual Review of Public Health, 32,* 381–398.

Braveman, P., & Gruskin, S. (2003). Defining equity in health. *Journal of Epidemiology & Community Health, 57,* 254–258.

Braveman, P., Sadegh-Nobari, T., & Egerter, S. (2011). *Early childhood experiences: Laying the foundation for health across a lifetime.* Robert Wood Johnson Foundation. Retrieved from http://www.rwjf.org

Brondolo, E., Hausmann, L. R., Jhalani, J., Pencille, M., Atencio-Bacayon, J., Kumar, A., ... Schwartz, J. (2011). Dimensions of perceived racism and self-reported health: Examination of racial/ethnic differences and potential mediators. *Annals of Behavioral Medicine, 42*(1), 14–28.

Carter-Pokras, O., & Baquet, C. (2002). What is a "health disparity"? *Public Health Reports, 117,* 426–434.

Caruso, C. C., Hitchcock, E. M., Dick, R. B., Russo, J. M., & Schmidt, J. M. (2004). *Overtime and extended work shifts: Recent findings on illness, injuries and health behaviors.* Cincinnati, OH: National Institute for Occupational Safety and Health, Centers for Disease Control and Prevention, U.S. Department of Health and Human Services.

Centers for Disease Control and Prevention (CDC). (2010). Adverse childhood experiences reported by adults: Five states, 2009. *Morbidity and Mortality Weekly, 59*(49), 1609–1613.

Centers for Disease Control and Prevention (CDC). (2013). CDC grand rounds: Public health practices to include persons with disabilities. *Morbidity and Mortality Weekly, 62*(34), 697–701.

Centers for Disease Control and Prevention (CDC). (2014). Vital signs: Disability and physical activity – United States, 2009–2012. *Morbidity and Mortality Weekly, 63*(18), 407–414.

Clougherty, J. E., Souza, K., & Cullen, M. R. (2010). Work and its role in shaping the social gradient in health: The biology of disadvantage; Socioeconomic status and health. *Annals of the New York Academy of Science, 1186,* 102–124.

Cohen, S., Deverts-Janicki, D., Chen E., & Matthews, K. A. (2010). Childhood socioeconomic status and adult health: The biology of disadvantage. *Annals of the New York Academy of Science, 1186,* 37–55.

Corso, P. S., Edwards, V. J., Fang X., & Mercy, J. A. (2008). Health-related quality of life among adults who experienced maltreatment during childhood. *American Journal of Public Health 98*(6), 1094–1100.

De Vogli, R., Ferrie, J., Chandola, T., Kivimäki, M., & Marmot, M. G. (2007). Unfairness and health: Evidence from the Whitehall II study. *Journal of Epidemiology and Community Health, 61*(6), 513–518.

Docteur, E., & Berenson, R. A. (June 2014). *In pursuit of health equity: Comparing U.S. and EU approaches to eliminating disparities.* Robert Wood Johnson Foundation and the Urban Institute. Retrieved from http://www.rwjf.org

Drum, C., McClain, M. R., Horner-Johnson, W., & Taitano, G (2011). Health disparities chart book on disability and racial and ethnic status in the United States. Durham, NH: Institute on Disability, University of New Hampshire.

Dube, S. R., Anda, R. F., Felitti, V. J., Edwards, V. J., & Croft, J. B. (2002). Adverse childhood experiences and personal alcohol abuse as a child. *Addictive Behavior, 27*(5), 713–725.

Dube, S. R., Fairweather, D., Pearson, W. S., Felitti, V. J., Anda, R. F., & Croft, J. B. (2009). Cumulative childhood stress and autoimmune diseases in adults. *Psychosomatic Medicine, 71*(2), 235–250.

Egerter, S., Braveman, P., & Barclay, C. (2011). *How social factors influence health: The role of stress.* Robert Wood Johnson Foundation. Retrieved from http://www.rwjf.org

Federal Interagency Forum on Child and Family Statistics. (2013). *America's children: Key national indicators of well-being, 2013.* Retrieved from http://childstats.gov

Felitti, V. J., Anda, R. F., Nordenberg, D., Williamson, D. F., Spitz, A. M., Edwards, V., ... Marks, J. S. (1998). Relationship of childhood abuse and household dysfunction to many of the leading causes of death in adults: The Adverse Childhood Experiences (ACE) Study. *American Journal of Preventive Medicine, 14*(4), 245–258.

Fitzpatrick-Lewis, D., Ganann, R., Krishnaratne, S., Ciliska, D., Kouyoumdjian F., & Hwang, S. W. (2011). Effectiveness of interventions to improve the health and housing status of homeless people: A rapid systematic review. *BMC Public Health, 11*(638), 1–14.

Frank, L. D., Andresen, M. A., & Schmid, T. L. (2004). Obesity relationships with community design, physical activity, and time spent in cars. *American Journal of Preventive Medicine, 27,* 87–96.

Gambone, M. A., Klem, A. M., Summer, J. A., Akey, T. M., & Sipe, C. L. (2004). *Turning the tide: The achievements of the First Things First education reform in the Kansas City, Kansas Public School District.* Youth Development Strategies, Inc. Retrieved from http://www.iree.org

Grosch, J. W., & Sauter, S. L. (2005). Psychologic stressors and work organization. In L. Rosenstock, M. MCullen, C. Brodkin, & C. Redlich (Eds.), *Textbook of clinical occupational and environmental medicine* (2nd ed., pp. 931–942). Philadelphia: Elsevier Saunders.

Herd, P., Goesling, B., & House, J. S. (2007). Socioeconomic position and health: The differential effects of education versus income on the onset versus progression of health problems. *Journal of Health Behavior and Social Behavior, 48,* 223–238.

Institute of Medicine (IOM). (2014). Applying a health lens to decision making in non-health sectors: Workshop summary. Washington, DC: National Academies Press.

Krieger, N. (2001). A glossary for social epidemiology. *Journal of Epidemiology & Community Health, 55,* 693–700.

Larson, N. I., Story, M. T., & Nelson, M. C. (2009). Neighborhood environments: Disparities in access to healthy food in the U.S. *American Journal of Preventive Medicine, 36*(1), 74–81.

LaVeist, T., Pollack, K., Thorpe, R., Fesahazion, R., & Gaskin, D. (2011). Place, not race: Disparities dissipate in southwest Baltimore when blacks and whites live under similar conditions. *Health Affairs, 30*(10), 1880–1887.

Lu, M. C., Kotelchuck, M., Hogan, V., Jones, L., Wright, K., & Halfon, N. (2010). Closing the black-white gap in birth outcomes: A life-course approach. *Ethnicity & Disease, 20*(Supple 2), 62–76.

Marmot, M. G., Rose, G., Shipley, M., & Hamilton, P. J. (1978). Employment grade and coronary heart disease in British civil servants. *Journal of Epidemiology and Community Health, 32*(4), 244–249.

Marmot, M. G., Stansfeld, S., Patel, C., North, F., Head, J., White I., ... Davey Smith, G. (1991). Health inequalities among British civil servants: The Whitehall II study. *Lancet, 337*(8754), 1387–1393.

McCann, B. (2005). *Designing for active recreation: A research summary* (Updated). Active Living Research, Robert Wood Johnson Foundation. Retrieved from www.activelivingresearch.org

McEwen, B. S., & Gianaros, P. J. (2010). Central role of brain in stress and adaptation: Links to socioeconomic status, health and disease. The biology of disadvantage: Socioeconomic status and health. *Annals of the New York Academy of Science, 1186,* 190–222.

National Alliance to End Homelessness. (2009). *Organizational change: Adopting a Housing First approach.* National Alliance to End Homelessness. Retrieved from http://www.endhomelessness.org/

National Center for Health Statistics (NCHS). (2013). *Health: United States, 2011 (with a special feature on socioeconomic status and health).* Hyattsville, MD: U.S. Department of Health and Human Services, Centers for Disease Control and Prevention.

National Center for *Health Statistics (NCHS). (2014). Health: United States, 2013 (with a special feature on prescription drug use).* Hyattsville, MD: U.S. Department of Health and Human Services, Centers for Disease Control and Prevention.

National Scientific Council on the Developing Child. (2014). *Excessive stress disrupts the architecture of the developing brain* (Working paper 3) (updated edition). Retrieved from http://www.developingchild.harvard.edu.

Patterson, M. L., Moniruzzaman, A., & Somers, J. M. (2014). Setting the stage for chronic health problems: Cumulative childhood adversity among homeless adults with mental illness in Vancouver, British Columbia. *BMC Public Health, 14*(1), 350–360.

Patterson, M .L., Rezansoff, S., Currie, L., & Somers, J. M. (2013). Trajectories of recovery among homeless adults with mental illness who participated in a randomized controlled trial of Housing First: A longitudinal, narrative analysis. *British Medical Journal (BMJ) Open, 10*(3), 1–8.

Robert Wood Johnson Foundation (RWJF). (2008). *Overcoming obstacles to health: Stories, facts and findings.* Retrieved from http://www.commissiononhealth.org

Robert Wood Johnson Foundation (RWJF). (2013). *Overcoming obstacles to Health in 2013 and beyond: Recommendations from the Robert Wood Johnson Foundation and the Commission to Build a Healthier America.* Retrieved from http://www.rwjf.org/commission.

Robert Wood Johnson Foundation, Commission to Build a Healthier America. (2009). *Beyond health care: New directions to a healthier America.* Retrieved from http://www.commissiononhealth.org/

Sadowski, L., Kee, R., VanderWeele, T., & Buchanan, D. (2009) Effect of a housing and case management program on emergency department visits and hospitalizations among chronically ill homeless adults: A randomized trial. *Journal of the American Medical Association, 301*(17), 1771–1778.

Salpolsky, R. M. (1998). *Why zebras don't get ulcers* (2nd ed.). New York: Freeman and Company.

Singh, G. K. (2010). *Child mortality in the United States, 1935–2007: Large racial and socioeconomic disparities have persisted over time.* Rockville, MD: U.S. Department of Health and Human Services, Health Resources and Services Administration, Maternal and Child Health Bureau.

Southern Education Foundation. (2008). *High school dropouts: Alabama's number one education and economic problem.* Retrieved from http://www.southerneducation.org

Thoits, P. A. (2010). Stress and health: Major findings and policy implications. *Journal of Health and Social Behavior, 51*(Supple 1), S41–S53.

Trust for America's Health. (2013). F as in fat: How obesity threatens America's future, 2013. Washington, DC: Robert Wood Johnson Foundation.

U.S. Department of Commerce, U.S. Census Bureau. (2012). *Median income of households by state: Two-year moving averages, 1984–2011.* Retrieved from http://www.census.gov/hhes/www/income/data/statemedian/

U.S. Department of Health and Human Services (USDHHS). (n.d.). *Healthy people 2020.* Retrieved from http://www.healthypeople.gov

U.S. Department of Health and Human Services (USDHHS). (2005). *The surgeon general's call to action to improve the health and wellness of persons with disabilities.* Washington, DC: U.S. Department of Health and Human Services, Office of the Surgeon General.

U.S. Department of Health and Human Services (USDHHS). (May 2014). *Healthy people 2020 leading health indicators: Social determinants.* Retrieved from http://www.healthypeople.gov

U.S. Department of Health and Human Services (USDHHS), Centers for Disease Control and Prevention (CDC), National Institute for Occupational Safety and Health (NIOSH). (2002). *The changing organization of work and the safety and health of working people.* Retrieved from http://www.cdc.gov/niosh/

U.S. Department of Health and Human Services (USDHHS), National Prevention Council (2011). *National prevention strategy.* Washington, DC: U.S. Department of Health and Human Services, Office of the Surgeon General.

U.S. Department of Labor, Bureau of Labor Statistics. (2013a). *A profile of the working poor, 2011* (Report 1035). U.S. Department of Labor. Retrieved from http://www.bls.gov/iif/

U.S. Department of Labor, Bureau of Labor Statistics. (March 2013b). *Census of fatal occupational injuries, 2012.* U.S. Department of Labor. Retrieved from http://www.bls.gov/iif/

U.S. Department of Labor, Bureau of Labor Statistics. (November 2013c). *Nonfatal occupational injuries and illnesses requiring days away from work, 2012.* U.S. Department of Labor. Retrieved from http://www.bls.gov/iif/

U.S. Department of Labor, Bureau of Labor Statistics. (March 2014). *Employment projections: Earnings and unemployment rates by educational attainment, 2013.* U.S. Department of Labor. Retrieved from http://www.bls.gov/EMP

Wilkinson, R., & Marmot, M. (2003). *Social determinants of health: The solid facts* (2nd ed.). Copenhagen, Denmark: World Health Organization.

Woolf, S., & Braveman, P. (2011). Where health disparities begin: The role of social and economic determinants, and why current policies make it worse. *Health Affairs, 30*(10), 1852–1859.

World Health Organization. (2008). *Closing the gap in a generation: Health equity through action on the social determinants of health.* Geneva, Switzerland: Commission on Social Determinants of Health. WHO Press. Retrieved from http://www.who.int/social_determinants/en

World Health Organization and World Bank. (2011). *World report on disability.* Geneva, Switzerland: WHO Press. Retrieved from http://www.who.int

Zaltman, G., & Zaltman, L. (2008). *Marketing metaphoria: What deep metaphors reveal about the minds of consumers.* Boston: Harvard Business School Press.

Health Behavior Theory

CHAPTER 4

Social Ecological Models and Health Behavior Theory

KEY TERMS

built environment	construct	intrapersonal	theory
community	model	system	variable
concept	interpersonal		

LEARNING OBJECTIVES

1. Describe the role of health behavior theory in understanding health behaviors.
2. Identify components of health behavior theories.
3. Identify multiple levels of influence within a social ecological model.
4. Assess factors of influence for personal health behaviors.
5. Assess attributes of place-based factors that influence health behavior.
6. Explain why social ecological models are used mainly as a long-term view of health promotion planning and are not often seen in short-term planning.

IN THE NEWS ...

In September 2012, the New York City Board of Health approved a ban on the sale of large sugar-sweetened beverages in select restaurant, retail, and entertainment venues. In March 2013, soda, sweetened tea and juice-flavored drinks larger than 16 ounces would not be allowed for sale within the city limits. Per the law, sugary beverages are those that contain more than 25 calories per 8 ounces and are less than 50 percent milk. Convenience store and grocery store sales were not included in the ban. Mayor Michael R. Bloomberg, with the support of the Board of Health, cited the high rates of diabetes, obesity, and other weight-related chronic diseases as a motivation for the measure. Over the next few months, the *New York Times* reported on support both for and against the measure. On March 11, 2013, one day before the ban was to take effect, the supreme court in Manhattan blocked the city ban on large sugary beverages. Judge

Milton A. Tingling called the limits "arbitrary and capricious." The city appealed the ruling; however, in July 2013, the First Department of the New York Supreme Court's Appellate Division upheld the lower court ruling, saying the ban "violated the state principle of separation of powers." Sugar-sweetened beverages won again. Mayor Michael R. Bloomberg, the ban's number one champion, retired from public office on December 31, 2013.

Introduction

In general, people must be motivated to act, must be able to act, and are cued and reinforced to act. The broad category of factors related to motivation are called predisposing factors and commonly include knowledge, beliefs, and demographic factors. Enabling factors include skills and resources. Cues nudge and encourage, whereas reinforcements are the outcomes after the behavior that influence future acts of the behavior.

Health behavior theory is useful for filling in the gaps and providing details within these broad categories. Health behavior theory can give insight into what type of beliefs predispose people to be ready to act. Health behavior theories also highlight the relationships, and sometimes sequences, of these behavioral mediators. The importance of health behavior theory in forming general understandings about health behaviors will be discussed in this chapter. It is through an understanding of the factors that influence behaviors that more effective interventions can be designed and implemented. The factors that influence motivation, ability, and reminders exert influence through multiple levels of a person's environment. The social ecological model is useful for understanding the multilevel layers of influence on a person's behavior.

Health Behavior Theory

Theories can help us understand the nature of health behaviors. They explain the factors that facilitate the behavior, but they also describe conditions under which the behavior is more or less likely to occur, hypothesize relationships among the factors and conditions, and can suggest processes for changing the behavior (Glanz & Bishop, 2010). Theoretical constructs explain and add details to general categories of factors. What types of knowledge or beliefs influence behavior? What resources are necessary to act? What kind of cues to act can encourage action, and are there times in the process of the behavior that certain factors are more influential?

All of these questions are answered through health behavior theory.

For example, self-efficacy is a widely addressed target of health promotion interventions. Self-efficacy is a belief, specifically one's confidence in successfully performing an action, and is a construct of the social cognitive theory. Self-efficacy is a strong predictor of numerous health behaviors (Bauman et al., 2012; Shaikh et al., 2008). Dr. Albert Bandura developed the theory, and through his initial work that was later confirmed through the work of others, health behaviorists have learned about a specific type of belief that is associated with health behavior execution (Bandura, 1977, 1986). From the social cognitive theory, it has also become known that one's confidence can be influenced by or have a relationship with external factors, namely observing the behaviors of others and the reinforcements given after the behaviors. Chapter 6 will discuss the social cognitive theory, along with self-efficacy and the related constructs, in detail.

A true understanding and appreciation of behavioral theory should improve one's health care–related practice. The utility of health behavior theory lies in its ability to explain, in great detail, possible factors that can influence behaviors. For instance, if self-efficacy improves behavioral action, then interventions should build self-efficacy. If trigger management skills aid in managing urges felt during the process of smoking cessation, then interventions should build trigger management skills. These factors then become the target for multilevel interventions.

Terminology

A **theory** is a set of interrelated concepts, definitions, and propositions that explain or predict events or situations by specifying relations among variables (Glanz & Bishop, 2010). The individual factors identified within health behavior theories vary, but different theories contain similar components. The components work together to collectively describe and organize the pieces within the theory. Three important components of health behavior theories are concepts, constructs, and, variables:

- *Concept.* Concepts are building blocks, the primary elements of a theory (NCI, 2005).

- *Construct.* The key concepts of a particular theory are its constructs. Constructs are given specific names within a theory, and thus, similar concepts can be named differently in different theories (NCI, 2005).

- *Variable.* Variables are constructs defined in a particular content area. They are the operational forms of constructs (NCI, 2005).

Constructs are the theory-specific elements of a health behavior theory. They are the individual factors that have hypothesized relationships with other factors. Constructs of the health belief model (see Chapter 5) include perceived susceptibility, perceived severity, perceived threat, perceived benefits and perceived barriers, and cues to act. Collectively, the constructs and relationships work to explain and predict the phenomenon of health behavior. **Concepts** are broader categories that can contain multiple specific constructs. For example, stages of change is a concept, and individual stages such as contemplation, action, and maintenance are included in the concept. Not all theories include broad concepts, but all theory includes constructs.

Finally, **variables** are the content-specific version of a construct. A construct is content neutral, and *variables are the working version of the construct.* When researchers explore or practitioners apply a construct to real-world situations, it is within a content area such as physical activity, preventive cancer screenings, or medication compliance. In a content area, the construct may be given a more specific term. For example, the construct of self-regulation (from social cognitive theory) becomes, in practice, goal setting and keeping a food journal.

Theory Properties and Practice

Like medicine, public health practice and health promotion initiatives are most efficacious when they are anchored in evidence-based practices. The process of building a body of evidence works through a cycle of observation, theory, and research (Brownson et al., 2009). For that reason, the importance of health behavior theory to improving practice cannot be overstated. Theory provides an initial framework for organizing thoughts about observed events. The beginning of theory development is triggered by an observation of a phenomenon. Researchers then make inferences about their patterns of observations to create a generalized theory of explanation. Without a theory of how smaller pieces fit together, those pieces of information often remain independent facts that may not be very useful to practitioners. With evidence of effectiveness and dissemination, some concepts that began as theoretical ideas are eventually adopted into general knowledge and practice. See the Behavioral Science in Action feature in Chapter 5 on the development of the health belief model as an example of how observations of health behaviors developed into one of the most widely referenced health behavior theories.

On a practitioner level, understanding concepts within health behavior theory alters the manner in which individuals think and behave in relation to planning health promotion programs. The deep factual knowledge within the various theories provides an organizing framework, or structure, that is synthesized and built upon. Through theory, planners also start to understand and hypothesize about relationships between behavioral factors and see opportunities for aligning interventions with antecedents.

Initially, the abstract nature of theories can be challenging. Health behavior theories are not organized around content areas; rather, they are often organized around levels of influence. Levels of influence beyond the self are other people, places, and societal systems. Dr. Karen Glanz, a leading scholar and author of works about health behavior theory, has described health behavior theory as a coffee cup. The cup provides valuable structure and form, but it starts out empty. Filling the coffee cup is what happens within content areas and through work with specific audiences (Glanz & Bishop, 2010; NCI, 2005). The abstraction can initially be difficult for new students of theory, but after mastering the concepts, the generalization becomes part of the usefulness of health behavior theory. Health behavior theories cut across population health disciplines and can serve as a framework in emerging areas of public health. For instance, as new target behaviors emerge, such as emergency preparedness or curtailing distracted driving, the core concepts of behavioral theory and the hypothesized relationships between behavioral factors serve as a method to organize initial observations, research, and practice.

Over time, concepts, constructs, and relationships that were once just theoretical postulates become ingrained in the general knowledge and practice of public health, health promotion, and medicine. Concepts that began as a theoretical idea and were validated through evaluation and research can become known as facts about behavior. Numerous examples of theoretical concepts are now widely accepted as generalized knowledge in health promotion practice. For example, most, if not all, individuals working in health promotion believe that behaviors develop and change through a gradual process. The process occurs over time and through a series of actions. Prochaska and DiClemente (1983) introduced this concept, called stages of change, as a theoretical conceptualization within the transtheoretical model. Prior to their theory, introduced in the early 1980s, behavior change was approached as an act that operates much like a light switch. With a single action, or flip of the switch, someone changes the status of a behavior. "I'm a smoker—flip—I'm a non-smoker." As will be discussed in Chapter 5, smokers often think about changing the behavior, may collect information for decision making, and enter trial periods of change, all before the act of giving up cigarettes. Based on this change in understanding of behavior change, evidence-based smoking cessation counseling is universally based upon a process of change (USPSTF, 2009).

Another example of health behavior constructs becoming ingrained into evidence-based practice comes from social cognitive theory. Self-regulation is a person's ability to set goals, track progress, and solve problems; it originated from social cognitive theory (Bandura, 1986). The shaping of self-regulation skills is a widely recommended and evidence-supported practice (Community Preventive Services Task Force, 2012). Furthermore, some practice guidelines within medicine—specifically guidelines for lifestyle management of obesity, hypertension, diabetes, and asthma—include recommendations for patients to set goals, keep records, and solve problems (self-regulation) (Lin et al., 2010; USDHHS & NHLBI, 1998; USDHHS & NHLBI, 2004; USDHHS & NHLBI, 2007). Risk perceptions, self-efficacy, and intention are other widely accepted intrapersonal constructs that have become generalized behavioral knowledge. All three constructs are specific individual beliefs from the health belief model, social cognitive theory, and theory of planned behavior, respectively, and will be discussed in Chapters 5 and 6.

Check for Understanding   List benefits of health behavior theory. Why might professionals not use theory to guide health promotion interventions?

Social Ecological Model

The social ecological model was introduced to health promotion practitioners two decades ago and is now a widely recommended framework for health behavior understanding and multilevel interventions of change. The Institute of Medicine, Public Health Foundation, Robert Wood Johnson Foundation, and Centers for Disease Control and Prevention have statements of support and significant works organized around the concept of the social ecological model (IOM, 2000; USDHHS, n.d.; Sallis et al., 2006; Warner, 2006). Social ecological models do not include specific constructs or relationships. **Models** are frameworks of larger concepts and often include information from across theories. In public health and health promotion, the social ecological model represents a picture of the individual and his or her relationship with surrounding multilevel factors. For this reason, the model is often represented as a series of spheres centered around the individual, where the rings represent the various levels of influence (see Figure 4-1). Specific variables can be identified within the various levels of the environment.

The basic idea represented in the pictorial model is that behaviors both shape and are shaped by the social and physical environment (Glanz & Bishop, 2010; McLeroy et al., 1988). People's actions create environments, *and* creating environments conducive to change in turn facilitates the adoption and maintenance of healthy behaviors. The model also depicts the various layers of environmental influence around individuals from a combination of people, places, and policies.

The levels of the environments represented around the individual are commonly labeled intrapersonal, interpersonal, community, organizations, and policy/systems (McLeroy et al., 1988). Because the framework is intentionally broad, the rings get personalized within content areas. The specific levels can be labeled in descriptive terms that represent the types of antecedents on that level of influence. The content-specific labels are more useful for sorting information and communicating to others. The following sections will define

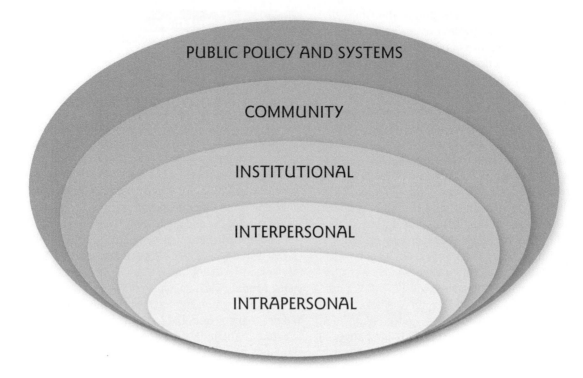

Figure 4-1 Social Ecological Model

the traditional labels of an ecological model and then give examples of more personalized versions.

Levels of Influence

The inner spheres of social ecological models are really about the individual and his or her relationships and interactions with others. The models have the individual at the innermost core, with one's closest interactions immediately surrounding the individual. The outer levels of ecological models represent community and societal systems in which a person operates and lives. The system levels are shown as distal from the person, often two levels removed from the individual. The factors represented in the outer rings are larger concepts such as neighborhood characteristics, systems within one's work and community organizations, and government policies.

The traditional definitions of the five levels of influence that were introduced by McLeroy and colleagues in 1988 and that are still in use today are:

1. *Intrapersonal factors.* Characteristics of the individual, such as knowledge, attitudes, behavior, self-concept, and skills, as well as socio-demographic factors and previous life experiences.

2. *Interpersonal processes and primary groups.* Formal and informal social networks and social support systems, including family, co-workers, and peer and friendship networks.

3. *Institutional factors.* Social institutions with organizational characteristics and formal and informal rules and regulations for operation. Institutions include schools, places of employment, places of worship, and civic groups.

4. *Community factors.* Communities are the groups (informal networks) to which individuals belong and the relationships among organizations and institutions.

5. *Policy.* Local, state, and national laws and policies that create built and social environments and systems related to the model's topic.

People

People are the common element of the innermost spheres of social ecological models. For all models, the individual is at the core, in the **intrapersonal** level. Health behaviors are influenced by a wide variety of factors, and a way to understand these factors is to examine their level of influence on the person. Characteristics of a person that may influence behavioral action include knowledge, beliefs, skills, demographic factors, and prior experiences (see Table 4-1).

The next level of influence, the interpersonal level, reflects the individual's social relationships. Individuals are connected to family, friends, peers, co-workers, and neighbors. Relationships are important sources of many behavior cues, resources, and reinforcements. Relationships, both formal and informal, provide emotional support, physical and financial resources, information, and opportunities to connect with others. Norms about acceptable behavior are also communicated, implied, and modeled through relationships. Properties of the networks that are reflected in the forthcoming examples can be size, structure, membership, and communication patterns. These two levels, intrapersonal and interpersonal, have collectively been called the attributes of people (Maibach, Abroms, & Marosits, 2007).

Places and Systems

After social networks, most social ecological models reflect settings that influence the behavior. Place-based influences come from the places individuals and networks move through in their lives: neighborhoods, work/school, health care, civic and community groups, and some of the resources in those settings (e.g., transportation). The physical properties of those settings are often reflected in models; however, these environments' products and services, rules, practices, and cultural messages also influence actions.

The systems level, sometimes also called the policy level, is the outermost level of influence in ecological models. **System** factors create large contexts of services, funding, physical environments, information, laws, and regulations that influence member practices (see Table 4-1). Service systems, such as education, social services, and transportation, consist of numerous elements that operate in a connected fashion to meet a function or purpose (IOM, 2013). The control of system-type factors tends to be somewhat distant from the individual and networks, but the influence is important to the actions of people in their daily places. For example, access to healthy food products comes from neighborhood grocery stores and farmers markets, whereas on a larger scale,

TABLE 4-1 Attributes by Levels of Influence

Person	Social Network	Places[a]	Systems
Knowledge	Family structures	Neighborhood	Physical structures
Beliefs	Peer and friendship relationships	Worksite and School	Funding systems
Abilities	Social support and resources	Health care resources and providers	Service systems
Demographics	Information and contacts	Civic and other community groups	Messages
Biology	Norms	Retail markets	Policy
Previous experiences		Places of worship	Laws
		Transportation	

a) In McLeroy and colleagues' original (1988) definitions, the places level reflects institutional and community factors.

system factors that influence access to products may be state or federal policies for retail incentives, farming subsidies, and Supplemental Nutrition Assistance Program (SNAP) policies. The policies, structures, and services of the outer ring radiate through and create many of the contexts described in institutions, communities, and networks. Chapter 7 will talk more about system frameworks and their influence on health behavior.

Preventive Cancer Screenings

Multilevel factors related to participation in preventive cancer screenings can be communicated in a social ecological model. The Colorectal Cancer Control Program funded by the Centers for Disease Control and Prevention uses an ecological model to communicate information about mediating factors and encourage communities to plan multilevel programs (USDHHS & CDC, n.d.b.). Intrapersonal factors related to intention and actual screening participation include a person's knowledge about the need for screening, screening options, how to access a screening, and beliefs (e.g., fear of the test). Demographic and personal history factors such as age, gender, and health history are other potential factors. Interactions with others and norms established with friends, family, health care providers, community health workers, and patient navigators represent potential sources of interpersonal messages and support. Provider prompts and encouragements are examples of evidence-based strategies implemented on this environmental level (Community Preventive Services Task Force, 2012).

Organizational systems that may influence screening participation include factors within health care, worksites, health care plans, local health departments, tribal and urban health clinics, and professional organizations. Specific factors operating on the organizational level can include on-site resources, physician access, and employer time-off practices. Community-level factors include community readiness, agency cooperation, and trust. These factors can be impacted by the work of comprehensive cancer control coalitions, tribal health departments, media, and community advocacy groups. The outermost level of the colorectal cancer prevention model is that of policy. The most notable and recent policy related to preventive cancer screenings is the inclusion of such screenings in all health insurance plans that is mandated by the Affordable Care Act. Not only are mammography, cervical cancer screenings, and colorectal cancer screenings now universally covered, since 2011, there has been no insurance co-pay for these preventive cancer screenings, which has created much greater access (USDHHS, n.d..)

Content-Specific Models

The traditional labels on the levels of influence within the social ecological model reflect groupings of factors that may impact health behavior. The groupings have similar qualities, as described earlier in this chapter. Within a content area or health behavior, sometimes a social, physical, or system environment can be more accurately described in different terms. A descriptive label can help individuals sort and understand the type of factors that operate on that level of the environment. The descriptive label can be derived by the type of antecedents reflected on that level of the environment, or the label can be influenced by the behavioral focus of the model.

A good descriptive label captures the unifying quality of most of the factors represented on that level of influence. Descriptors can reflect the types of social networks (relationships), types of antecedents (perceptions), a setting (health care), and/or types of systems (local food system). As with all theoretical concepts, not all individual factors may align perfectly within the concept's descriptive label. In the following violence prevention and physical activity examples, the descriptive labels attached to the levels of influence have been changed to clarify the types of factors on a particular level of influence.

Violence Prevention

The Centers for Disease Control and Prevention has adopted a four-level social ecological model to understand violence and guide prevention activities. The environment levels of influence have been renamed to more accurately describe the broad types of antecedents operating on levels of the environment. The four levels in this model are individual, relationship, community, and society (Dahlberg & Krug, 2002; WHO, 2002). Biological and personal history factors that increase the likelihood of becoming a victim or perpetrator of violence make up the first level. These factors include age, education, income, and substance use or a history of abuse. Substance abuse and a history of abuse increase the likelihood of most types of violence, especially intimate partner violence, suicide, gang violence, child abuse, and elder abuse (Chiu et al., 2013; Krug et al., 2002a; Rutherford, 2008; Stöckl et al., 2013). For example, in a recent study in Boston, children who experienced a single type of childhood abuse (physical, sexual, or emotional) were five times more likely to report abuse as adults. The magnitude of the relationship was even higher for women; adult women who experienced a single type of abuse in childhood were seven times more likely to report abuse in adulthood (Chiu et al., 2013). Early life experiences create powerful trajectories into adult relationships.

The second level represents one's close relationships, often with peers, partners, and family members. Most acts of violence occur within established relationships (Rutherford, 2008; Stöckl et al., 2013; WHO, 2002). The properties of an individual's relationships make violence more or less likely (Figure 4-2). Relationship attributes—such as family structure, levels of conflict, communication styles, level of supervision, and emotional support—may influence the risk of experiencing violence as a victim or being a perpetrator of violence (Krug et al., 2002b; Rutherford, 2008; WHO, 2002). For example, having friends that encourage violence increases a young person's risk of being a victim or perpetrator (Espelage & De La Rue, 2011; WHO, 2002). However, positive social networks and neighborhood connections have been reported as attributes that protect children and young people from violence (WHO, 2002). For intimate partner violence, the most consistent relationship marker for violence is the level of conflict and disagreement within the relationship (Krug et al., 2002b; WHO, 2002). Conflict over money, child care, domestic roles, infidelity, sex, and "obeying" are common triggers for acts of partner violence (WHO, 2002). Similarly, strained family relationships and relationships in which an elderly person is dependent on family for support increase the likelihood

of elder abuse (WHO, 2002). Certainly, conflict is part of both healthy and unhealthy relationships, but communication skills, networks of support, and resources can help reduce the likelihood of violence and abuse.

Communities, the third level of the environment, are the places where relationships occur, including home, school, and work. The structures, resources, and practices of the places people frequent can create or encourage protective or risky environments. One of the most consistent community-level factors associated with abuse is poverty (Chiu et al., 2013; Krug et al., 2002b; Rutherford, 2008; WHO, 2002). Income levels of a neighborhood influence a community's structures and resources, for example, resident occupancy and transient rate, resident connectedness, and recreational opportunities. The general income level can also impact the physical layout of the neighborhood, such as sidewalks, lighting, and green space. Organizational practices are also important community-level attributes that can discourage violence. School and workplace policies on bullying, supervision, and equal opportunities tend to create cooperative and peaceable climates and limit opportunities for violence.

On the fourth level, societal factors can create levels of acceptance of violence. Social norms toward women, children, minorities, and other groups can create a context in which violence is more likely (Rutherford, 2008; USDHHS & CDC, n.d.a; WHO, 2002). Specific norms related to rigid gender roles, access to education, economic equality, and sexuality can create climates that make abuse toward others more acceptable and therefore more likely to occur. Other societal factors include policies on and the availability of firearms, home visitation in early childhood, and housing policies. Collectively, individual traits along with attributes of relationships, community, and the formal and informal codes of conduct work synergistically to decrease or increase the risk for being involved in an act of violence.

Physical Activity

Physical activity, specifically activity through recreation; transportation (walking and biking); and occupation have been studied extensively using the levels of the social ecological model. Based on their work and the contributions of others, Sallis and colleagues (2006) developed a model of people and systems that influence physical activity in the following manner: individual, environmental perceptions, built environment,

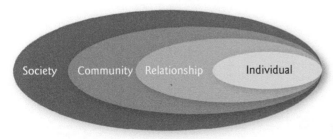

Figure 4-2 CDC Violence Prevention Model
Source: Centers for Disease Control and Prevention

and activity policy and systems. Intrapersonal factors include demographics, beliefs (most notably self-efficacy), and situational intentions (see Figure 4-3).

A unique level in the physical activity model is a person's perceptions (beliefs) of his or her environment. How one perceives the properties of his or her environment may differ from the objectively measured walking environment assessed by researchers and therefore has its own level of influence. Perceptions of safety, attractiveness, comfort, convenience, and accessibility have consistent relationships to the likelihood of someone walking for transport or enjoyment (Carlson et al., 2012; Owen et al.,

2004; Saelens et al., 2012). Attractiveness and perceived comfort are reliable correlates for adult walking behaviors, whereas parents' beliefs about neighborhood safety, traffic safety, and distance have a relationship with children walking to and from school (Davison, Werder, & Lawson, 2008).

The actual functional and aesthetic qualities of one's environment, called the **built environment**, represent the third level of the model. This level of community is commonly referred to as built environment because of the types of factors included in the category. Human-made properties of neighborhoods, schools, workplaces, retail spaces,

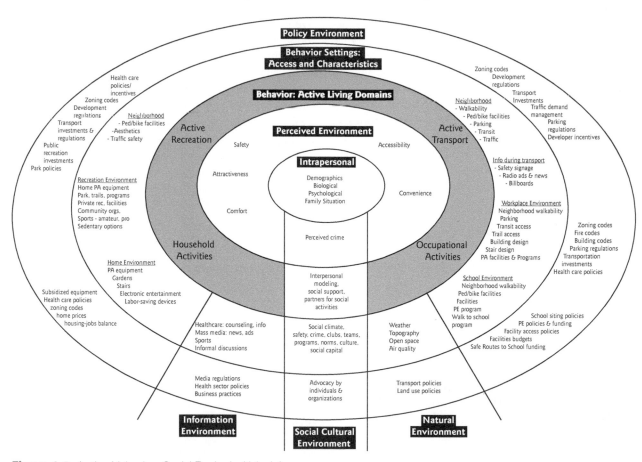

Figure 4-3 Active Living in a Social Ecological Model
Source: Reproduced with permission of Annual Reviews

and public places can significantly influence activity levels. Sidewalks, crosswalks, mixed land use, recreation facilities, accessible stairways, and comfort qualities—including shade, art, green space, and landscaping—improve rates of walking. Conversely, high traffic speed, high traffic density, property vacancies, and crime all lower rates of walking and active recreation (Bauman et al., 2012; Ding et al., 2011; Sallis et al., 2006; Sallis & Glanz, 2009). In addition to the environment's functional and aesthetic qualities, services such as public transportation may also be associated with walking and biking. Adults with access to public transportation, such as a bus or subway, report higher levels of activity (Besser & Dannenberg, 2005).

Finally, policies that create built and perceived environments represent the outermost level of the model. Governmental policies that regulate zoning, land use, and street connectivity influence the creation of built attributes. Policies also mandate resources for environmental features, including bike paths, parks, recreation opportunities, and art (Bauman et al., 2012). Worksite and school policies can operate in a similar regulatory manner and provide resources. School policies regulate physical education time and instruction, recess, and school busing. Worksite policies regulate fitness facilities or incentives, break times, and environmental conditions.

> **Check for Understanding** Networks are relationships with other people. Networks are a source of information, emotional support, resources, and contact with others. Pick one of the following behaviors: eating, driving, or immunizations. List and explain three network-based factors that influence this behavioral action. Refer to Table 4-1 as needed.

From Framework to Practice

The social ecological model is a generic framework for thinking about and seeking greater understanding about health behaviors and environmental risk factors. In addition to the various levels of influence, social ecological models that influence health promotion practices are also behavior specific, reflect a reciprocal relationship of person to environments, and contain specific variables on each level of the environment.

To put social ecological models into practice, the models need to be health behavior specific. Numerous specific factors influence health behaviors, and the factors vary by behavior. For instance, the factors that influence healthy eating are different from the factors that influence physical activity (Sallis & Glanz, 2009). Thus, the models that represent these two phenomena (healthy eating and activity) should communicate the differences. There are similarities in the factors; both include broad topical categories (e.g., neighborhood opportunities) as well as specific factors within the model (e.g., parental role modeling). Despite the similarities, there are a greater number of unique factors, which creates the need for behavior-specific models.

Models for specific versions of a behavior may also be more useful in community programming. A model that applies to a more general health behavior can be tailored to address a particular aspect of the behavior or a specific group. For example, the World Health Organization and the Centers for Disease Control and Prevention put forth the broad model for violence prevention discussed earlier in this chapter (see Figure 4-2). Figure 4-4 shows a conceptual model, which was developed by a public health professional, that more specifically addresses bullying and the relationship among the factors by the levels of influence. The bullying model builds from the violence prevention framework, using the person, relationships, and setting levels of influence; however, the narrowed focus on a specific act of violence—youth bullying—more clearly identifies factors that mediate such violence and serve as targets of change.

Another fundamental aspect of social ecological models is that behaviors both shape *and* are shaped by the social and built environment. The contextual factors of one's environments do influence behavior, but a person's behavior can also influence the environment. The violence prevention model highlights this bidirectional relationship in which a person can be represented as "potential victim" or "potential aggressor," but he or she also can also be an agent of change within the ecosystem. The behaviors modeled by others, the advocacy actions taken, and the resources championed can alter factors within the social and system context of violence and other behaviors. Furthermore, some of these relationships between factors and behaviors are direct, whereas some of the relationships of influence operate indirectly. For instance, governmental policy change can indirectly influence workplace policies,

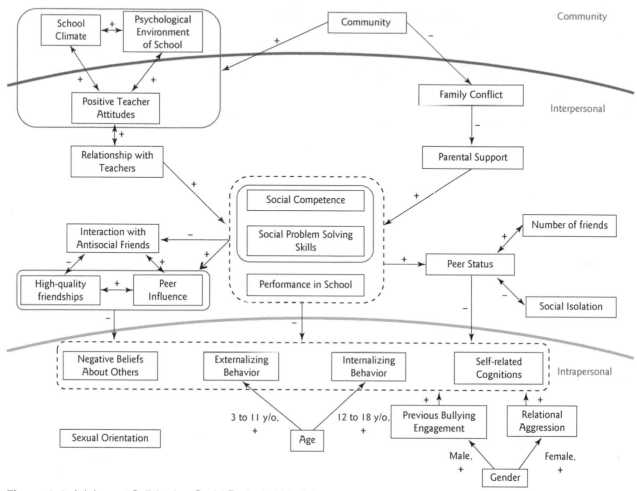

Figure 4-4 Adolescent Bullying in a Social Ecological Model
Source: Courtesy of Dustin Ratliff, Clark County Combined Health District Registered Sanitarian

which in turn change norms and shared beliefs over time, leading to individual adoption of those beliefs.

Social ecological models of behaviors contain specific variables on each level of the environment. The identification of behavioral antecedents on each environmental level comes from a variety of sources, most often health behavior theory, the research work of others, and a practitioner's own work with an audience and behavior. The physical activity model (see Figure 4-3), for instance, contains 100 entries within the model and represents at least 20 years of research (Barker & Gutman, 2014; USDHHS, 1996). The social ecological model is an organizing framework for the types of factors, but many

actual entries within the model come from decades of research and the work of numerous researchers. Early studies, guided by health behavior theory, identified intrapersonal characteristics and interpersonal networks that influenced physical activity. Active individuals could identify benefits of activity, enjoyed activity, reported support from friends and family, and were able to set goals and adhere to structured program (USDHHS, 1996). More recent works, guided by social ecological conceptual models, have established evidence of specific factors and relationships of outer level factors. As discussed previously, properties of one's environment, access to recreational opportunities, and policies that regulate transportation, street connectivity, and school wellness have been added to the understanding of promoting physical activity levels (Bauman et al., 2012; Sallis et al., 2006; USDHHS, 2008).

Identifying the specific factors is paramount to health promotion practice because *they* (the factors represented within the levels of the environment) become the target of interventions and strategies of change. The elaborate activity model exists because of the observations, theoretical hypothesizing, and research of many professionals in a variety of settings interested in active living. The purpose of identifying these correlates is to link understanding to intervention development (Green, Richard, & Potvin, 1998; Stokols, 1992). Tobacco control initiatives and physical activity initiatives have made this link. Evidence of other multidisciplinary, multilevel ecological programming in other content areas, however, is not yet as common in health promotion literature (Golden & Earp, 2012). Intervention outcomes are commonly reported as change in the innermost spheres of the model, that is, the intrapersonal and interpersonal levels (Golden & Earp, 2012).

> **Check for Understanding** Take the behavior you chose from the prior Check for Understanding exercise: eating, driving or immunizations. List and explain three place-based factors and three system-based factors that influence this behavioral action. Refer to Table 4-1 as needed.

The Long-Term Approach to Health Promotion

Social ecological model–based programming is a long-term approach to population health and involves the work of many researchers and practitioners. Implementing multilevel interventions takes time to gather an understanding of the various factors that influence behavior and then implement strategies of change on the various levels of influence. With both physical activity and tobacco, understanding of the behavior grew by levels of understanding, starting with what motivates people. From there, understanding about networks, places, and systems has grown, but deep understanding takes time. Tobacco control studies have been in place for over 50 years and continue today. Similarly, work on identifying the outer levels of environmental influence (built and policy) on physical activity began 10 years ago and is now entering a third phase (Barker & Gutman, 2014).

It is also important to note that work on the outer level of influence can take more time than examinations of change on the individual and network levels. Policy development within a community can take years. For instance, to gather support for the idea, draft legislation, inform voters, and pass the Ohio statewide smoking ban took 2 to 3 years (Tung & Glanz, 2007). After passage of the ban, enforcement responsibilities and processes to enforce the ban continued for years.

Second, working on various levels of influence also involves different sectors of the population and professional

> **Model for Understanding** Tobacco control has been the work of a variety of disciplines: health care, public health, education, law enforcement, substance abuse, media, and business. It has been the work of coalitions, nonprofits, groups of parents, state legislators, lobbyists, researchers, chief executive officers (CEOs), insurers, and many more. Tobacco use has truly been addressed through multilevel interventions that have reached across population segments. Some have called it a model to be applied to other population-level improvements in health behaviors and health status (Brownell & Warner, 2009; Mercer et al., 2003; NCI, 2007).
>
> Tobacco control efforts began with awareness and education interventions, progressed to behavioral and social interventions, and along the way have included numerous policy actions. Individuals learned about the ill effects and the addictive nature of tobacco; individuals were taught methods to quit, including involving the support of others; institutions encouraged and resourced members to quit, adopted policies that restricted tobacco use, and built norms around tobacco; and organizations developed policy statements on use and advocated for change. Governments implemented clean air policies, taxed tobacco, restricted advertising, and regulated retail sales (IOM, 2007; Warner, 2006). This widened system approach to tobacco control has had documented success. The number of adults in this country who smoke cigarettes and use other tobacco products has been cut in half, from over 50% of the adult population in the 1960s to around

20% of the current adult population (American Lung Association, 2011).

Can healthy eating be the next tobacco? Can place- and system-level changes in food access, messaging, and pricing promote changes in population-level food and beverage intakes? Medical, public health, and nutrition experts say the answer is "yes" (IOM, 2013; Kumanyika et al., 2008; Sallis & Glanz, 2009; Story et al., 2008).

The *In the news* feature at the beginning of the chapter discussed how the New York City Board of Health attempted to pass legislation limiting access to sugar-sweetened beverages. Sugar-sweetened beverages can be a significant source of "empty calories" (calories that add to one's daily intake with little to no nutritional value). To some readers, the attempt to regulate soda may seem far reaching, if not crazy. These so-called crazy policies may be exactly what is needed to combat the consumption of unhealthy food and beverages. Similar measures were used successfully in tobacco control initiatives. Access-related legislation included minimum age of purchase, location in retail stores, and minimum pricing for tobacco products. Communities may be unwilling to tax junk food and beverages, but schools and select worksites have adopted policies that limit soda access, set guidelines for vending machine items, and charge more for unhealthy items.

Further, there is momentum for more favorable pricing of fruits, vegetables, and other healthier choices. These early natural experiments of place and system changes to promote healthy eating imply that the strategies may look a bit different than what was used with tobacco, but experts and researchers remain optimistic. As a note, the New York City Board of Health was able to ban the use of trans fat in restaurants and encourage restaurants to post calories of menu items.

disciplines. The skills and resources required to implement system changes or policy development are different than the skills necessary to implement awareness and education programming. Likewise, the interventions targeting health care providers to facilitate change come before the implementation of health care system–based interventions. Each level of influence involves different interventions, different target audiences, different agents of change, and varying resource requirements. Adopting a social ecological model becomes a long-term view of health promotion—a body of work by many, for many.

SUMMARY

Social ecological models are a way of thinking about the numerous factors that influence health behaviors and health status. The social and built environment has various levels of influence, traditionally labeled intrapersonal, interpersonal, community, organizations, and policy/systems. Social ecological models are most useful in practice when they are behavior specific and when they include specific factors on each level of the model. Health behavior theory is useful for providing details within these broad categories. Health behavior theory consists of factors (called constructs) and hypothesized relationships among the factors. Health behavior theory is a critical part of the process of building evidence-based public health practice.

The future of population-level health improvements will come through the simultaneous work of many disciplines addressing multiple levels of influence. Social ecological models have guided the research agendas, strategic plans, and funding offered by national and state organizations. As a result, there will likely continue to be more content-specific models and additional evidence of the impact of outer-level–based interventions. The policy, system, and environment (PSE) agenda of the Centers for Disease Control and Prevention, among others, also has a role in smaller agencies of schools, worksites, and neighborhoods. School wellness committees, employee wellness coalitions, regional health care organizations, and community coalitions are encouraged to adopt a multilevel framework for understanding and impacting change.

BEHAVIORAL SCIENCE IN ACTION

The Ecology of Human Development

Urie Bronfenbrenner, who was born in the Soviet Union in 1917, was a pioneer in the field of child psychology. After serving as a military psychiatrist during World War II, Bronfenbrenner eventually ended up as a professor and researcher at Cornell University. Throughout his tenure, he authored and edited over 300 articles and book chapters and 14 books (Lang, 2005). He was incredibly influential in the fields of child psychology and development, sociology, and anthropology. *The Ecology of Human Development*, written by Bronfenbrenner in 1979, is credited as the first social ecological model of public health.

In 1965, Bronfenbrenner was appointed to a federal panel tasked with examining development in poor underprivileged children. He believed that the key to the development of children into adults was a strong family, so he advocated for programs to counteract the increasing rates of drug use, violence, teen pregnancies, high school dropouts, and divorce. The federal panel created the foundation for the Head Start program, which continues to provide programming aimed at school readiness for low-income children.

It was widely thought in the 1960s and 1970s that child development was entirely a biological process. Child psychology experiments focused on how children reacted in carefully controlled settings that allowed for the influence of only one particular variable. Bronfenbrenner realized that this was unnatural and hypothesized that children are impacted by the people and environmental influences around them. He theorized that the environment could play a vital role in a child's development and that a person reaches his or her potential through a combination of biological, environmental, and social forces. This became known as the ecological systems theory, or human ecology model, and was published in *The Ecology of Human*. Bronfenbrenner later added the concept of the chronosystem, which took into account the idea that a person and his or her environments change over time. To observe children in their own complex environments, Bronfenbrenner conducted his research over extended periods of time in places such as homes, day cares, and schools. Bronfenbrenner continued to tweak and add to his theory until his death in 2005.

IN THE CLASSROOM ACTIVITIES

1) Describe the role of health behavior theory in understanding health behaviors.
2) Compare concepts, constructs, and variables.
3) Take the list of factors that influence one of your health behaviors (see Chapter 2, activity 5). Classify the factors into the corresponding levels of the social ecological model. Knowing the levels of influence, add additional factors to each level.
4) Visit the Pedestrian and Bicycle Information Center and download the Walkability Audit.

Complete a walkability audit of a section of a campus or off-campus location. Take two photos that capture key features of the environment. Compare your walking scores with those of other students. Observe walking for transportation in the area; do perceived walking rates vary? What system- and policy-level factors may be associated with the walking score?

WEB LINKS

Active Living Research: http://www.activelivingresearch.org/

Pedestrian and Bicycle Information Center: http://www.pedbikeinfo.org/

World Health Organization: http://www.who.int/en/

REFERENCES

American Lung Association. (July 2011). *Trends in tobacco use*. New York: Author.

Bandura, A. (1977). Self-efficacy: Toward a unifying theory of behavior change. *Psychological Review, 84*(2), 191–215.

Bandura, A. (1986). *Social foundations of thought and action*. Englewood Cliffs, NJ: Prentice Hall.

Barker, D. C., & Gutman, M. A. (2014). Evaluation of active living research: Ten years of progress in building a new field. *American Journal of Preventive Medicine, 46*(2), 208–215.

Bauman, A. E., Reis, R. S., Sallis, J. F. Wells, J. C., Loos, R. J., & Martin, B.W. (2012). Correlates of physical activity: Why are some people physically active and others not? *Lancet, 38*, 258–271.

Besser, L. M., & Dannenberg, A. L. (2005). Walking to public transit: Steps to help meet physical activity recommendations. *American Journal of Preventive Medicine, 29*(4), 273–280.

Brownell, K.D., & Warner, K.E. (2009). The perils of ignoring history: Big tobacco played dirty and millions died; How similar is big food? *Milbank Quarterly, 87*(1), 259–294.

Brownson, R. C., Fielding, J. E., & Maylahn, C. M. (2009). Evidence-based public health: A fundamental concept for public health practice. *Annual Review of Public Health, 30*, 175–201.

Carlson, J. A., Sallis, J. F., Conway, T. L., Saelens, B. E., Frank, L. D., Kerr, J., et al. (2012). Interactions between psychosocial and the built environment factors in explaining older adults' physical activity. *Preventive Medicine, 54*(1), 68–73.

Chiu, G. R., Lutfey, K. E., Litman, H. J., Link, C. L., Hall, S. A., & McKinlay, J. B. (2013). Prevalence and overlap of childhood and adult physical, sexual, and emotional abuse: A descriptive analysis of results from the Boston Area Community Health (BACH) survey. *Violence and Victims, 28*(3), 381–402.

Community Preventive Services Task Force. (2012). *2012 Annual report to Congress and to agencies related to the work of the task force*. Retrieved from http://www.thecommunityguide.org/annualreport/index.html

Dahlberg, L. L., & Krug, E. G. (2002). Violence: A global public health problem. In E. Krug, L. L. Dahlberg, J. A. Mercy, A. B. Zwi, & R. Lozano (Eds.), *World report on violence and health* (pp. 1–56). Geneva, Switzerland: World Health Organization.

Davison, K. K., Werder, J. L., & Lawson, C. T. (2008). Children's active commuting to school: Current knowledge and future directions. *Preventing Chronic Disease, 5*(3), 1–11.

Ding, D., Sallis, J. F., Kerr, J., Lee, S., & Rosenberg, D. E. (2011). Neighborhood environment and physical activity among youth: A review. *American Journal of Preventive Medicine, 41*(4), 442–455.

Espelage, D. L., & De La Rue, L. (2011). School bullying: Its nature and ecology. *International Journal of Adolescent Medicine and Health, 24*(1), 3–10.

Glanz, K., & Bishop, D. B. (2010). The role of behavioral science theory in development and implementation of public health interventions. *Annual Review of Public Health, 31*(1), 399–418.

Golden, S. D., & Earp, J. L. (2012). Social ecological approaches to individuals and their contexts: Twenty years of health education & behavior health promotion interventions. *Health Education & Behavior, 39*(3), 364–372.

Green, L. W., Richard, L., & Potvin, L. (1996). Ecological foundation of health promotion: An introduction to the ecological approach in health promotion; Historical and intellectual roots, applications, strengths, and limitations. *American Journal of Health Promotion, 10,* 270–281.

Institute of Medicine (IOM). (2000). *Promoting health: Intervention strategies from social and behavioral research.* Washington, DC: National Academies Press.

Institute of Medicine (IOM). (2013). *Evaluating obesity prevention efforts.* Washington, DC: National Academies Press.

Institute of Medicine (2007). *Ending the tobacco problem: A blueprint for the nation.* Washington, DC: National Academies Press.

Krug, E. G., Dahlberg, L. L., Mercy, J. A., Zwi, A. B., & Lozano, R., (2002a). *World report on violence and health.* Geneva, Switzerland: World Health Organization.

Krug, E. G., Mercy, J. A., Dahlberg, L. L., & Zwi, A. B. (2002b). The world report on violence and health. *Lancet, 360,* 1083–1088.

Kumanyika, S. K., Obarzanek, E., Stettler, N, Bell, R., Field, A. E., Fortmann, S. P. ... Hong, Y. (2008). Population-based prevention of obesity: The need for comprehensive promotion of healthful eating, physical activity, and energy balance; A scientific statement from American Heart Association Council on Epidemiology and Prevention, Interdisciplinary Committee for Prevention. *Circulation, 118,* 428–464.

Lang, S. S. (2005). Renowned bioecologist addresses the future of human development. *Human Ecology, 32(3),* 24–25.

Lin, J. S., O'Connor, E., Whitlock, E. P., & Beil, T. L. (2010). *Behavioral counseling to promote physical activity and a healthful diet to prevent cardiovascular disease in adults: A systematic review for the U.S. Preventive Services Task Force* (AHRQ Publication No. 11-05149-EF-3). Retrieved from http://www.uspreventiveservicestaskforce.org/uspstf11/physactivity/physart.htm

Maibach, E. W., Abroms, L. C., & Marosits, M. (2007). Communication and marketing as tools to cultivate the public's health: A proposed 'people and places' framework. *BMC Public Health, 7*(88), 88–103.

McLeroy, K. R., Bibeau, D., Steckler, A., & Glanz, K. (1988). An ecological perspective on health promotion programs. *Health Education Quarterly, 15*(4), 351–377.

Mercer, S. L., Green, L. W., Rosenthal, A. C., Husten, C. G., Khan, L. K., & Dietz, W. H. (2003). Possible lessons from the tobacco experience for obesity control. *American Journal of Clinical Nutrition, 77*(4 Supp), 1073S–1082S.

National Cancer Institute (NCI). (2007). *Greater than the sum: Systems thinking in tobacco control* (Tobacco Control Monograph No. 18; NIH Pub. No. 06-6085). Bethesda, MD: U.S. Department of Health and Human Services, National Institutes of Health, National Cancer Institute.

National Cancer Institute (NCI). (2005). *Theory at a glance: A Guide to health promotion practice* (U.S. Department of Health and Human Services, Pub. No. 05-3896). Retrieved from www.cancer.gov/cancertopics/cancerlibrary/theory.pdf.

Owen, N., Humpel, N., Leslie, E., Bauman, A., & Sallis, J. F. (2004). Understanding environmental influences on walking: Review and research agenda. *American Journal of Preventive Medicine, 27*(1), 67–76.

Prochaska, J. O., & DiClemente, C. C. (1983). Stages and processes of self-change of smoking: Toward an integrative model of change. *Journal of Consulting and Clinical Psychology*, 51, 390–395.

Ratliff, D. (2013). *Adolescent bullying in a Social Ecological Model: Theoretical logic model* (Unpublished graduate project). Dayton, OH: Wright State University.

Rutherford, A. (2013). Violence/intentional injuries: Epidemiology and overview. *International Encyclopedia of Public Health,* 500–508.

Saelens, B. E., Sallis, J. F., Frank, L. D., Cain, K. L., Conway, T. L., Chapman, J. E., Slymen, D. J., & Kerr, J. (2012). Neighborhood environment and psychosocial correlates of adults' physical activity. *Medicine & Science in Sports & Exercise, 44*(4), 637–646.

Sallis, J., Cervero, R., Ascher, W., Henderson, K., Kraft, K., & Kerr, K. (2006). An ecological approach to creating active living communities. *Annual Review of Public Health,* 27, 297–322.

Sallis, J. F., & Glanz, K. (2009). Physical activity and food environments: Solutions to the obesity epidemic. *Milbank Quarterly, 87*(1), 123–154.

Shaikh, A. R., Yaroch, A. L., Nebeling, L., Yeh, M. C., & Resnicow, K. (2008). Psychosocial predictors of fruit and vegetable consumption in adults: A review of the literature. *American Journal of Preventive Medicine 34*(6), 535–543.

Stöckl, H., Devries, K., Rotstein, A., Abrahams, N., Campbell, J., Watts, C., & Moreno, C. G. (2013). The global prevalence of intimate partner homicide: A systematic review. *Lancet, 383*(9895), 859–865.

Stokols, D. (1992). Establishing and maintaining healthy environments: Toward a social ecology of health promotion. *American Psychologist, 47*(1), 66–22.

Story, M., Kaphingst, K. M., Robinson-O'Brien, R., & Glanz, K. (2008). Creating healthy food and eating environments: Policy and environmental approaches. *Annual Review of Public Health, 29,* 253–272.

Tung, G., & Glantz, S. (2007). *Clean air now, but a hazy future: Tobacco industry political influence and tobacco policy making in Ohio, 1997–2007.* Retrieved from http://repositories.cdlib.org/ctcre/tcpmus/Ohio2007.

U.S. Department of Health and Human Services (USDHHS). (n.d.). *Health care reform.* Retrieved from www.healthfinder.gov/HealthCareReform/.

U.S. Department of Health and Human Services (USDHHS). (1996). *Physical activity & health: A report of the surgeon general.* Rockville, MD: National Center for Chronic Disease Prevention and Health Promotion, Office on Smoking and Health.

U.S. Department of Health and Human Services (USDHHS). (2008). *2008 physical activity guidelines for Americans.* Rockville, MD: U.S. Department of Health and Human Services, Office of the Surgeon General.

U.S. Department of Health and Human Services (USDHHS), Centers for Disease Control and Prevention (CDC). (n.d.a). *The social-ecological model: A framework for prevention.* Retrieved from http://www.cdc.gov/violenceprevention/overview/social-ecologicalmodel.html

U.S. Department of Health and Human Services (USDHHS), Centers for Disease Control and Prevention (CDC). (n.d.b). *Colorectal Cancer Control Program (CRCCP).* Retrieved from http://www.cdc.gov/cancer/crccp/sem.htm.

U.S. Department of Health and Human Services (USDHHS), National Health Lung and Blood Institute. (1998). *Clinical guidelines for the identification, evaluation and assessment treatment of overweight and obesity in adults*. Retrieved from www.nhlbi.nih.gov/guidelines/obesity.

U.S. Department of Health and Human Services (USDHHS), National Health Lung and Blood Institute. (2004). *The seventh report of the Joint National Committee on Prevention, Detection, Evaluation, and Treatment of High Blood Pressure: Complete report*. Retrieved from www.nhlbi.nih.gov/guidelines/asthma.

U.S. Department of Health and Human Services (USDHHS), National Health Lung and Blood Institute. (July 2007). *Guidelines for the diagnosis and management of asthma (EPR-3)*. Retrieved from http://www.nhlbi.nih.gov/health-pro/guidelines/current/asthma-guidelines/.

U.S. Preventive Services Task Force (USPSTF). (2009). Counseling and interventions to prevent tobacco use and tobacco-caused disease in adults and pregnant women: U.S. Preventive Services Task Force reaffirmation recommendation statement. *Annals of Internal Medicine, 150*, 551–555.

Warner, K. E., (Ed.). (2006). *Tobacco control policy: Robert Wood Johnson Foundation Series on Health Policy* (S. L. Issacs & J. R. Knickman, J. R, series editors). San Francisco: Jossey-Bass.

World Health Organization (WHO). (2002). *World report on violence and health: Summary*. Geneva, Switzerland: World Health Organization.

CHAPTER 5

Theories of Intrapersonal Influence

KEY TERMS

action	maintenance	perceived susceptibility	subjective norm
attitude	modifying factors	perceived threat	temptation
contemplation	perceived barriers	precontemplation	variable
cues to action	perceived behavioral control	preparation	
decisional balance	perceived benefits	self-efficacy	
intention	perceived severity	stages of change	

LEARNING OBJECTIVES

1. Describe health behavior theories at the individual level of influence.
2. Identify the constructs of the health belief model.
3. Explain the stages of change in the behavioral process of change.
4. Give examples of behavioral intention and describe factors that influence a person's intention to act.
5. Compare predisposing factors that motivate an individual to act.

IN THE NEWS ...

On May 20, 2013, an EF5 tornado hit Moore, Oklahoma. Based on wind estimates and damage, tornados are assigned a score from zero to five on the Enhanced Fujita Scale (EF). With winds in excess of 200 miles per hour, the tornado created a path of destruction over 17 miles long and a mile and a half wide. Buildings, structures, and roads were destroyed, including the collapse of two schools, a medical center, and entire neighborhoods. Twenty-four people were killed. Local officials and politicians expressed empathy and support for the community. In news reports and media interviews, response workers reminded residents that "this is tornado season," and everyone should be prepared. This naturally occurring event, and the media coverage of it, prompted many people to create or revisit their emergency plan and kit of provisions.

One year later, news outlets revisited the event on the anniversary of the EF5 tornado. Residents of Moore discussed an increase in emergency preparedness. Specifically, families reported the creation of kits and family communication plans and often the inclusion of a shelter in their rebuilding efforts.

Introduction

The individual is at the heart of social ecological models of health behavior. It is the individual who makes decisions to act or not to act. It is the individual who interacts with others, develops skills, seeks resources, and advocates for change. While other levels of influence are important to an individual's actions, the behavior ultimately originates from the individual. In this chapter, health behavior theories that explain factors of the intrapersonal level of influence will be discussed (see Figure 5-1). The health belief model, the theory of planned behavior, and the transtheoretical model are established theories that identify an individual's specific attitudes and actions. Theory explains the factors that facilitate the behavior, describes conditions under which the behavior is more or less likely to occur, hypothesizes relationships among the factors and conditions, and finally, suggests processes for changing the behavior (Glanz & Bishop, 2010).

The health belief model suggests that individuals who perceive a threat of illness are more likely to take action. Cues to act and perceived benefits and barriers can further influence behavioral action. The theory of planned behavior also suggests that individual attitudes toward a behavior mediate action. The theory of planned behavior introduces the important construct of intention—does the person plan to change? Intention is a cognitive factor influenced by one's attitudes, the social norm, and a factor similar to self-efficacy. Intention to act can be an important milestone in behavioral change.

The concept of stages of change, from the transtheoretical model, states that change is a process that occurs over time. People progress from phases of thinking about change to exploring change with small actions and then to actually performing the action of change. The final stage is working to maintain the behavior change. All five stages of change are significant in the process. Mediating factors and strategies

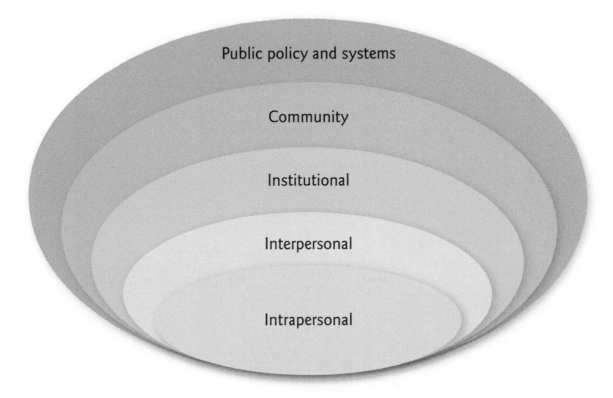

Figure 5-1 Social Ecological Model

of change vary by the individual's stage of change. Later, Chapter 8 will discuss a process for combining the rich detail provided by these theories into general concepts and principles of practice.

Health Belief Model

The health belief model (HBM) is one of the most widely used intrapersonal models for explaining health behavior. The primary concept of the HBM is that a person's likelihood of taking a health-related action is influenced by his or her perceived threat for injury, illness, or disease (Rosenstock, 1974). If an individual perceives a personal threat of illness, then he or she is more likely to engage in a health behavior related to the health issue. Conversely, if a person perceives little to no likelihood of illness, disease, or injury, then he or she is unlikely to engage in the preventive action. Simply put, if a person is worried about his risk of a certain type of cancer, then he or she is more likely to engage in a preventive cancer screening.

This concept of perceived threat of illness is central to the health belief model. A person must perceive risk and/or threat in order to act (see Figure 5-2). Perceived threat is a product of the interaction of other types of beliefs and conditions. In general, a person's likelihood of adopting a health-related behavior can be predicted by four beliefs (Rosenstock, 1974):

1. A person thinks his or her health is at risk, which is known as perceived susceptibility.

2. The individual develops an idea of the perceived severity of the illness or condition, which may include pain, death, and/or negative consequences at work or home.

3. The individual must be able to identify the pros and cons, known as perceived benefits and perceived barriers. When he or she believes that the benefits of making a behavior change outweigh the negative aspects, it is probable that he or she will attempt to change the health behavior.

4. The individual feels a need to take action due to external influences or reminders, known as cues to action.

Perceived Susceptibility

Perceived susceptibility refers to how strong an individual's belief is that he or she is at risk for illness or injury (Janz & Becker, 1984). Does a person believe that he will or will not develop the illness or disease? As discussed in Chapters 1 and 2, risk for disease and disability can come from modifiable and

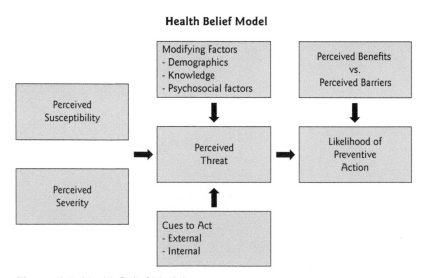

Figure 5-2 Health Belief Model

nonmodifiable traits and behaviors. Risk can stem from biological, environmental, and lifestyle factors (e.g., age, gender, water source, and smoking status). Furthermore, susceptibility is disease specific and person specific. A woman may perceive her risk for breast cancer as higher or lower than her risk for heart disease based on family history and understanding of the diseases.

Throughout the health belief model, *perception* is a repeated and important term. One's interpretation or perception of personal risk is the theoretical construct. Risk can be objective and based on scientific research and statistics, but it also includes the person's own subjective interpretation of his or her risk. Perception can vary from an objective measure of risk for a variety of reasons. A language barrier or poor health literacy may mean that a person does not fully understand his or her risk for a particular disease or condition (Garcés-Palacio & Scarinci, 2012). Furthermore, a woman who has regular visits with a health care professional and feels healthy in general may believe that she is doing everything necessary to prevent and protect against a health problem, regardless of whether she is actually protecting herself from the disease (Garcés-Palacio & Scarinci, 2012). The strength of an individual's perceived susceptibility plays a role in the likelihood of taking preventive action. Perceived susceptibility has a relationship with the next construct of perceived severity—how bad is it going to be?

Perceived Severity

The degree of seriousness an individual associates with contracting a particular illness, disease, or injury is known as **perceived severity**. Perceived severity includes concepts such as an individual's expectations about the scope and duration of symptoms and the possibility of a cure associated with a given disease. In the case of cancer, an individual's perception of severity may include how serious he considers the symptoms, the effect the disease and treatment might have on himself and his family, the chances of being cured, and the possibility of death. An individual's perception of severity is not a fixed idea because it can change over time as knowledge, treatment options, and stigmas change. Many diseases that were once untreatable are now curable with antibiotics. The perceived severity of these diseases, such as tuberculosis and syphilis, is often much lower now than in the past because of effective treatment options.

Expected outcomes of a disease or disability are not restricted to just symptoms and medical outcomes. Financial, emotional, and social outcomes are also categories of outcomes considered by an individual. For some individuals, the consideration of nonhealth outcomes may be even more concerning than symptoms or health outcomes. For example, individuals perceive the severity of human immunodeficiency virus (HIV) as very high because of its associations with cancer, dangerous infections, and death. Research has shown, though, that the stigma tied to having a specific illness or disease, as well as a fear of isolation, can be as much of a consideration as illness and/or death and may prevent some from seeking proper treatment or lead to self-isolation (Mahajan et al., 2008). The perceived stigma associated with being HIV-positive may cause an even higher perceived severity.

> **Check for Understanding**   Evacuation prior to a natural disaster, such as a tornado or hurricane, can be a target health behavior. Individuals who evacuate are safer and less likely to experience an injury. Draw the HBM core with evacuation as the target behavior and threat of injury and illness as the threat. What are three factors that may influence a person's perceived susceptibility and severity?

Perceived Threat

Perceived threat is the combination of perceived susceptibility and perceived severity, making it a **variable** and ever-changing concept. **Perceived threat** varies based on one's perceived susceptibility and/or severity. These three constructs represent the core of the health belief model (see Figure 5-3). If susceptibility is high and severity is high, perceived threat is high. Similarly, if susceptibility is low and severity is low, perceived threat is low. A moderate level of threat can develop through a combination of conditions: If an individual believes herself to be at a low risk for a disease but the perceived severity of the disease is high, then she is said to have a moderate perceived threat for the disease or health condition. Conversely, she may perceive the severity as low but believe she has a high likelihood of developing the disease (susceptibility), which again implies a moderate degree of threat. Researchers have not established a minimum level of universal threat needed to take action, but numerous studies have found that a moderate level of threat seems necessary to increase the likelihood of action.

Health Belief Model—Core

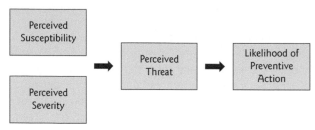

Figure 5-3 Health Belief Model: Core

Model for Understanding: Influenza Influenza among college students is an excellent example of how variable perceived threat can be. Students may believe they are susceptible to the flu, but most students do not believe the flu's severity is very high. A college student who gets the flu may be ill for about a week and may miss some classes, but the perceived severity does not rise to a level at which the college student believes he or she may die. Thus, moderate to high susceptibility and low severity means the perceived threat of the flu is reduced, and the likelihood of college students getting flu shots is lower than in other populations (Byrne et al., 2012). This specific group has not been studied as much as other subpopulations, but a study conducted at several universities in Minnesota found that only 30.2% of students were vaccinated against the flu during the 2002–2006 study period (Nichol, D'Heilly, & Ehlinger, 2008).

The recent HINI flu epidemic, on the other hand, was known to cause serious illness and to greatly impact those less than 35 years of age. It was thought that this would lead to high perceived susceptibility and high perceived severity, and according to one study, this increased perceived threat caused more college-aged students than usual to intend to get vaccinated (Byrne et al., 2012). Another study, however, found that despite frequent media coverage of the novel HINI strain, only 20% of students at eight North Carolina universities actually received a seasonal flu shot during the 2009–2010 flu season (Poehling et al., 2012). Researchers continue to examine the complex reasons behind why college students do or do not seek out a flu shot.

Perceived Benefits and Perceived Barriers

Perceived benefits are the positive expected outcomes an individual believes exist if he or she undertakes a certain behavior necessary to avoid illness or disease (Rosenstock, 2005). Perceived benefits include positive treatment outcomes, symptom relief, and support or reward from others. **Perceived barriers** refer to the anticipated obstacles or challenges an individual believes exist when engaging in the behavior or preventive health action. Expected costs when undertaking a particular course of action are also included in perceived barriers. Perceived negative outcomes may include monetary expenses, time and resources required, emotional distress (such as embarrassment), and physical pain or unpleasantness (Rosenstock, 2005).

In the framework of the health belief model, an individual evaluates the pros and cons associated with engaging in the proposed preventive behavior. To increase the likelihood of the person engaging in the health behavior, the benefits should outweigh the barriers (Rosenstock, 2005). For example, researchers observed that women often found the idea of performing a breast self-examination (BSE) to be upsetting due to the possibility of finding a lump. Studies have shown that women with higher levels of perceived benefits for performing the monthly self-exam and higher levels of health motivation were more likely to begin and continue monthly BSEs because they believed the potential for early breast cancer detection outweighed the negative aspects of the exam (Hajian-Tilaki & Auladi, 2014; Norman & Brain, n.d.). Barriers tend to be stronger predictors of behavior. An individual who cannot find a way to weigh the benefits more heavily than the barriers may constantly vacillate between action and inaction or simply refuse to continue thinking about making a behavior change—both of which result in the person not undertaking the desired action (Rosenstock, 2005).

Again, perception is an important concept for understanding individual behavior. Perceived barriers can differ from actual barriers, and the strategies to overcome a perceived barrier may differ from those for an actual barrier. For example, access to a screening facility can be both a real and a perceived barrier to a mammogram. In the first example, a woman may not live near a facility providing mammograms, or she may lack health insurance that covers mammograms. In a second scenario, a woman may have access to a facility, but she may not know that she has that access. In this case, a woman might need to be made aware of the facility and/or a screening voucher program. Both categories of benefits and barriers, perceived and actual, are important for understanding health behavior.

Cues to Action

Cues to action are simple actions or events that nudge or remind an individual to engage in a specific health behavior. A person may have the readiness to act due to his or her perceived susceptibility and severity, but a cue to act is often the little push necessary to actually take action (Rosenstock, 2005). Cues to act can come from other people, the media, witnessing an event, and even from within the individual. Common external cues to action include prompts from a family member, reminder postcards from a physician or dentist, and media reports. Symptoms, like fever or pain, are internal cues to act. For example, recurring headaches that appear for no apparent reason might prompt an individual to schedule an appointment with a physician. The patient is then more likely to agree to proposed tests or screenings because of the painful headaches.

Much like an elbow to the side, cues to act can have different strengths. Not all cues are equal. For a selected group of people, one form of a cue to act may be more meaningful or influential than another. For example, women may find messages, reminders, or encouragement from other women to be a more powerful reminder to act than if those same messages were to come from a man. Further, the important and meaningful cues in one population may differ in another population. Health care provider prompts are one such example. A physician or other health care provider reminding a patient to participate in a screening has been shown to increase the likelihood of mammography, cervical cancer screenings, and colorectal screenings (Baron et al., 2010). However, physician prompts for prostate screenings for African American males do not lead to an increased likelihood of screenings. There is ongoing research to see if clergy and other spiritual leaders may provide more powerful prompts to members of this community.

Modifying Factors

Modifying factors are a person's characteristics that influence his or her perceived threat. **Modifying factors** can be demographic, social, and/or psychological. Demographic factors that may influence one's perception of threat include age, sex, race, and ethnicity. Psychological factors that may influence one's perception of threat include personality, motivation, and knowledge. Social variables include the perceived social norm, religion, culture, and socioeconomic status. Some of these factors, such as knowledge, are changeable, while others (e.g., race and sex) remain fixed.

Modifying factors can be confused with factors related to risk and susceptibility. Modifying factors tend not to be disease specific but more global, like personality traits, socioeconomic status, past experiences, and education level. For example, cancer fatalism is a broad belief about the unalterable, likely death that is associated with all cancer. It can influence the perceived threat for many cancers and other diseases (Powe, 2003). However, someone who has had cancer in the past and survived may perceive the severity of the disease to be lower than others do because of his or her history of survival (Powe, 2003; Smith-Howell et al., 2011). Another example is socioeconomic status (SES). As a modifying factor, women with higher SES tend to use preventive screening services more often than women of lower SES (Katz & Hofer, 1994; Sambamoorthi & McAlpine, 2003). As a result, a perceived threat for a specific illness and disease may be more likely to be acted upon by someone with certain modifying factors.

Self-Efficacy

Like many theories, the HBM has been modified as researchers and practitioners learn more about human behavior. The model was modified in 1974 to include the construct of self-efficacy. **Self-efficacy** is an individual's confidence in his or her ability to perform specific tasks or behaviors in order to reduce or prevent the likelihood of contracting a particular health issue (Glanz & Bishop, 2010). Self-efficacy is a strong predictor of behavior. Even though self-efficacy was a later addition to the HBM, the construct is important and helps explain why some individuals are more likely than others to undertake a new health behavior (Rosenstock, Strecher, & Becker, 1988). Table 5-1 summarizes the constructs of the HBM.

Applications of the Health Belief Model

The basis of the HBM is that an individual's perceived threat of a disease, condition, or injury determines the likelihood that the individual will engage in a preventive behavior or action. A practitioner using the HBM as the foundation of a community-based health program will develop a program

TABLE 5-1 Constructs of the Health Belief Model

Construct	Definition
Perceived susceptibility	An individual's beliefs about his or her personal likelihood of developing a health issue or being injured.
Perceived severity	A person's beliefs regarding the seriousness of a particular condition and the possible consequences.
Perceived threat	The overall perception of the risk associated with a specific health issue or disease, developed as a combination of perceived susceptibility and perceived severity.
Perceived benefits	The anticipated outcomes from engaging in a particular behavior or preventive health action.
Perceived barriers	The obstacles or challenges an individual believes exist to engaging in a particular behavior or preventive health action.
Cues to action	Simple actions or events that remind or nudge an individual to act.
Modifying factors	Individual characteristics of a person that influence his or her perceived threat.
Self-efficacy	An individual's confidence in his or her ability to engage in a particular preventive behavior and the resulting likelihood that the preventive behavior will reduce the likelihood of contracting the health issue.

Source: Adapted from Champion & Skinner, 2010

focused on increasing the perceived threat within the target population. The HBM also provides an excellent structure for studying a health behavior before designing and implementing an intervention. To develop interventions designed to decrease perceived barriers or increase perceived susceptibility, it is necessary to first know the perceived barriers and levels of perceived susceptibility in the target demographic group.

Breast and cervical cancer screenings have been the focus of numerous studies in recent decades in an effort to increase the number of women obtaining these preventive cancer screenings. The health belief model has been used by many researchers because it allows them to explore the complex reasons that determine whether women will obtain these screenings. Initial applications of the HBM focused on women in general to determine why the number of women obtaining screenings as recommended was so low.

In 1987, the National Health Interview Surveys found that only 16% of American women over the age of 40 had had a mammogram in the previous year, and the Behavior Risk Factor Surveillance Survey found that 29% of women over the age of 50 had had a breast cancer screening in the past 12 months (Fulton et al., 1991). Fulton and colleagues (1991) wanted to use the HBM, already shown to be successful when applied to prevention activities, to discover why the number of women receiving mammograms was so low. Their research, which involved conducting telephone interviews of women over the age of 40 in Rhode Island, showed that low income and low educational attainment were linked to a decreased likelihood of being screened for breast cancer (Fulton et al., 1991). They also observed that previously having had a mammogram, regularly seeing a gynecologist, and perceiving mammograms to be safe were predictive of women obtaining a yearly mammogram (Fulton et al., 1991). Women who did not receive mammograms were less likely to have a medical provider recommend a mammogram and more likely to not have a regular physician, believe that they were not very susceptible to breast cancer, believe that breast cancer was not an especially serious disease, and/or believe that mammography was not effective or safe (Fulton et al., 1991). Following this study, health care providers were urged to recommend mammograms to all women according to current guidelines, and messages about mammography were altered to focus on the safety and efficacy of the screening. Rhode Island also began covering breast cancer screenings through Medicaid to enable women with low incomes to obtain mammograms (Fulton et al., 1991).

Cervical cancer screening behavior and beliefs became important in the United Kingdom when it was discovered that over 80% of women dying from cervical cancer had never received cervical cancer screening (Gillam, 1991). Using the HBM as a framework, researchers compiled answers to questionnaires to develop interventions designed to increase cervical cancer screening rates. It was observed that many women did not perceive themselves to be susceptible to developing cervical cancer due to misconceptions, for example, cervical cancer is linked to taking oral contraceptives or smoking and that women after menopause are not at risk of contracting cervical cancer (Gillam, 1991). It was also observed that many women in the study perceived cervical cancer to be a very serious disease and were often reluctant to undergo screening due to anxiety or fear (Gillam, 1991). When women were asked why they received a recent screening, 60% stated they scheduled the procedure on their own initiative and were not prompted by a physician or other cue to action (Gillam, 1991). Following this study, physicians were counseled to encourage women to obtain screenings, reminder letters were rewritten to better explain the risk of cervical cancer, and abnormal result letters were rewritten to decrease the anxiety associated with receiving such a result while still providing important information on follow-up treatment (Gillam, 1991). Laboratories around the United Kingdom reported that the number of Pap smear samples submitted increased after these changes were implemented (Gillam, 1991).

The number of women receiving breast and cervical screenings in the United States peaked around 2000 for most racial and ethnic groups and has decreased since then (NCHS, 2014). Healthy People 2020 objectives include goals of a 10% increase in women receiving these screenings, with targets set at 81.1% of women between the ages of 50 and 74 receiving a breast cancer screening and 84.5% of women between the ages of 21 and 65 receiving a cervical cancer screening based on current recommendations (USDHHS, 2014). To reach the objective, studies often focus on specific groups with low

adherence, such as Spanish-speaking immigrants or women with low incomes living in a particular area.

One such study examined why Korean American women have low rates of cervical cancer screenings. Fang and colleagues (2007) conducted a literature review to determine the perceived risk, perceived barriers, and other health beliefs this particular subgroup associated with cervical cancer screening. They found that Korean American women cited embarrassment, poor English skills, and a cultural belief that one seeks medical care and treatment only when actively showing symptoms of illness as some of the reasons for not obtaining a cervical cancer screening (Fang et al., 2007). The researchers then used the HBM to create an intervention designed to address the perceived barriers to obtaining cervical cancer screenings. The women participated in bilingual education sessions that addressed cervical cancer risk factors, the efficacy of screening methods, and the prevalence of cervical cancer among Asian Americans (Fang et al., 2007). In an effort to increase self-efficacy, the researchers addressed goal setting and used role-playing to improve the participants' confidence in handling a potentially awkward visit to a physician (Fang et al., 2007). Following this multiprong intervention, cervical cancer screening rates among participants increased from 12% to 83% within 6 months (Fang et al., 2007).

The cost of obtaining preventive screenings is often cited as a reason for women in the United States not participating, and this perceived barrier does not apply to Canadian women, who benefit from universal healthcare (Austin et al., 2002). Austin and colleagues (2002) used the HBM to explore why Hispanic women living in Canada had low levels of mammograms and cervical cancer screenings despite widespread access to free screenings. Their findings included perceived barriers such as embarrassment of discussing and/or exposing private body parts, especially in front of a male physician; a cultural belief that cancer is a punishment from God that one is powerless to avoid; and limited English language skills (Austin et al., 2002). The researchers also noted that Hispanic women often have a low perceived susceptibility because they typically do not consider themselves at risk for breast or cervical cancer if there is no family history and/or they are currently asymptomatic (Austin et al., 2002). Suggestions for future interventions include culturally sensitive pamphlets available in Spanish, working with leaders and churches in the Hispanic communities to promote screenings, and using community health workers to educate women on the importance of cancer screenings (Austin et al., 2002).

To increase perceived threat, some interventions use fear. Fear tends to impact behavior, though what sort of impact is still unclear. Some studies have found that arousing a fear of death is more effective than appeals that are less severe (Cooper, Goldenberg, & Arndt, 2014). Cooper and colleagues (2014) observed that study participants who received a fear appeal message that connected sun damage with cancer and possible death were more likely to use sunscreen than participants whose fear appeal message discussed less severe appearance related side effects. Other studies have noted that fear appeals may cause someone to undertake any action to reduce the feeling of fear or threat regardless of whether it is effective, or it may push people into denial or avoidance if they are unable or unsure of how to reduce their threat (Witte & Allen, 2000).

One of the common conclusions of researchers and practitioners using the HBM is the importance of tailored messaging, reminders, and interventions. One way to increase perceived threat is through cues to action that focus on the modifying factors of your target population. For instance, sexually active college students are at risk for a variety of sexually transmitted infections (STIs). Many students are not aware of the risk they face, nor are they always knowledgeable about signs and symptoms (or lack thereof) that might signal an STI. Cues to action for this subgroup could include informational brochures tailored to the target group at the student health center and in common areas in the dormitories. Peer health educators at campus health-related events could increase awareness of STI prevalence on campus, discuss methods of prevention, and demonstrate proper condom use. Physicians at student health services could communicate directly with patients and discuss individual risk factors and prevention methods. Practitioners could also use social media to get brief informative messages to target audiences in an effort to increase the number of students getting routine STI testing.

Transtheoretical Model

The transtheoretical model (TTM) is another intrapersonal theory used to explain how individuals adopt a new behavior or change a current behavior. It is a more recent theory that emerged through extensive research of smoking cessation programs. In observing individuals trying to quit smoking, it became clear that people trying to quit moved through stages of the quitting process, which researchers called the stages of change (Prochaska & DiClemtene, 1983). Unlike the HBM, which is best suited to examine single event actions such as getting a flu shot or participating in a cancer screening, the TTM incorporates time as a new dimension in behavior change. This makes it ideal for changes that occur over a period of time or require continual effort, like losing weight or correct and consistent condom use. In addition, researchers identified 10 common skills that appear in people who successfully quit smoking, which they called processes of change (Prochaska & DiClemente, 1983).

Stages of Change

The stages of change concept is the main organizational structure in the transtheoretical model. The concept posits that individuals go through a *process* of change, the process consists of various **stages of change**, and these stages occur over time. People adopting (or stopping) a behavior think about changing the behavior, experiment with the behavior change, actively change the behavior, and then work to maintain the behavior change. Although it may now seem obvious that big changes require a lot of smaller changes over time, researchers used to view behavior change as a single event (Velicer et al., 1998). Change is now viewed as a continuum of factors and actions, not a single act. Stages of change have been documented for a number of behaviors. Individuals go through stages for smoking, alcohol, and drug cessation; changing eating habits to conform to a specific diet; adopting an exercise regimen; sunscreen use; and condom use (Prochaska et al., 1994; Zimmerman, Olsen, & Bosworth, 2000).

There are five stages of change: precontemplation, contemplation, preparation, action, and maintenance (see Figure 5-4). Stage names express the overall theme of what is occurring in that stage. For example, people in precontemplation are not yet contemplating a behavior change, whereas in contemplation, they are considering the behavior change. Stages of change is important to understanding behavior because the factors that influence health behaviors vary by stage of change. Therefore, understanding a health behavior means understanding factors across the stages of change. The following sections describe the continuum of stages in more detail and conclude with a newly suggested possible sixth stage.

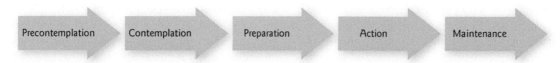

Figure 5-4 Stages of Change

Precontemplation

Individuals in the **precontemplation** stage have no intention of changing their behavior. They are not considering the change and do not expect to change within at least the next 6 months. Individuals may be in this stage because they are unaware of the risks of their behavior or inaction, or they may have tried and failed to change in the past and are discouraged from trying again (Prochaska, Redding, & Evers, 2008; Prochaska & Velicer, 1997). Regardless of the reason they are in this stage, individuals in precontemplation usually avoid any mention of their currently risky behavior or the healthier behavior. Many interventions are not designed to deal with individuals in this stage, as they may be seen as resistant to change or completely unmotivated (Prochaska et al., 2008).

Contemplation

The **contemplation** stage encompasses individuals who are considering making a positive behavior change within the next 6 months. In this stage, people are weighing the pros and cons of behavior change. To reach the contemplation stage, individuals tend to know of the benefits of change, but they are also very aware that there may be negative aspects associated with the change (Prochaska & Velicer, 1997). If the balance does not swing more heavily toward the benefits of changing, individuals may be stuck in limbo for an extended period of time while they continue to weigh the pros and cons (Prochaska et al., 2008). While in this stage, most individuals will not be ready for interventions typically designed for people more prepared to actively change their behavior. Building a person's efficacy for successful change is a more appropriate stage-matched target of change.

Collectively, preparation and contemplation are considered cognitive and affective stages of change. Many of the factors driving or influencing the behavior are located in the brain, and individuals debate the value of change as well as their ability to change.

Preparation

After contemplating behavior change, individuals will move into the **preparation** phase. At this stage are people who plan to actively make a change in their behavior within the next month. They have spent time developing a plan for the impending change, whether that is signing up for a class, talking to a physician or other health professional, or purchasing books or other necessary equipment (Prochaska et al., 2008). Whether the goal is losing weight, quitting smoking, or overcoming an eating disorder, these individuals are ready to be recruited into interventions focusing on active behavior changes.

Preparation is often recognized by small actions of change. Individuals "play with" the behavior in an attempt to develop a plan of action. Smokers cut down on the number of cigarettes, they restrict the places where they smoke, and/or they switch brands. All these activities are part of the preparation for action. Similarly, individuals may also try different versions of a behavior, again in an attempt to build efficacy and identify action strategies. A future exerciser may try an exercise class at a recreation center or walk during lunch. From this trial of behaviors, a movement to action can occur.

Action

At the **action** stage are those individuals who have made measurable changes in their behavior within the past 6 months. This action must occur at a risk-reducing level, however, so people making very minor changes may not be in this stage but rather in preparation (Prochaska et al., 2008). For example, individuals seeking to lose weight must decrease caloric and fat intake while increasing the number of fruits and vegetables consumed. If the only dietary change the addition of one apple per day, the individual is trialing a healthy behavior (preparation) but has not fully committed to a lifestyle change necessary to move into the action stage. Individuals in this stage are vulnerable to relapsing or regressing to an earlier stage, so it is important that they receive adequate support and encouragement.

Participation in the action phase of change requires skills, resources, and social support. For example, smokers require trigger management skills, are often aided by nicotine replacement products, and benefit from the emotional support of others.

Maintenance

In the **maintenance** stage, individuals continue the behavior changes they adopted in the action stage. As individuals become more confident in their ability to maintain the change, the behavior becomes more second nature and there is less reliance on change processes when compared to the action stage. Because temptations and the possibility of relapse still exist, individuals are often permanently in the maintenance stage. Recently, some experts have suggested that an additional stage, known as termination, is the sixth stage of change. Termination occurs when people experience no temptation and their self-efficacy is at 100% (Prochaska et al., 2008). There is no consensus on this proposed stage, however, and many researchers and practitioners continue to use a five-stage transtheoretical model.

In Figure 5-4, the five stages are shown as a linear model with forward progressive movement. Real-world behavior change occurs in both directions: the forward movement into stages is depicted in the figure, as is movement backward to one or more previous stages. Regression refers to any backward move in the stages, while relapse occurs when an individual moves from action or maintenance to an earlier stage. Relapse and regression are common in behavior change, and it is important to understand that this is a natural part of behavior change and should not be considered a failure (Zimmerman et al., 2000). Someone can regress or relapse for any number of reasons, including temptations, a change in or lack of social support, or moving to a new environment. It is important to monitor individuals in a behavior change program for signs of possible regression or relapse and offer the support necessary to keep them actively progressing or maintaining their lifestyle changes (Zimmerman et al., 2000).

Temptation

Temptation is the one of the challenges faced by an individual making a behavior change. It refers to the strength of the impulse to return to previous unhealthy behaviors when in a challenging or stressful situation. Although it is not always considered a construct of the TTM, it is relevant to the stages of change because people struggling with temptations may relapse or regress. Temptations can be broken down into three categories: cravings, emotional stress or anxiety, and positive or encouraging social situations (Prochaska et al., 2008). Someone striving to reduce overeating tendencies may struggle with temptation at sad events, such as a funeral, or at a birthday party when everyone else is eating a lot of pizza and cake. A person in the process of quitting smoking may run into problems with temptation when hit with cravings for nicotine and a strong urge to smoke a cigarette.

Additional TTM Concepts

While stages of change is a widely accepted and applied concept in health behavior and health promotion, the transtheoretical model contains other important concepts and activities. Since the TTM explores behavior change as a continuous process occurring over many months and years, it is necessary to be able to determine where an individual falls on the spectrum of change. The model uses the constructs of decisional balance, self-efficacy, and the processes of change as ways of examining an individual's readiness and location in the stages of change (Prochaska et al., 2008). Processes of change are also described in the TTM, where processes of change are the behavioral strategies (activities) that people use to move through the stages. Decisional balance, is the activity of weighing the pros and cons of behavior change. Finally, as with the health belief model, self-efficacy was added as a construct in a later revision of the TTM.

Processes of Change

The processes of change (see Table 5-2) are activities that individuals use in the process of moving through the stages of change (Prochaska & DiClemente, 1983). Consciousness raising, dramatic relief, environmental reevaluation, social liberation, and self-evaluation are cognitive processes used mainly in the early stages of change. These cognitive and affective activities, coined experiential processes by Prochaska and DiClemente (1983), impact an individual's knowledge and emotional readiness. These processes are emphasized most in the precontemplation, contemplation, and preparation stages (Prochaska et al., 2008). Reinforcement management, helping relationships, counterconditioning, stimulus control, and self-liberation are considered behavioral processes. These activities

TABLE 5-2 Processes of Change

Process of Change	Definition
Consciousness raising	Greater knowledge of underlying causes, side effects, and cures or treatments for a health problem. This can be accomplished through classes, media campaigns, and other educational programs.
Dramatic relief	The purpose of dramatic relief is to elicit an emotional response in individuals and then offer a solution to the feelings. Personal stories or testimonies of those suffering from an illness, media campaigns, and health screenings are all effective activities that can initiate the process.
Environmental reevaluation	This process of change involves an assessment of how someone's habit affects those around him or her, such as how smoking affects family members and friends. Environmental reevaluation may also include learning about how one is a positive or negative role model for others.
Self-liberation	An individual needs to believe that he or she is capable of changing and will continue to be committed to the change, also known as self-liberation. People who make their commitment to changing public by sharing with friends and family are often the most successful. Individuals who have multiple choices in how to change a behavior are also very successful. For example, a smoker should be offered nicotine replacement patches, gum, or going cold turkey so that he or she can make the best self-liberated decision.
Self-reevaluation	This process of change requires an individual to imagine his or her self-image with and without a particular unhealthy habit, such as picturing oneself as a smoker and a nonsmoker.
Stimulus control	Removing objects or cues that trigger unhealthy habits and inserting reminders and cues for healthy actions is known as stimulus control. Examples include avoidance, reengineering or reorganizing environments, and self-help or support groups.
Helping relationships	Creating positive relationships that are built on trust, caring, honesty, and acceptance is an important process of change. These relationships can take the form of a workout buddy, a counselor, or a support group.
Counterconditioning	Counterconditioning is the substitution of healthier behaviors or habits for unhealthier ones. This can take the form of taking soda out of the fridge and replacing it with bottled water and low-fat milk, or it may be trying relaxation techniques to counteract stress.
Reinforcement management	Adding rewards for positive behavior change and reducing rewards for unhealthy behaviors. Reinforcements can be public, such as certificates of achievement for reaching milestones in a group, or private, such as positive statements and affirmations.
Social liberation	Social opportunities for groups to demonstrate population-level support of a behavior. Typical interventions focus on advocacy, empowerment, and policy formation. These interventions often impact the health of a wider audience, such as smoke-free areas and freely accessible condoms.

Source: Adapted from Prochaska et al., 2008 Velicer et al., 1998

are applied in the later stages of change (action and maintenance) and tend to focus on behavioral skills and actions (Prochaska & DiClemente, 1983).

Decisional Balance

Decisional balance is the cognitive process of weighing the pros and cons of change. People weigh the pros and cons of various decisions on a daily basis, but a long-term behavior change requires people to frequently reassess the positive and negative aspects of their decision (Prochaska et al., 1994). Individuals may choose to look at the pros and cons of their unhealthy behavior, or they may choose to focus on the positives and negatives of the new healthy behavior. For example, a smoker may weigh the pros and cons of smoking (the unhealthy behavior) and say that she enjoys smoking with her friends at parties but does not like how all of her clothes smell like smoke. Another smoker may weigh the pros and cons of quitting smoking (the new healthy behavior). He might list saving money by not buying cigarettes as a positive outcome of quitting and the difficulties and frustration he experienced the last time he tried quitting as a negative outcome.

Individuals in the same stage often view the pros and cons in a similar manner, regardless of the health behavior in question. People in precontemplation see the cons of changing their behavior as greatly outweighing the benefits of changing or adopting a new behavior (Prochaska et al., 1994). In contemplation, the balance between the pros and cons is about equal. This explains why people in the stage are now considering making a change some time in the future, as the idea of making a lifestyle change no longer seems impossible or overwhelmingly negative. Individuals in preparation, action, and maintenance view the pros of the new healthy behavior as outweighing the cons (Prochaska et al., 1994).

Self-efficacy

Self-efficacy refers to an individual's belief that he or she is capable of engaging in a new health behavior. In the context of the TTM and the stages of change, this more specifically refers to a person's confidence that he or she can stick to a new health behavior in difficult, stressful, or unfamiliar situations (Glanz & Bishop, 2010). For example, someone trying to eat a low-fat diet with lots of fruits and vegetables may feel confident in his or her ability to eat healthfully at home. Self-efficacy in this case refers to confidence in maintaining a healthy diet while faced with many unhealthy foods on vacation. Again, self-efficacy is a strong predictor of behavior and is often added to behavioral theories for that reason.

Application of the Transtheoretical Model

The transtheoretical model is a very useful model of behavior change for practitioners involved in the development and planning of health interventions. Unlike other models, the TTM can recruit individuals of all stages of readiness for change instead of just those individuals ready to undertake an immediate change in behavior. By tailoring interventions to reach individuals in all stages, many behavior change programs using the TTM see high participation rates (Prochaska et al., 2008). Retaining individuals in behavior change interventions is challenging regardless of the target behavior change. Correctly classifying and working with individuals in their current stage places more reasonable demands and expectations on individuals and may help decrease dropout rates (Prochaska et al., 2008).

The stages of change in the TTM allow for an individual's change to be measured. It is possible to identify a person's progress throughout the course of a lifestyle and behavior change instead of relying on one single benchmark. The TTM allows for all changes related to the behavior to be measured, whether the change is cognitive, behavioral, or emotional. This enables practitioners to reinforce all changes along the way and remain vigilant for signs of possible relapse or regression.

Theory of Reasoned Action and the Theory of Planned Behavior

The theory of reasoned action (TRA) (see Figure 5-5) and the theory of planned behavior (TPB) (see Figure 5-6) are related theories that focus on an individual's intentions regarding a behavioral change. The TRA was first developed in 1967, and it attempts to explain the relationship between someone's attitude and his or her resulting behavior (Ajzen, 2012). The theory proposes that the proximal predictor of successful behavior change is the intention to change, and intention is influenced by attitudes toward that behavior and the subjective norm (see Table 5-3) (Fishbein & Ajzen, 1975).

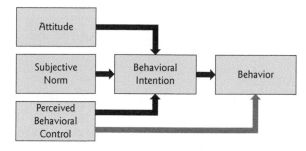

Theory of Reasoned Action

Figure 5-5 Theory of Reasoned Action

Theory of Planned Behavior

Figure 5-6 Theory of Planned Behavior

TABLE 5-3 Constructs in the Theory of Reasoned Action and the Theory of Planned Behavior

Determinant or Construct	Definition
Behavioral intention	Someone's readiness to undertake a specific behavior change. This is the construct that immediately precedes a behavior change.
Attitude toward the behavior	Outcomes that a person anticipates from the performance of a behavior.
Subjective norm	The pressure an individual perceives to be coming from others to perform or not perform a certain behavior. A form of social pressure.
Perceived behavioral control	The ease or difficulty one associates with carrying out a specific behavior.

Source: Adapted from Azjen, 1991

Attitude toward the Behavior and Subjective Norms

Attitudes toward a behavior are the outcomes that a person anticipates from the performance of that behavior. Attitudes can be positive or negative, and expected outcomes can be emotional, psychological, or physical in nature. Psychologically, one could expect success or embarrassment as an outcome. Emotionally, one might expect something such as praise or punishment. Physically, one might expect to receive a reward or to make friends, or get a punishment or experience withdrawal. Attitudes are behavior specific and cognitions of the individual.

A **subjective norm** is the pressure an individual perceives to perform or not perform a certain behavior. It has been described as the perceived acceptability of a behavior. As one might imagine, the subjective norm can vary by networks or peer groups. Within a network of friends, a particular behavior, such as binge drinking, may be the norm. This same behavior may have a lesser degree of perceived acceptability among family and co-workers. Individuals will have different motivations to comply with the various referent groups. Thus, an important step in understanding the influence of subjective norm on intention is to understand the networks of groups that influence the individual.

Attitudes and norms are beliefs, and beliefs come in different strengths. Attitudes exist on a continuum from a super-strong emotion to an indifferent shoulder shrug. It is also possible for a person to have simultaneous conflicting attitudes about a particular behavior, with the attitudes having differing strengths. For example, one's desire to fit into peer groups or be seen as "cool" can be an outcome that is strongly associated with adolescent risk behaviors such as tobacco and alcohol use. Adolescents may also believe that there are consequences to the behavior, but the desire for the positive outcomes influences intention much more than perceived negative outcomes.

Intention

The theory of reasoned action and the theory of planned behavior work hand in hand to explore the relationship between a health behavior and an individual's intention to change. As noted by Ajzen in a recent reflection on the theory, "At its core, TPB is concerned with the prediction of intentions" (2011, p. 1115). Someone's intention to change or adopt a behavior is the greatest determinant of actually carrying out the behavior (Ajzen, 1991; McEachanm et al., 2011). **Intention** is an indicator of motivation and willingness to change. Intention signals a positive attitude, a valued outcome and the belief that others approve of the behavior. Therefore, these theories are most effective at predicting behavior change for behaviors that are largely under the control of the individual (Albarracín et al., 2001; McEachanm et al., 2011).

Intention to perform a behavior can vary in the form of the behavior and the conditions of the behavior, and it can vary over time. First, there may be some versions of a behavior that are more appealing to individuals than other forms. Because of the expected outcomes (attitudes), the norm, and/or one's confidence in performing the behavior, a person's intention can vary. For example, there are forms of physical activity that people are more and less like to participate in. People report a lower intention to participate in moderate to vigorous activity. Common attitudes related to this intention are the expected sweat and discomfort, and the low perceived likelihood of success. Similarly, intention changes over time. Because of changing cultural attitudes, changing norms, and/or change in perceived behavioral control, a mother's intention to breastfeed an infant can change. The intention to breastfeed can change across numerous time periods: prior to birth, in the hospital, on returning home, and when returning to work.

> **Check for Understanding** Using the constructs of (1) attitudes, (2) subjective norm, and (3) perceived behavioral control, give three specific reasons that a mother's intention to breastfeed her newborn or infant could change from prior to birth, while in the hospital, on returning home, and when returning to work.

Perceived Behavioral Control

The TPB expands on the TRA to suggest that one's intention is formed by a third belief: perceived behavioral control. **Perceived behavioral control** is the ease or difficulty one associates with carrying out a specific behavior (Ajken, 1991; Albarracín et al., 2001). It is a reflection of confidence and ability, as well as opportunity. In that sense, perceived behavior control is similar to the concept of self-efficacy—it is one's confidence in performing a specific skill (Ajzen, 1991). Unlike attitudes and subjective norm, though, perceived behavioral control can be a predictor of actual behavior (Ajzen, 1991, 2011; McEachanm et al., 2011).

Collectively, the theory of planned behavior suggests that three different beliefs impact an individual's behavior: behavioral, normative, and control (Ajzen, 1991, 2011). Behavioral beliefs are an individual's expected outcomes with regards to a behavior or behavior change. These beliefs can paint the health behavior in a positive or negative light and influence an individual's opinion on the behavior. Normative beliefs are other people's expectations and the desire or motivation to fulfill these expectations. They may be construed as social pressure, also known as the subjective norm. Control beliefs are external factors that may improve or impede the individual's ability to carry out a health behavior, and they influence one's perceived behavioral control (Ajzen, 1991; Fishbein & Ajzen, 1975, 2010).

Applications of the Theory of Planned Behavior

The TPB model has been applied to many different types of health behaviors. With a nationwide increase in the prevalence of HIV contracted by the heterosexual partners of drug users, Bowen and colleagues (2001) used the TPB to develop interventions intended to increase condom use by crack cocaine users. One of their interventions focused on reshaping normative beliefs related to condom use and increasing the intention to use condoms. Before emergency contraception (EC) became available over the counter, Sable and colleagues (2006) used the TPB as a framework to understand why physicians prescribed EC at varying rates to different groups of women. Their research found that a physician's beliefs and the subjective norm greatly impacted his or her intention to prescribe EC, which led the researchers to recommend interventions that incorporated the subjective norm and other attitudes while working to encourage physicians to prescribe the medication. Other researchers have also used the models to explore the relationship between intention and behavior in the context of diet, exercise, donating blood, using various contraceptive methods, getting a flu shot, injury prevention, and adhering to practice guidelines. The model has also been used to explore many nonhealth-related behaviors, such as voting, purchasing products, and going to church (Albarracín et al., 2001; Glanz & Bishop, 2010; Sheppard, Hartwick, & Warshaw, 1988).

The strength of the intention-behavior relationship varies and at times can be quite weak. A person may have the intention to change many times but be unsuccessful in actually changing. Rather, for many behaviors, intention is a milestone in the adoption of a behavior; one must intend to change in order to initiate the process of change (Ajzen, 2011). Intention, and the understanding of what influences intention, is an important contribution to health promotion practice. One of the most direct ways of determining an individual's beliefs or intentions is through administering a questionnaire. Respondents use a Likert scale (e.g., extremely likely, likely, neutral, unlikely, extremely unlikely) to answer questions such as, "How likely are you to tell your partner to use a condom during the next month?" After a thorough study of the factors influencing people's beliefs and intentions to carry out a health behavior, practitioners can develop interventions designed to target these normative, behavioral, and control beliefs (Ajzen, 2011).

SUMMARY

Health behavior theories at the intrapersonal level deal with the individual and his or her personal characteristics. Personal characteristics include knowledge, beliefs, previous experiences, and socio-demographic attributes. Collectively, intrapersonal factors influence one's motivation to take action. The core of the health belief model states that individuals who perceive a threat for illness are more likely to take action. The perception of threat is created through a combined influence of perceived susceptibility to and perceived severity of a disease or condition.

The theory of planned behavior added intention as an important predictor of behavior. Someone's intention is influenced by his or her attitude toward the behavior, the subjective norm, and perceived behavioral control. Because attitudes, norms, and perceived control change, intention also varies. Finally, the transtheoretical model introduced the idea that a health behavior change does not occur following a single action. Individuals move through stages of change and develop a set of cognitions and skills to achieve long-term behavior change.

BEHAVIORAL SCIENCE IN ACTION

Development of the Health Belief Model.

The health belief model was developed in the 1950s by a group of researchers working with the U.S. Public Health Service (USPHS). During this decade, the USPHS was involved mainly with preventive services rather than providing medical care to patients. In addition to screening for polio, dental diseases, rheumatic fever, and cervical cancer, one of the program's main goals was to prevent the spread of tuberculosis (TB)

(Rosenstock, 1974). Even though these preventive screenings were widely available and free or low cost, they were greatly underutilized. Numerous studies were conducted to figure out why people were not using these free services, but the studies yielded conflicting and inconclusive results (Rosenstock, 2005). The USPHS researchers worked to develop a model that would explain why Americans were not utilizing free or inexpensive TB screening services.

Researchers faced a paradox—the members of the public stood to benefit a lot from the control of TB, yet they were not very interested in participating in screenings to help prevent the spread of the disease (Hochbaum, 1958). Tuberculosis was a widespread disease that posed a serious threat to those infected, so researchers were puzzled as to why people did not take advantage of well-advertised, easily accessible, free X-ray screenings (Hochbaum, 1958). There was a group of individuals, however, who did take advantage of the X-ray program. This group seemed to be very similar to those who opted not to obtain X-rays (Hochbaum, 1958). Researchers wanted to find out what separated those who used the preventive services from those who did not.

The researchers determined that their key audience was made up of people who were not showing signs or symptoms of disease, as people with symptoms of active TB were much more likely to seek medical attention (Rosenstock, 1974). They wanted to examine the various variables of someone obtaining an X-ray, when he or she would get an X-ray done, what type of X-ray facility he or she chose, and which type(s) of educational or promotional influences factored into the decision. Following a study in three U.S. cities, the researchers found that individuals must be psychologically ready to take action, and conditions must be favorable in order for one to take action (Hochbaum, 1958). They determined that "readiness" was comprised of knowledge, emotions, and previous experiences. Also important to the decision to seek an X-ray were the beliefs that one could contract TB at any time, that one could currently be infected with TB, and that early detection and treatment were beneficial (Hochbaum, 1958). Researchers also noted that study participants differentiated between the possibility that they *could* contract TB and the likelihood that they *would* contract the disease (Hochbaum, 1958).

Basing a lot of their model on the ideas of social psychologist Kurt Lewin, the USPHS researchers realized that all behavior starts with some form of intention (Rosenstock, 2005). The data they collected from study participants helped them add the constructs of perceived susceptibility, perceived seriousness, perceived benefits, and perceived barriers to taking action, and cues to action (Rosenstock, 1974). Although the terms used today are slightly different, it is clear that the groundbreaking research conducted by members of the USPHS was a major step in the development of health behavior theory.

IN THE CLASSROOM ACTIVITIES

1. List five attributes of people related to motivation to take action.
2. List constructs of the health belief model and explain the role of perceived benefits and barriers and modifying factors on perceived threat.
3. Track cues to act for a day. Share your list of cues with others students. As a small group, create lists of common behavioral targets and the corresponding cues.
4. As a class, pick one or two specific health behaviors. Informally interview five people about the behaviors. From the interview information, can you determine a stage of change for the person? Support your answer with at least one statement.
5. Intention is an important behavioral milestone. Explain how a college student's intention to smoke cigarettes may change as he or she starts college or explain how a young person's intention to practice safer sex may vary by the social context.

WEB LINKS

Cancer Prevention Research Center: http://www.uri.edu/research/cprc/transtheoretical.htm

Centers for Disease control and Prevention Center for Emergency Preparedness and Response: http://emergency.cdc.gov/

REFERENCES

Ajzen, I. (1991). The theory of planned behavior. *Organizational Behavior and Human Decision Processes, 50*(2), 179–211.

Ajzen, I. (2011). The theory of planned behaviour: Reactions and reflections. *Psychology & Health 26*(9), 1113–1127.

Ajzen, I. (2012). Martin Fishbein's legacy: The theory of reasoned action. In M. Hennessy (Ed.), *Advancing reasoned action theory* (pp. 11–27). Thousand Oaks, CA: Sage.

Albarracín, D., Fishbein, M., Johnson, B. T., & Muellerleile, P. A. (2001). Theories of reasoned action and planned behavior as models of condom use: A meta-analysis. *Psychological Bulletin, 127*(1), 142–161.

Austin, L. T., Ahmad, F., McNally, M.-J., & Stewart, D. E. (2002). Breast and cervical cancer screening in Hispanic women: A literature review using the health belief model. *Women's Health Issues, 12*(3), 122–128.

Baron, R. C., Melillo, S., Rimer, B. K., Coates, R. J., Kerner, J., Habarta, N.,... Jackson-Leeks, K. (2010). Intervention to increase recommendation and delivery of screening for breast, cervical, and colorectal cancers by healthcare providers: A systematic review of provider reminders. *American Journal of Preventive Medicine, 38*(1), 110–117.

Bowen, A. M., Williams, M., McCoy, H. V., & McCoy, C. B. (2001). Crack smokers' intention to use condoms with loved partners: Intervention development using the theory of reasoned action, condom beliefs, and processes of change. *AIDS Care, 13*(5), 579–594.

Byrne, C., Walsh, J., Kola, S., & Sarma, K. M. (2012). Predicting intention to uptake H1N1 influenza vaccine in a university sample. *British Journal of Health Psychology, 17,* 582–595.

Champion, V. L., & Skinner, C. S. (2008). The health belief model. In K. Glanz, B. K. Rimer, & K. Viswanath (Eds.), *Health behavior and health education: Theory, research, and practice* (4th ed., pp. 45–65). San Francisco: John Wiley and Sons.

Cooper, D. P., Goldenberg, J. L., & Arndt, J. (2014). Perceived efficacy, conscious fear of death and intentions to tan: Not all fear appeals are created equal. *British Journal of Health Psychology, 19*(1), 1–15.

Fang, C. Y., Ma, G. X., Tan, Y., & Chi, N. (2007). A multifaceted intervention to increase cervical cancer screening among underserved Korean-American women. *Cancer Epidemiology, Biomarkers & Prevention, 16,* 1298–1302.

Fishbein, M., & Ajzen, A. (1975). *Beliefs, attitudes, intentions, and behavior: An introduction to theory and research.* Reading, MA: Addison-Wesley.

Fishbein, M., & Ajzen, A. (2010). *Predicting and changing behavior: The reasoned action approach.* New York: Psychology Press.

Fulton, J. P., Buechner, J. S., Scott, H. D., DeBuono, B. A., Feldman, J. P., Smith, R. A., & Kovenock, D. (1991). A study guided by the health belief model of the predictors of breast cancer screening of women ages 40 and older. *Public Health Reports, 106*(4), 410–420.

Garcés-Palacio, I. C., & Scarinci, I. C. (2012). Factors associated with perceived susceptibility to cervical cancer among Latina immigrants in Alabama. *Maternal and Child Health Journal, 16,* 242–248.

Gillam, S. J. (1991). Understanding the uptake of cervical cancer screening: The contribution of the health belief model. *British Journal of General Practice, 41*(353), 510–513.

Glanz, K., & Bishop, D. B. (2010). The role of behavioral science theory in development and implementation of public health interventions. *Annual Reviews in Public Health, 31,* 399–418.

Hajian-Tilaki, K., & Auladi, S. (2014). Health belief model and practice of breast self-examination and breast cancer screening in Iranian women. *Breast Cancer, 21*(4), 429–434.

Hochbaum, G. M. (1958). *Public participation in medical screening programs: A socio-psychological study.* Washington, DC: U.S. Department of Health, Education, and Welfare.

Janz, N. K., & Becker, M. H. (1984). The health belief model: A decade later. *Health Education Quarterly, 11*(1), 1–47.

Katz, S. J., & Hofer, T. P. (1994). Socioeconomic disparities in preventive care persist despite universal coverage: Breast and cervical cancer screening in Ontario and the United States. *JAMA (Journal of the American Medical Association), 272*(7), 530–534.

Mahajan, A. P., Sayles, J. N., Patel, V. A., Remien, R. H., Ortiz, D., Szekeres, G., & Coates, T. J. (2008). Stigma in the HIV/AIDS epidemic: A review of the literature and recommendations for the way forward. *AIDS, 22*(Suppl 2), S67–S79.

McEachanm, R. R. C., Conner, M., Taylor, N., & Lawton, R. J. (2011). Prospective prediction of health related behaviors with the theory of planned behavior: A meta-analysis. *Health Psychology Review, 5*(2), 97–144.

National Center for Health Statistics (NCHS). (2014). *Health: United States, 2013; With special feature on prescription drugs.* Hyattsville, MD: U.S. Department of Health and Human Services.

Nichol, K. L., D'Heilly, S., & Ehlinger, E. P. (2008). Influenza vaccination among college and university students: Impact on influenzalike illness, health care use, and impaired school performance. *Archives of Pediatrics & Adolescent Medicine, 162*(12), 1113–1118.

Norman, P., & Brain, K. (n.d.). *An application of the health belief model to the prediction of breast self-examination in a national sample of women with a family history of breast cancer.* Institute of Medical Genetics, University of Wales College of Medicine, UK. Retrieved from http://userpage.fu-berlin.de/~health/materials/normanb.pdf

Poehling, K. A., Blocker, J., Ip, E. H., Peters, T. R., & Wolfson, M. (2012). 2009–2010 seasonal influenza vaccination coverage among college students from 8 universities in North Carolina. *Journal of American College Health, 60*(8), 541–547.

Powe, B. D. (2003). Cancer fatalism: The state of the science. *Cancer Nursing, 26*(6), 454–467.

Prochaska, J. O., & DiClemente, C. C. (1983). Stages and processes of self-change of smoking: Toward an integrative model of change. *Journal of Consulting and Clinical Psychology, 51,* 390–395.

Prochaska, J. O., Redding, C. A., & Evers, K. E. (2008). The transtheoretical model and stages of change. In Glanz, K., Rimer, B.K. & Viswanath K. (Eds.), *Health behavior and health education* (4th ed., pp. 97–121). San Francisco: John Wiley & Sons, Inc.

Prochaska J. O., & Velicer, W. F. (1997) The transtheoretical model of health behavior change. *American Journal of Health Promotion 12*(1), 38–48.

Prochaska, J. O., Velicer, W. F., Rossi, J. S., Goldstein, M. G., Marcus, B. H., Rakowski, W., ... Rossi, S. R. (1994). Stages of change and decisional balance for 13 problem behaviors. *Health Psychology, 13*(1), 39–45.

Rosenstock, I. M. (1974). Historical origins of the health belief model. *Health Education Monographs, 2*(4), 328–335.

Rosenstock, I. M. (2005). Why people use health services. *Millbank Memorial Fund Quarterly, 83*(4), 1–32.

Rosenstock, I. M., Strecher, V. J., & Becker, M. H. (1988). Social learning theory and the health belief model. *Health Education Quarterly, 15*(2), 175–183.

Sable, M. R., Schwartz, L. R., Kelly, P. J., Lisbon, E., & Hall, M. A. (2006). Using the theory of reason action to explain physician intention to prescribe emergency contraception. *Perspectives on Sexual and Reproductive Health, 38*(1), 20–27.

Sambamoorthi, U., & McAlpine, D. D. (2003). Racial, ethnic, socioeconomic, and access disparities in the use of preventive services among women. *Preventive Medicine, 37,* 475–484.

Sheppard, B. H., Hartwick, J., & Warshaw, P. R. (1988). A comparison of three behavioral intention models: The case of Valentine's Day gift-giving. *Journal of Consumer Research, 15,* 325–343.

Smith-Howell, E. R., Rawl, S. M., Champion, V. L., Skinner, C. S., Springston, J., Krier, C., ... Myers, L. J. (2011). Exploring the role of cancer fatalism as a barrier to colorectal cancer screening. *Western Journal of Nursing Research, 33*(1), 140–141.

U.S. Department of Health and Human Services (USDHHS). (2014). *Healthy people 2020: Topics & objectives, Cancer.* Retrieved from http://www.healthypeople.gov/2020

Velicer, W. F., Prochaska, J. O., Fava, J. L., Norman, G. J., & Redding, C. A. (1998) Smoking cessation and stress management: Applications of the transtheoretical model of behavior change. *Homeostasis, 38,* 216–233.

Witte, K., & Allen, M. (2000). A meta-analysis of fear appeals: Implications for effective public health campaigns. *Health Education & Behavior, 27*(5), 591–615.

Zimmerman, G. L., Olsen, C. G., & Bosworth, M. F. (2000). A "stages of change" approach to helping patients change behavior. *American Family Physician, 61*(5), 1409–1416.

CHAPTER 6

Theories of Interpersonal Influence

KEY TERMS

behavioral capability	goal	physiological arousal	social support: emotional,
cognitions	incentive motivation	procedural knowledge	instrumental,
collective efficacy	intrinsic	received social support	informational, and
dynamic	knowledge	reciprocal determinism	appraisal
enactive attainment	mastery	reinforcements	verbal persuasion
environment	observational learning	self-efficacy	vicarious experiences
extrinsic	outcome expectations	self-regulation	
facilitation	perceived social support	social integration	

LEARNING OBJECTIVES

1. Describe health behavior theories at the interpersonal level of influence.
2. Identify the constructs of the social cognitive theory.
3. Explain how self-efficacy impacts behavior both directly and indirectly.
4. Give examples of reciprocal determinism in terms of personal, environment, and behavior factors.
5. Identify four types of social support.
6. Assess instances where social support is a behavioral antecedent.

IN THE NEWS ...

All states now offer some form of graduated driver licenses (GDL) for teen drivers. Through state legislation, driving privileges for drivers under age 18 are phased in, as compared to older models that largely granted full driving privileges after a short education and waiting period. Full driving licenses are phased in through a progression of stages, beginning with a minimum supervised learner's period, then a provisional period with limits on unsupervised driving in high-risk situations, and finally to full driving privileges. Programs and conditions vary widely by state; however, high-risk situations are commonly defined as evening driving and driving with passengers. In Kansas, during the first 6 months of the provisional period, new drivers cannot be on the road after 9 p.m. In Connecticut, Georgia, and Massachusetts, new drivers cannot have a peer as a passenger for the first 6 months of driving. Learners may begin supervised driving at age 14 in some states, such as Iowa and Kansas, but teens must wait until age 16 in New York, Pennsylvania, and other states. The National Highway Traffic Safety Administration reports that automobile crashes involving young drivers drop by 10–50% when GDL programs are implemented.

Introduction to Interpersonal Theories

Individuals must be motivated to act, be able to act, and be reinforced and reminded to act. This chapter will discuss the factors that often enable one to act and how reinforcements impact action. Information in this chapter builds on the concepts of the previous chapter. The person, and his or her motivation, is still at the center of the social ecological model of action (see Figure 6-1). Interpersonal factors, from the second level of influence, will be added. Interpersonal models incorporate individual attributes along with other factors and people that influence the individual's behavior. Interpersonal factors come from a person's formal and informal social networks and social support systems, including family, co-workers, and friendship networks. In addition to the social environment, one's physical environment also influences his or her behavior by presenting barriers, benefits, and nudges.

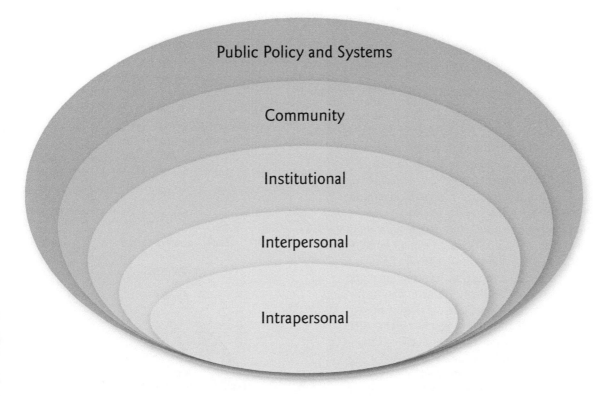

Figure 6-1 Social Ecological Model

The social cognitive theory (SCT) states that health behavior arises from the dynamic interaction of cognitions, the environment, and one's behaviors. As the name implies, cognitive factors of knowledge and beliefs interact with personal skills such as self-regulation, and with reinforcements and resources from the environment. Through this reciprocal interaction of factors, behavioral actions become a learned phenomenon. Self-efficacy, a construct in most intrapersonal and interpersonal theories, is a strong predictor of behavior and originates from SCT. Social support theory also provides rich information about important factors on the interpersonal level of influence. Social support explains why some relationships have more powerful influences on an individual's actions. Relationships with others can facilitate and reinforce behavior through the resources and responses provided through the interaction. Social support theory describes four specific types of support received from networks: emotional, instrumental, information, and appraisal. Emotional support is the act of caring. Instrumental support is the sharing of resources and goods that are related to behavioral action. Informational support is the sharing of knowledge and advice that can facilitate change. Finally, appraisal support provides constructive feedback for future action. Support can facilitate and reinforce behavioral action.

Social Cognitive Theory

The social cognitive theory is the most widely referenced theory in health promotion literature and practice (Glanz & Bishop, 2010). The basic concept of SCT is that behavior is learned, and it is learned through a person's **dynamic** interaction with his or her environment. The social environment, in particular, serves as a source of information about behaviors, procedures, and outcomes. Information from the environment is taken in by the person via cognitions and then influences the person's thoughts, expectations, and abilities. The popularity of the theory is due in part to this "learned behavior" concept as well as the origins of self-efficacy. First, if behavior is learned, it can be taught. After explaining how behavior is learned, practitioners can shape those factors and teach target behaviors. In this regard, SCT lends itself well to designing person-focused interventions. Second, self-efficacy originates from SCT (Bandura, 1986). By now, readers have seen numerous times that self-efficacy

is a consistent predictor of behavioral action. The idea that a person's confidence in performing actions is an important predictor of action was developed by Dr. Albert Bandura as part of this learned behavior phenomenon and will be discussed in this chapter.

Central to SCT is the idea that because the individual interacts in various social and physical environments, factors of these environments influence a person's ability to act. The interactions with factors outside the individual also influence the individual's cognitions and future actions. The resources available in an individual's environment influence his or her own behavior. For example, the availability of fruits and vegetables influences one's intake of fruits and vegetables. In addition, observing others and their consumption of fruits and vegetables also influences one's beliefs about fruits and vegetables, as well as knowing how to and being able to prepare and store foods.

The interaction and influence of the various categories of factors is a construct known as **reciprocal determinism**. Behavior, cognitions, and environmental influences all operate interactively as determinants of each other (Bandura, 1986). These three categories of influences can be imagined as forming a triangle, with arrows denoting bidirectional interactions (see Figure 6-2). In this feedback loop of information and influence, there is mutual action between the factors (reciprocal) and the production of effects (determinism). Relationships between factors of influence are a fundamental component of all health behavior theory. For example, the previous chapter discussed how attitudes toward a behavior and subjective norm influence one's intention to complete a behavior. Likewise, the perceived threat of an illness

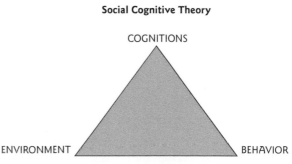

Figure 6-2 Social Cognitive Theory

is influenced by perceived susceptibility and severity. The described relationships were linear. Reciprocal determinism differs because the feedback loops are multidirectional between factors. A can influence B, and B can influence A; both A and B can influence and be influenced by C.

Reciprocal determinism also characterizes relationships of constructs by the types and number of potential relationships. First, many factors are often needed to produce an effect or action. The same factor, then, can be involved in different combinations of relationships that produce different effects (Bandura, 1986). For example, cognitions can be determined by a particular situation. The situation that one is in influences particular beliefs. Self-efficacy is one of those beliefs; in certain environments, one's confidence in the ability to perform an action (self-efficacy) may be higher or lower. As a result of changes in the context and self-efficacy, behavioral performance may vary. Second, relationships between factors are not fixed in a sequential order. In a behavioral chain, influence can originate with any behavioral factor. For example, a belief about a behavior (outcome expectations) can influence intention to act (goal). If that outcome occurs after performing the behavior (reinforcement), then the belief becomes more cemented, and there is an impact on future behavior.

Because of the three categories of factors, the numerous concepts within each category, and the potential interaction among the factors, the social cognition theory can be quite comprehensive. Social cognitive theory's most common and useful constructs related to health promotion are introduced in the following sections. To aid the reader, the following sections are organized by the three domains of potential interactions: personal factors, environment, and behavior.

Personal Factors

Interpersonal theories of behavior change differ from intrapersonal theories because of the inclusion of social and physical environmental factors of influence. In interpersonal models, cognitions and other personal factors still play a significant role in learning and maintaining a health behavior. Albert Bandura (1986), the developer of SCT, notes that if "human behavior always co-varied closely with the occurrence of external events, there would be no need to postulate any internal determinants" (p. 454). People in the same environments exhibit different behaviors, though. An individual's

knowledge, beliefs, and other cognitive factors remain an important influence on behavior. **Cognitions** are at the core of ecological models and are important to a person's motivation to act. People are able to think about actions before carrying them out, and this forethought plays a major role in determining future actions. Further, individuals interpret others' and their own actions along with environmental feedback and incorporate these influences into future behavior. Some of the important cognitive processes include setting personal goals, appraising personal capabilities (also known as self-efficacy), determining motivation felt toward carrying out a behavior or achieving a goal, problem solving, and inferring possible outcomes of behaviors (Bandura, 1989).

Self-efficacy

A key construct of SCT is self-efficacy. **Self-efficacy** is an individual's perceived confidence that he or she is capable of carrying out a specific action (Bandura, 1997). The belief that one can overcome obstacles and stick with a task is vital to any sort of behavior change. Someone who believes in his or her capabilities is usually able to overcome temporary failures or setbacks, whereas individuals with low self-efficacy are more likely to give up or settle for results that are below their original goals (Bandura, 1989). A person with a strong sense of self-efficacy is able to visualize positive outcomes, which in turn increases his or her motivation to persevere with the target behavior (Bandura, 1986). As a result, self-efficacy can be the missing link between knowing what to do and being able to perform the skill in a given situation. People must have the skill and think that they can use the skill before they can use it effectively. Programs teach and shape skills through education and modeling, but an individual's personal judgment about using that skill is just as important (if not more so) to "real-world" behavioral action.

Self-efficacy is unique in that it has a variety of documented relationships to behavioral action. First, self-efficacy has many indirect relationships to behavioral action. Self-efficacy influences constructs such as skills and outcome expectations related to action, so the relationship is indirectly related to behavioral action (Bandura, 2004). But self-efficacy has also been shown to have direct relationships with a target behavior (Bandura, 2004). One's confidence in performing the target behavior can itself predict performance of the target behavior. For example, confidence in exercising has a relationship with the amount of exercise a person performs (Bauman et al., 2012). Confidence in remaining a nonsmoker is related to cessation success (Gwaltney et al., 2009). Finally, behavioral action and self-efficacy have a strong reciprocal relationship. Confidence influences actions, *and* successful action influences confidence.

Self-efficacy is skill and situation specific. Confidence in performing a skill is linked to a specific skill. Efficacy for healthy eating is different from efficacy for exercising. Similarly, confidence in performing that skill can vary based on environmental context. People may feel more or less confident about their ability in certain situations. Situations can vary by the complexity of the skill needed, by the social influencers, and by the outcome expectations. For example, keeping a food diary is an important skill for balancing caloric intake. It can be a simple behavior: record the foods eaten, the amounts eaten, and the associated calories. When eating out, during holidays, and over weekends, the skill can become a bit more complex and, therefore, confidence and behavioral action may drop.

Skill progressions and context variations affect self-efficacy. People need to be able to perform the skill in various situations and be confident in their ability to perform. Think about the ability to drive a car and its relationship to self-efficacy. Driving a car is a skill that many adults use on a daily basis. Driving situations tend to progress in complexity, and if a driver is successful in a more complex situation, the result is an increase in self-efficacy. **Mastery** occurs through practice and successful experience in a variety of situations. Early driving experiences likely involve the new driver and a single adult passenger, with the driver keeping both hands on the wheel. Following success in that experience, the driver may progress to multiple passengers, evening driving, and listening to the radio while driving. The level of skill and self-efficacy can eventually progress to driving on a curvy road, highway driving, driving in snow, and other challenging contexts. The ability to drive in a variety of situations and the confidence to drive in those situations reflects the concept of mastery. Graduated driving license programs, referenced in the In the News feature at the beginning of this chapter, restrict new teen drivers' privileges to more introductory environments and ease drivers into more difficult driving situations.

Self-efficacy can develop in a variety of ways. The two most common ways to build feelings of self-efficacy are through one's own experiences and through **vicarious experiences** (Bandura, 1986). Developing efficacy through one's own experiences is called **enactive attainment**. Simply carrying out a behavior successfully one time may be enough to develop an individual's sense of self-efficacy. Mastery, however, is improved confidence in a skill through the successful completion of the action in a number of situations and contexts (Bandura, 1997). The more difficult the skill and/or situation, the greater the potential increase in efficacy. Self-efficacy can also develop vicariously, through observing others. Watching others perform a task can teach the skill, which in turn can introduce efficacy. For example, after watching a peer cook a meal, swing a golf club, or exercise on a piece of equipment, an individual may walk away from the experience thinking, "I can do that!" In SCT-based interventions, role-playing or other behavioral practice exercises target performance-based efficacy, and peer modeling targets vicarious development of skills and efficacy.

Two other sources of information related to self-efficacy development are verbal persuasion and emotional/physiological arousal. **Verbal persuasion** is widely used to talk people into believing they have the necessary capabilities related to a desired action (Bandura, 1986). Like vicarious experiences, the source of learning is from other people. But with verbal persuasion, the information is not observed; rather, it is communicated via directions, encouragement, and feedback. Verbal persuasion, also called social persuasion, improves confidence, particularly when the action is within one's skill level. The effects on efficacy can be more short term than effects gained through one's own performance and vicarious learning, but this remains a target of many interventions for early stage action (Bandura, 1977). Finally, one's **physiological arousal** can also influence the perception of skill ability. Fear, anxiety, and similar emotions can inhibit successful behavioral action. For example, experiencing upsetting news prior to driving may affect one's ability to perform the behavior. When individuals are in fearful or stressful states, those emotions affect their confidence. Fear arousal may be a natural part of some skill execution; increased the heart rate, blood pressure, and respirations are natural arousal responses. Teaching individuals to manage arousal so that they do not decrease efficacy and skill ability is the target of interventions. Modeling and behavioral rehearsal are two means of removing dysfunctional fears (Bandura, 1997, 1977).

Collective efficacy is a specific type of efficacy related to the shared beliefs of a group or population of people. **Collective efficacy** is the group's shared belief in its shared capabilities to organize and execute the courses of action required to produce given levels of attainments (Bandura, 1997, 2000). Perceived collective efficacy fosters group motivational commitment to their missions, resilience to adversity, and performance accomplishments.

Outcome Expectations

Individuals develop ideas about what they believe will occur if they act a certain way. These are known as outcome expectations. **Outcome expectations** are judgments of the likely consequences that a behavior will produce (Bandura, 1986). Like self-efficacy, outcome expectations are important to one's motivation to act. People who believe that good things will occur as a result of their action are more likely to act. Conversely, individuals who anticipate a negative outcome are less likely to take action. If a person expects to fail every time she performs a behavior, how often will she try? Expectations can be positive or negative as well as psychological/emotional, social, or physical. Emotionally, one might think about success and pride as outcome expectations. Socially, making friends, connecting to others, and enjoyment are possible expectations. Physically, one might develop expectations of a reward, a hug, or another physical benefit.

> **Check for Understanding** Pick a health behavior and list its negative outcome expectations. Sort the expectations into the following categories: emotional, social, and physical.

Outcome expectations are developed by observing others and through one's own experiences. First, a person develops expectations by watching others. In the course of a day, one observes others performing a variety of health-related behaviors. Eating, physical activity, driving, sleeping, alcohol use, contraception use, health care use, and communication are a few examples. In addition to observing the behavior, one also observes outcomes of the behavior. This pattern of action and outcome develops expectations for one's own future behavior. Family, friends, co-workers, neighbors, and service providers are all sources of observed actions and related outcomes.

Media can have a strong influence on outcome expectations. Advertising, television shows, and books contain stories of numerous behaviors and actions. People can develop ideas of acceptable behavior by witnessing the types of actions that receive favorable responses or approval from others, as well as unacceptable behavior by paying attention to what is ridiculed or punished. Watching others receive desirable outcomes from health-related behaviors develops expectations for one's own actions. In some instances, the behavior-outcome pattern shown in media can be inaccurate and can include mixed messages. A teenager can learn about the legal consequences of drunk driving by watching the evening news but change the channel and see a television show depicting the fun social interactions associated with underage drinking.

Other people are one source of outcome expectations; self is the second source. Through prior experiences with behaviors, a person develops outcome expectations for future behavior. The behavioral outcome that one experienced previously is likely to occur again. Outcome expectations are also partly influenced by an individual's level of self-efficacy, that is, someone with strong self-efficacy is more likely to imagine positive outcomes because she is confident in her abilities to carry out the activity (Bandura, 1989). As a person's experiences with behaviors change, in time and/or context, the outcome expectations can also change.

Knowledge

Knowledge is the third cognition that influences behavioral action. **Knowledge** implies the possession of information, sometimes a large category of information. In social cognitive theory, two specific types of knowledge are helpful to facilitate behavioral action. First, being able to identify health risks and benefits creates interest in change (Bandura, 2004). Needing the benefits of change and having the opportunity to effect that change begin to motivate an individual to act. Without knowing that change is warranted, people are unlikely to initiate action.

A second type of knowledge, called **procedural knowledge**, is knowing *how* to do something. The premise of SCT is that behavior is learned, and part of learning behavior and the related skills involves information about how to act. All skills, whether related to health or other areas, have an element of procedural knowledge. Knowing what to do and in what order are the steps to the behavioral action. Procedural knowledge related to behavioral skills can vary in complexity. Some skills can be very simple, like how to schedule preventive cancer screenings. Other skills can be more complex, like the preparation work for a colonoscopy. Identifying environmental resources also has an information component. Being able to identify what resources are available, where the resources are located, and how they can be accessed prepares a person for action.

Knowledge is an important part of the change process, but by itself is insufficient to produce and sustain behavioral change. Bandura notes, "It is not enough to convince people that they should alter risky habits. . . . People also need guidance on how to translate their concerns into efficacious actions" (1994, p. 36). Consider again the information about driving in this chapter's In the News feature . . . knowledge enables an individual to start the car engine and provides some operating instructions to the driver, but the driver still needs to be able to drive the car in a variety of conditions. Table 6-1 summarizes the SCT constructs.

Environment

The **environment** is external to one's self and is made up of physical surroundings as well as other people, cultural influences, and media. The environment influences outcome expectations and feelings of self-efficacy, presents challenges on a daily basis, provides tangible and emotional resources, and presents examples of various types of behaviors for observation.

Observational Learning

A person learns by watching others. In the process of observing others, one sees a behavior and observes the outcome. Individuals do learn through the process of trial and error but are also are able to learn by watching others. This learning by observation is known as vicarious learning, and it is a significant source of learning throughout one's life span. Through **observational learning**, children learn language and social skills, adolescents learn about risk behaviors like alcohol and tobacco use, and adults learn about financial

TABLE 6-1 Constructs of Social Cognitive Theory

Construct	Definition
Knowledge	Information related to risk or benefit. Procedural knowledge is how to perform an action.
Self-efficacy	A person's confidence in performing an action.
Collective efficacy	A group's belief in its shared capabilities to organize and execute the courses of action required.
Outcome expectations	Beliefs about the likely consequences of a behavior.
Observational learning	The process of watching the actions of others and the outcomes associated with the actions.
Reinforcements	The actions or consequences that occur after a behavior is performed. Positive reinforcements increase the likelihood of future action; negative reinforcements decrease the likelihood of future action.
Incentive motivation	The use of rewards and punishments to modify behavior.
Behavioral capability	A person's ability to perform a given action.
Facilitation	The provision of resources, tools, or environmental change.
Self-regulation	The ability to set goals, track progress, and problem solve toward a behavioral target.
Reciprocal determinism	The dynamic interaction of personal, behavioral, and environmental factors.

management, conflict resolution, and health care utilization. Being able to anticipate outcomes through observing others tremendously increases the capacity for learning and acting. One's abilities and confidence would be far less, and slower to develop, if trial and error were the only method of behavioral development. Of course, many skills, like speaking a second language or playing an instrument, are too complex to be learned or understood simply through observation. The combination of learning through one's own experiences and vicarious learning increases the capacity for behavioral development.

Observational learning is basically the processing of information. The information being processed is the skill that is, "What do I do, how do I do it, and in what sequence?" The outcomes associated with the observed actions are a second part of information processing. For example, if someone has seen a friend successfully quit smoking, he or she has also probably seen the friend cope by chewing nicotine gum or using nicotine patches and avoiding social situations where smoking is prevalent. The individual can use these observations and positive testimony from the friend about improved health to think about how quitting may impact his or her own life. Someone else may consider quitting smoking too difficult while working in a job with a lot of co-workers who smoke, but he or she may reevaluate this difficulty after moving to a new company that encourages employees to quit smoking.

Not all observed behaviors are effectively learned. Factors involving both the model and the learner can play a role in the degree of observational learning. For learning to occur, the learner must be able to pay attention and retain the information, as well as be able to reproduce the action (Bandura, 1986). Attributes of the model also affect the amount of learning and motivation. Watching people similar to oneself, in terms of demographic traits (e.g., age, gender) and abilities, tends to be more meaningful. For example, female novice athletes demonstrate a stronger sense of physical ability and efficacy after exposure to abilities modeled by other non- or new athletes (Bandura, 1997). The ability to relate to the model improves motivation, attention, and the transfer of information. Observational learning, through those similar to self, is called peer modeling. It becomes both a behavioral target and an intervention tool in health promotion interventions.

Reinforcements

Reinforcements are the actions or consequences that occur after a behavior is performed (Bandura, 1986). Reinforcements increase or decrease the likelihood of future behavior. If something desirable happens as the result of an action, a person is more likely to repeat the behavior (positive reinforcement). If something undesirable happens as the result of an action, one is less likely to repeat the behavior (negative reinforcement). Reinforcements are central in behavioral development, the construction of outcome expectations, and the repeated performance of behaviors.

Reinforcements and outcome expectations are closely related. Outcome expectations are present *before* one acts, whereas reinforcements come *after* the behavior is completed. Based on the reinforcements seen or experienced, individuals modify their original outcome expectations or create new ones. Thus, outcome expectations and reinforcements have a bidirectional relationship and are moderated by behavioral action. In this relationship, outcome expectations also influence the interpretation of reinforcements. For instance, sometimes a person engages in a behavior and has concerns about the outcome, for example, participating in a health screening and worrying about embarrassment or discomfort. If those feared outcomes do not happen, the occurrence of "nothing" can be a positive reinforcement. Similarly, if someone expects to hate all forms of exercise but ends up enjoying a kickboxing class, he might interpret it as positive reinforcement despite his sore muscles.

Reinforcements come from the person performing the action as well as from the environment. **Intrinsic** factors originate from within the person, and **extrinsic** factors are external to the person. Extrinsic reinforcements tend to be sensory, social, monetary, or activity in nature (Bandura, 1986). Sensory feedback appeals to sight, sound, smell, and touch. Infants repeatedly perform acts that produce sounds and sights. An infant may hit a button on a toy and the button lights up and makes noise, so she hits the button again. Adults can also be moved by sensory feedback. For example, when walking on a treadmill or riding an exercise bike, the bars on the screen that are tracking and encouraging continued action are sensory reinforcements. Social reinforcements come from other people in the form of interest, approval, and reactions. Social reactions can take many forms, for example, an expression, a physical act, or withholding. They can be as simple as a smile or a thumbs-up, or as extravagant as a large cash prize. Monetary incentives, both money and goods, can be used as a reward or as a punishment to reinforce action. Activity feedback and reinforcements are the last category of extrinsic reinforcements. As the name implies, activity reinforcements pair select activities with another action. Parents use activity-type reinforcements frequently. Offering video game time, television watching, snacks, and delayed bedtimes are examples of activity reinforcements possibly paired with behaviors such as homework, chores, or "behaving."

By contrast, intrinsic factors originate from one's self and are biologically and psychologically based. Psychologically, an action may give a person a sense of accomplishment or a sense of pride. In a negative direction, an action may produce feelings of shame or embarrassment. Both the positive psychological states and the negative states alter the likelihood of future action. Actions that bring positive feelings are more likely to be repeated. Biologically, behavioral action can produce physical outcomes such as soreness, enhanced energy, or weight loss.

Not all positive reinforcements support healthy behavioral development. Positive reinforcements increase the likelihood of a future behavioral action, whether or not the behavior is healthy or socially acceptable (Bandura, 1986). With tobacco use, many intrinsic and extrinsic reinforcements increase the likelihood of future action. The "kick" smokers report from that first drag and the cessation of withdrawal symptoms are two examples of intrinsic reinforcements. The feelings from the first inhale tend to reinforce future action; by contrast, the anxiety of withdrawal also reinforces smoking. Extrinsically, being included in peer smoking breaks and bonding with others can reinforce the unhealthy behavior.

Incentive Motivation

Incentive motivation is an extension of the construct of reinforcements to reflect *the process* of using rewards and punishments to modify behavior. Incentive motivation is often a target for interventions. For example, behavioral contracts for change prompt people to set a goal, track progress, and include a reward. The reward may be time for a hobby, a material object, or an activity with a loved one. Identifying a forthcoming reward requires the process of managing reinforcements to encourage behavior. Conversely, removing activities that provide undesirable reinforcements is another example of incentive motivation. For example, time with peers is a reinforcement for smoking while at work. A smoke break is a time to chat with others and is one of the positive reinforcements of the behavior. Scheduling a replacement activity that allows a person to continue spending time with peers, such as a walking break or a juice break, proactively uses the system of reinforcements to support cessation.

> **Check for Understanding** List three behaviors that you learned by observing others. Explain the role of observational learning and reinforcements to the development of the behavior.

Facilitation

Behavior change would be easy if there were no impediments to overcome. Perceived facilitators and obstacles are another determinant of health behaviors (Bandura, 2004). **Facilitation** is the provision of tools, resources, or environmental change necessary to facilitate behavioral action. Like incentive motivation, facilitation is a *process* and a target of health promotion interventions. For example, in safer sex education programs, students are provided with condoms and other modes of contraception. The provision of these resources facilitates execution of the desired action. Having condoms, as well as the skill and efficacy to use them, are necessary to use them consistently and correctly (Kirby, Laris, & Rolleri, 2007). Environmental structures can also be manipulated through interventions to promote and facilitate the target behavior. Environmental facilitation involves both the addition and the subtraction of resources or attributes. In the physical activity example in Chapter 4, sidewalks, crosswalks, and comfort features of an environment facilitate walking for transportation.

Facilitation is a multilevel process. Facilitators and barriers operate on every level of social and physical environments (Bandura, 2004). Individual behavior is enabled, or dissuaded, by tools, resources, and environmental properties of families, social networks, organizations, and health care systems.

Behavior

Behavior is ultimately influenced by both cognitive and environmental factors. While people need to react to environmental influences and conditions, that reaction is not automatic and out of a person's control. Furthermore, although a person may be able to fully think about how he intends to act, the goals he plans to stick to, and the coping skills he is going to use, the environment he finds himself in at a certain point in time may render part or all of his forethought and planning useless (Bandura, 1989). Behavior change is often viewed as a feedback loop in which the positive reinforcements one receives confirms that he is making the right choices and negative reinforcements encourage him to make changes to achieve the desired positive result (Bandura, 1989).

Behavioral Capability

The execution of health behaviors over time involves the ability to perform skills related to the action. **Behavioral capability** is the construct name for skills related to health behavior. What does a person need to be able to do to execute the behavior? Within content areas, the skills take on specific names. For example, reading labels, planning menus, and estimating portion size are three skills related to the health behavior of caloric balance to maintain a healthy weight. There are skills involved in quitting behaviors, too. Trigger management skills and coping skills are two skill sets related to successful tobacco cessation (Fiore et al., 2008). For some health behaviors, the skills might seem much simpler. Participating in preventive cancer screenings involves the sub-skills of making an appointment and accessing information about testing facilities. These skills may not require as much practice as other skills but are nonetheless necessary to carry out the health behavior.

Skills are content specific, for example, reading labels and meal preparation within nutrition content areas. There are also general skills that have relationships across health behaviors. Self-regulation is one of those skills sets.

Self-Regulation

Self-regulation is the ability to set goals, track progress, and solve problems to meet those goals. It is an umbrella term for describing the process of pursuing and attaining goals (Mann, de Ridder, & Fujita, 2013). Self-regulation is a self-directed process that involves cognitive and behavioral processes that are involved in the adoption of new behaviors and the long-term maintenance of behaviors. Like self-efficacy, the concept of self-regulation is widely adopted and has strong relationships with health behaviors (Bandura, 1986, 2004; Glanz & Bishop, 2010).

Self-regulation begins with goal setting. **Goals** are statements of desired outcomes to which people intend to commit action. Goal setting works by focusing one's attention. By setting standards of behavior (goal statements), individuals create self-inducements to act until their action equals the standard of performance. A discrepancy between behavior and desired state increases motivation to perform (Bandura, 1986; Mann et al., 2013). Goals can target various objects. In health promotion, behavioral targets work best to influence action. Behavioral goals include behavior targets, not behavior-related outcomes, for example, exercising, not losing weight. Goal setting involves being able to identify modifiable targets and setting realistic and attainable levels of performance (Bandura, 1986).

The ability to track progress toward the goal is another skill involved in self-regulation. Tracking mechanisms provide an accurate assessment and information about current actions. Without logs or diaries, people have a tendency to overestimate their fruit and vegetable intake as well as activity levels. Goal setting and tracking mechanisms such as logs work synergistically throughout the process of change. First, logs identify areas for which to set goals for improvement. A log will identify intake and activity levels across a period of time and as a result, trends that may go unnoticed without a record become visible. Logs can also shape behavior through the process of recording the behavior. There is a level of immediate ownership to a behavior when it is written down, and diaries may contribute to fewer bites, snacks, and second helpings. Finally, logs serve as a source of positive reinforcement once the goal is achieved. Numerous studies have found that when people keep journals, caloric intake can go down by several hundred calories and physical activity can increase by 35% (Burke, Wang, & Sevick, 2011; Guide to Community Preventative Services, 2014).

Setting goals and tracking progress forms a feedback loop with behavior. Long-term continuation of action also involves the cognitive and behavioral processes of making behavioral and strategy adjustments. The process of changing or adopting a new behavior is often full of setbacks, plateaus, and struggles, so it is imperative for an individual to develop ways of dealing with these challenges. Interventions planned by using SCT to model behavior change often concentrate on self-regulation skills such as setting attainable goals and keeping a journal of the target behavior (healthy eating, exercising, etc.), as well as skills and efficacy to aid a person in solving problems (Bandura & Wood, 1989). A new exerciser may encounter environmental challenges, such as bad weather, lack of sidewalks, or injury, that require him to use problem-solving skills to overcome challenges and continue working toward his goal. He may perceive positive feedback (losing weight, feeling stronger, support from family members) and negative feedback (injury, stress due to time commitment) that will impact his motivation and determination.

Self-regulation has been a recommended practice for a number of health behaviors. The shaping of self-regulation skills is a widely recommended and evidence-supported practice (Community Preventive Services Task Force, 2012). Practice guidelines within medicine, specifically guidelines for lifestyle management of obesity and overweight, hypertension, diabetes, and asthma, all include recommendations for patient goal setting, record keeping, and problem-solving coaching (self-regulation) (Lin et al., 2010; USDHHS, 1998, 2004, 2007).

> **Check for Understanding** What skills are involved in driving an automobile? How might situational efficacy influence those skills?

Application of the Social Cognitive Theory

SCT has been applied to a variety of fields, including public health, marketing, and education. Researchers have used SCT to explain behavior and plan interventions in areas such as childhood nutrition, STI and pregnancy prevention, physical activity, HIV treatment compliance, and bullying in high schools (Lopez et al, 2013; Nokes et al., 2012; Plotnikoff, 2013; Prati, 2012; Rinderknecht & Smith, 2004). Most skill-based health promotion interventions are formed using the social cognitive theory.

Safer sex programs emerged in the late 1980s as part of the national plan to address the alarming increases in HIV infections. These new health education programs were based on the social cognitive theory framework and taught safer sexual practices. The programs represented a significant paradigm shift from the information- and pledge-based education of the time (Merson et al., 2008). Correct and consistent condom use was the targeted outcome behavior. The behavior was shaped through building procedural knowledge, efficacy, and the skills of correct usage. The person- and network- (interpersonal) focused education was also supported by massive awareness campaigns that targeted the norms of condom use. Figure 6-3 shows a campaign poster from the Maryland Department of Health and Mental Hygiene.

Backed by federal funding, these HIV prevention programs were the first large wave of interventions based on health-related skill building and reciprocal determinism. The foundation of facilitating safer sexual practices through social cognitive means continues today. In a 2013 review of theory-based contraception use interventions, SCT interventions were most common, followed by the health belief model (Kirby et al., 2007; Lopez et al., 2013).

Safer Choices is an SCT-based STI and pregnancy prevention program. Program evaluations have documented increased condom use, delayed age of sexual initiation, and fewer unprotected sexual partners (Advocates for Youth, 2012; Coyle et al., 2001; Kirby et al., 2004). The curriculum builds specific skills related to condom use and delayed/reduced sexual activity. Correct condom use, condom negotiation, refusing unwanted sex, setting personal limits, purchasing contraception, and communication are skills built in the lessons. Students learn the procedural knowledge for the skills, practice the skills via role-playing and peer modeling, and build efficacy and develop positive outcome expectations through these activities (Coyle et al., 1999; Kirby et al., 2004; Kirby et al., 2007). Knowledge of STIs and pregnancy, awareness of personal risks, and perceived norms are other common changes credited to the program (Kirby et al., 2007).

Of the four behavioral targets (delayed initiation, condom use, contraception use, and number of sexual partners), Safer Choices had the greatest impact on condom use. Sexually experienced students who participated in the program and who reported having sexual intercourse during the prior 3 months were 1.68 times more likely to have used condoms than students who did not participate in the program (Coyle et al., 2001). Program impacts were larger for males than females (Kirby et al., 2004). Students also reported 25% fewer sexual partners with whom they had sexual intercourse without a condom. In a review of Safer Choices and similar skill-based curriculum, positive behavioral changes were demonstrated across a variety of groups, regardless of their gender, ethnicity, or sexual experience (Advocates for Youth, 2012; Kirby et al., 2007).

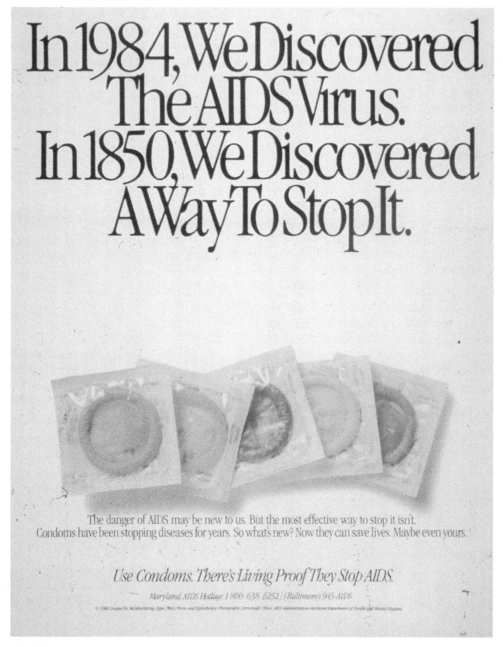

Figure 6-3 AIDS Public Health Poster.

Source: the U.S. National Library of Medicine: www.nlm.nih.gov/index.html

Social Support

People play a large role in influencing the actions of others. As explained in the previous section, social environments provide opportunities to observe others and receive feedback from others. Through observation and interaction, people develop ideas about their own actions, efficacy, and outcomes. Another person-based product facilitated through engagement within a social environment is that of social support. **Social support** consists of the various types of assistance exchanged through social relationships (House, 1981; Bandura, 2004). Social support is positive in nature; it is intended by the contributor to be helpful and/or supportive. It is not intended to be harmful or disingenuous. The person's offer of support is also intentional, as opposed to accidental or unconscious. He or she purposefully takes action in support of another; whether the recipient perceives the support as positive or helpful is a different story (Bandura, 1986).

Social support is an environmental resource. People give advice, goods, and/or feedback in a manner that can facilitate behavior change. Support can enable action through the provision of tangible or informational resources as well as motivate one to take action through the enhancement of self-efficacy (Bandura, 1997). Social support "theory" comes from not only social cognitive frameworks but also from across works in attachment theory, exchanges theory, and attribution theory (Bandura, 1997; Berkman et al., 2000; Umberson, Crosnoe, & Reczek, 2010). Thus, social support is more accurately labeled as a theoretical concept that fits multiple places within the body of health behavior theory knowledge. It is not a stand-alone theory. The construct of support, its various subtypes, and hypothesized relationship with other factors of behavior will be discussed.

Social networks differ from support. Networks are the structure, or the frame, of social relationships. Networks have been described as webs, with the dots representing people and the lines representing relationships (Berkman 1984; Smith & Christakis, 2008). Social network analysis is the study of the properties of those dots, those lines, and the larger web. Social networks look different for different people. Networks can be large, small, and every size in between; further, the relationships that surround a person can differ across life stages (Uchino, 2009; Umberson et al., 2010). Regardless of size or structure, social support is one of the primary functions of a social network. Within the ties, people offer and receive support. A network's influence on health and behavior, though, extends well beyond the provision of social support (Berkman et al., 2000; House, Umberson, & Landis, 1988). The structure and secondary purposes of networks will be one of the topics in the next chapter. For now, the discussion is about social support, a property that is provided through social ties with others.

Types of Support

Social support refers to various types of assistance that people receive from and offer to others. A bus pass, a phone number, the name of a physician, and a hug are a few examples of such support. Broadly, people share resources and information within their social ties, and there are countless types of support, which can be organized into four categories: emotional, instrumental, informational, and appraisal (see Table 6-2). The subtypes of support are discussed in distinct categories, though they rarely exist independently. People who are invested enough in an individual to provide social support typically offer more than one type of support. A family member who provides encouragement and love along with rides to weight loss meetings is providing emotional and instrumental support. A friend who offers nutritional advice and cheers on an individual to continue making his own healthy eating choices contributes information and appraisal support.

Emotional support consists of communicating feelings of love, caring, empathy, and trust (House, 1981). **Emotional support** refers to the things that people do to make us feel loved and cared for and bolster a sense of self-worth. Talking over a problem, providing encouragement, or just listening

TABLE 6-2 Types of Social Support

Type of Support	Definition
Emotional	Expressions of kindness, love, and empathy
Instrumental	The provision of goods or services
Informational	Advice, suggestions, or information
Appraisal	A specific type of information that aids in self-evaluation

Source: House, 1981; House & Kahn, 1985.

and nodding are examples of emotional support. Emotional support is most likely to occur in primary relationships, where an intimate partner or close tie often provides emotional support (Thoits, 2011). Other less intimate ties can also provide emotional support; however, emotional support from secondary ties tends to occur under specific conditions (Thoits, 2011). For example, a co-worker encourages another co-worker on a specific work issue, or a neighbor steps in to express support of a family issue.

People who offer physical or tangible aid and services are said to supply **instrumental support**. Instrumental support refers to the various types of physical goods or services that others may provide; help with child care or housekeeping and providing transportation or money are examples of instrumental support. Instrumental support can also be called tangible support because the aid offered is a material, physical, or service good.

Informational support represents a third type of social support and refers to the delivery of advice or information (House, 1981; House & Kahn, 1985). Gathered facts and/or opinions can help another person develop procedural knowledge, build skills, or locate resources. Again, people learn quite a bit from one another; informational support is another mechanism for learning. The fourth category of support also is information based, but the information aids in self-evaluation and is called **appraisal support**. Appraisal support is constructive or corrective in nature. "If I were you, I would . . ." can be the introductory clause to appraisal support. It can aid in decision making or help someone decide which course of action to take. Appraisal support is similar to the broader category of informational support and at times, the two categories are discussed as one category—informational support.

Perceived versus Received Support

An interesting wrinkle in the workings of social support is the distinction between what a person perceives versus what they actual experience. **Perceived social support** is one's potential for accessing social support (Uchino, 2009). Perceived support is a person's anticipation of future potential aid. Perceived support is general and tends to be anticipated across situations; statements such as "She would do anything for me" reflect the concept of perceived social support. Perceived support is not called upon and has great value. Whether one

actually needs the support or not, it is perceived support that tends to have the documented relationship with health benefits (Thoits, 2011; Uchino, 2009).

Received social support, by contrast, is the actual receipt of support resources. Received support is more situational and is triggered by stressful circumstances such as a job issue, childrearing, or a health event (Barrera, 2000; Thoits, 2011; Uchino, 2009). Perceptions, once again, can differ from actual events or information. By definition, received support is an exchange of actual resources between persons and is an interpersonal factor. Perceived support, though, is an intrapersonal factor, that is, it is a belief inside someone's head. Perceived support may or may not occur. *Both* versions of support are important to health, coping, and behavior. They are different constructs, reflecting different attributes. Because the two types of support reflect different attributes, the relationship between the two versions may or may not be related (Thoits, 2011). The contrast of perception to actual experiences has been a common distinction in constructs of intrapersonal theories.

> **Check for Understanding** Reflect on your interactions with others over the past 24 hours. List at least one example of social support received or offered from each support category (emotional, informational, instrumental, and appraisal).

Mechanisms of Social Support

Social support contributes to health outcomes through a variety of mechanisms. In reviews of social support, three consistent pathways to health emerge across the varied lists. Social support can directly impact health and mortality; indirectly, social support can buffer the impact of stress on health, and social support can also serve as an antecedent that facilitates health behavior (Anderson et al., 2003; Berkman et al., 2000; House et al., 1988; Stansfeld, 2006; Thoits, 2011; Uchino, 2009; Umberson et al., 2010).

Reduce Mortality

In general, people need connections to other people. Connections to others lead to psychological, physiological, and functional benefits; the lack of social relationships can negatively impact mental and physical health.

Social integration is participation in a broad range of relationships (Berkman et al., 2000). Social integration promotes positive psychological states (identity, purpose, self-worth, and positive effect) that induce health-promoting physiological responses (Berkman et al., 2000; Cohen, 2004; Uchino, 2009). Relationships provide opportunity and purpose. There is the opportunity to engage in a wide range of social activities or relationships and a sense of communality and identification with one's social roles.

One of the most cited studies on the subject of social relationships and health was that of the life expectancy of residents of Alameda County, California. Researchers found that healthy adults were more socially integrated. People who lacked social and community ties were more likely to die in the follow-up period than those with more extensive contacts. The group of men with the fewest social connections had an age-adjusted mortality rate 2.3 times higher than men with the most social connections. Women who had the lowest number of social connections had an age-adjusted mortality rate 2.8 times higher than the mortality rate for women with the most social connections. Close relationships were achieved through marriage, close family and friends, and meaningful social and religious groups (Berkman & Syme, 1979; Berkman, 1984).

Stress Buffering

The second mechanism by which social support contributes to health outcomes is indirectly through buffering. Social support may intervene between a stressful event and a person's stress response; the support buffers the impact of the event. Buffering eliminates or reduces effects of stressful experiences by promoting less threatening interpretations of adverse events and effective coping strategies (Berkman et al., 2000; Cohen, 2004). The belief that others will provide helpful resources may increase one's perceived ability to cope with demands, changing the appraisal of the situation and lowering its effective stress (Cohen & Wills, 1985; Stansfeld, 2006; Thoits, 2011; Uchino, 2009; Wethington & Kessler, 1986). The belief that support is readily available may also improve emotional and physiological responses to the event or alter unhealthy behavioral responses (Cohen, 2004). For example, Cohen and colleagues found that both student and adult groups reported more symptoms of depression and of physical ailments under stress but that these associations were lessened among those who perceived that support was available from their social

networks (Cohen et al., 1985). The receipt of actual support also plays a role in buffering the impact of stress. Support may provide a solution to the stressful problem, reduce the importance of the problem, or provide a distraction (Cohen, 2004).

Health Behavior Antecedent

A second indirect relationship of support to health outcomes is through health behaviors. Social support is a construct whose presence can increase the likelihood of behavior action. Relationships provide information and are a source of motivation and social pressure to care for oneself. Like other theoretical constructs, it is the variation of antecedents that then explains the variation in behavior. Individuals can provide information or resources that help another perform or quit a behavior. Without the information or resources, individuals are less likely to be motivated or able to take action. Informational support can help another person develop procedural knowledge, perform skills, or locate resources. Social support can also reinforce action through appraisal support or emotional support. Likewise, the fourth type of support, instrumental aid in the form of resources and services, can facilitate action.

There is consistent evidence that social support has a reciprocal relationship with another behavioral antecedent, self-efficacy. First, social support can enhance self-efficacy. The provision of emotional, informational, and tangible resources can increase a person's cognitions and expectations for positive outcomes (Bandura, 1997; Berkman et al., 2000; Umberson et al., 2010). A person has the resources he or she needs to be successful, so he or she believes he or she will be successful. Self-efficacy may also alter perceived social support. It is hypothesized that if a person expects to be successful, part of his or her confidence is in the ability to gather the necessary resources to be successful as well (Bandura, 1997). For this reason, social support is particularly important during the early periods of behavioral change (Bandura, 1997, 2004).

Application of the Social Support to Interventions

Social support is a common component of health promotion interventions. Evidence-based programs from physical activity, nutrition, violence, tobacco cessation, sexual risk, breastfeeding, medical treatment adherence, and chronic disease management include social support components (Cotter et al., 2014; DiMatteo, 2004; Guide to Community Preventive Services, 2014; Renfrew et al., 2012). For example, community-wide campaigns and organizational clubs that foster support and shared experiences are effective in getting people to be more physically active, as measured by various means such as blocks walked or flights of stairs climbed daily, frequency of attending exercise sessions, or minutes spent in physical activity (Task Force on Community Preventive Services, 2002). People are more likely to be physically active when they are in the companionship of another. Similarly, new mothers are more likely to initiate and continue breastfeeding an infant when they receive peer support (CDC, 2013; Renfrow et al., 2012). Support includes elements such as reassurance, praise, information, and the opportunity to discuss and respond to the mother's questions.

As an intervention target, social support can be facilitated much like development of skills. Participants can be taught how to develop supportive relationships, whether in an existing network or through the building of new social ties (Anderson et al., 2003; Hogan, Linden & Najarian, 2002; Uchinio, 2009). First, individuals can work with their existing social structures (families, neighborhoods, or organizations) and learn how to support one another. Home visit programs in which trained personnel offer information about child health, development, and care; offer support; provide training; or deliver any combination of these services have demonstrated positive outcomes for child health as well as reductions in child abuse and neglect (Bilukha et al., 2005). Parish health programs also operate within establish networks—the organization of the church. Members of the church, using existing skills or newly acquired skills, offer support to one another through visits, errand running, health screenings, and education.

Some people need to develop or enhance social networks. Building new social ties improves opportunities for support. A number of health promotion programs, by design, provide a forum for building relationships—and therefore, support. Self-help groups and peer-to-peer programs link people with similar goals. To lose weight, to abstain from using harmful substances, or to be a good parent are common goals that can bring people together. Meetings, whether professionally led or peer led, become a forum for information sharing, instruction, and emotional support (Hogan et al., 2002). Face-to-face interactions are the traditional method of many support-based groups; however, new technology-enhanced techniques have emerged as effective mechanisms for social support. Tobacco quit lines and online groups are two examples of social support. In general, cessation rates are 3% higher for individuals who use a quit line and almost 10% higher when the support calls are coupled with the use of nicotine replacement products (Civljak et al., 2010; Guide to Community Preventive Services, 2014; Stead, Hartmann-Boyce, Perera, & Lancaster, 2013).

Model for Understanding: Social Relationships and Health

Social relationships have numerous pathways to health, and new learners can easily get lost in the rich amount of information. In the previous section alone, three broad mechanisms of social influence were summarized: one primary pathway to health and two indirect relationships were presented. The amount of literature on social influences and health is growing quickly and is full of detailed information for practitioners. For example, one of the referenced reviews introduced seven detailed pathways of social support to health (Thoits, 2011). The author took the three primary relationships (direct, buffering, and behavioral antecedent) and broke them down further into subcategories. Adding to the possible confusion, terms such as "social networks," "social support," "social cohesion," and "social capital" sound similar but have different roles in relationships between behaviors and health.

Throughout the text, the disease prevention model has been a way to organize facts, information, and relationships. The model can help categorize information related to social relationships and health. Social relationships that alter life expectancy or risk for disease are a risk factor or protective factor. This relationship moves directly from the social factor to the health outcome (see Figure 6-4). Changing the risk factor alters the likelihood of disease. Examples of behaviors or traits that influence this level of the model are social connectedness, social isolation, proactive coping, and healthy relationship.

Attributes of social relationships that facilitate or inhibit behavior action are behavioral antecedents. This relationship is between attributes on the third level of the model and risk factors of the second level. Operating on the third level, social support is a resource, reinforcement, or information that facilitates or hinders behavioral action. It precedes an action, and the action alters risk for disease. Across a life course, the sources of support vary as social ties grow and change. Over

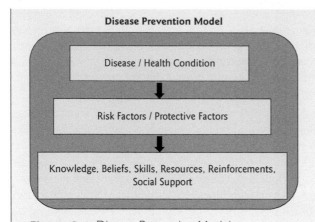

Figure 6-4 Disease Prevention Model

a life course, primary support comes from parents, peers, and then an adult partner (Uchino, 2009; Umberson et al., 2010).

It is important to understand the fundamental relationship in order to develop appropriate interventions. Interventions change behavioral antecedents, which are the third level of the disease prevention model. Interventions seek to change specific knowledge, beliefs, resources, and social support. As understanding of specific social relationships continues to emerge, using the disease prevention model to sort, categorize, and place information will aid in understanding how certain relationships fit into the body of information.

SUMMARY

People learn health behaviors, and a great deal of learning occurs through observation of and interaction with one's social environment. In observing others, people develop ideas about behavior, skills, and outcomes. Individuals also have the ability to influence their own behavior via cognitions and self-regulated action. Self-efficacy, the confidence in completing an action, is important to one's motivation to act and the resolve for continued effort. Self-efficacy also develops through interactions with others and self-experiences. Social support is another environmental resource that enables people to act through the offering of goods and information; support can also enhance self-efficacy and motivation to act. Reciprocal determinism is the social cognitive theory term to describe the multidirectional interactions between behavioral, environmental, and personal factors.

BEHAVIORAL SCIENCE IN ACTION

Violence as a Learned Behavior.

As described earlier in this chapter, people develop a behavior-consequence pattern through observational learning. On a larger scale, the social environment influences people by shaping beliefs on what is and is not socially acceptable behavior. Bandura and colleagues (1961) conducted a series of experiments involving children watching others interact with a doll called a bobo doll. The bobo dolls were inflatable toys usually painted to look like clowns that stood about 5 feet tall and were weighted so that they would return to a standing position after being knocked over.

The group conducted several different versions of the experiment, the first of which occurred in 1961. The children were all between 3 years 6 months and 5 years 11 months old and included an equal number of boys and girls. The first version of the experiment had the children alone in a playroom with one adult and a bobo doll. Some of the children observed an adult physically abusing the doll, including punching, hitting, and striking the doll with a toy mallet while shouting aggressive phrases such as "Sock him!" and "Throw him in the air!" The other children observed an adult quietly playing with other toys while ignoring the bobo doll.

Afterward, the children were taken to a different playroom and allowed to play with any of the toys for a few minutes. An adult then told them these toys were reserved for other children, and they could no longer play with them. With the children now experiencing some frustration, they were led back into the playroom with the bobo doll and allowed to play freely for 20 minutes. Researchers found that the children who had seen the aggressive adults were far more like to engage in aggressive play with the bobo doll than those who had observed the nonaggressive adult (Bandura, Ross, & Ross, 1961). They also found that children were more likely to act aggressively after observing an adult of the same sex acting aggressively and that boys in general were more likely to act aggressively than girls regardless of the sex of the adult model.

In another version of the experiment, conducted in 1963, all groups of children were shown a film of children acting aggressively toward a doll. The control group saw only the child's aggressive behavior, whereas the control groups saw either an adult reward the aggressive behavior with candy or punish the behavior with a scolding (Bandura, Ross, & Ross, 1963). These results showed that the children who had viewed the film ending in punishment showed less aggressive behavior when allowed to play with a bobo doll than the children in the control group or those who saw the child receive candy.

The work of Bandura and colleagues has received a fair amount of criticism. The children used as subjects all attended the nursery school at Stanford University, a prestigious university that was at the time attended by mostly upper middle- and upper-class white students. Although Bandura does not explicitly state the ethnicity or income level of the children, it can be assumed that the majority of the children were from wealthier white families. Some critics have claimed that using children from only one nursery school led to selection bias, and the results do not apply to children of all races and socioeconomic statuses. Others have claimed that the children were too young at the time and were still in a stage of mental development in which they could not always distinguish fantasy from reality, while others claim the children were essentially manipulated into responding in an aggressive manner (Committee on Public Education, 2001; Wortman, Loftus, & Weaver, 1998).

The basic idea of the bobo doll experiments has been adapted by other researchers interested in the behavior of children, college students, and adults. They have studied the impact of violent television, films, and video games, and the majority of studies have found increased aggression or emotional arousal in those assigned to observe the more violent media. Health behavior researchers and practitioners continue to learn more about how observational learning social modeling impacts all manner of health behaviors, and it is likely that Bandura's work will remain influential in future studies.

IN THE CLASSROOM ACTIVITIES

1. List constructs of the social cognitive theory by the three domains of personal factors, environment, and behavior. Once again, take the behavior and list of factors created in Chapter 2 activity #5 homework. Identify factors of influence on the list that reflect constructs of the social cognitive theory and/or social support.

2. How might self-efficacy impact test-taking abilities?

3. Using the link in the Web Link section, visit the Visual Culture and Public Health Posters of the U.S. National Library of Medicine. Select one poster and identify the target audience and the specific belief or norm that is being targeted.

4. Pick one health behavior that tends to change during college years, for example, sleeping, coping, eating, alcohol consumption, and sexual behaviors. Explain potential sources of observational learning for the behavior. Finally, identify four other social cognitive theory constructs that might influence the behavior.

5. Online, access the Centers for Disease Control and Prevention HIV/AIDS Evidence-Based Behavioral Programs. Review one of the programs from either the risk reduction or the medication compliance chapter. Identify the following elements: target audience, outcome behavior(s), skills, and other behavioral mediators.

6. Track your social interactions with others for a period of two days. For each day, record the different types of social support and the sources. Summarize trends in the types of support, the sources of support, and perceived verses received differences.

WEB LINKS

Centers for Disease Control and Prevention HIV/AIDS Evidence-Based Behavioral Programs: http://www.cdc.gov/hiv/prevention/research/compendium/index.html

U.S. National Library of Medicine: www.nlm.nih.gov/index.html

REFERENCES

Advocates for Youth. (2012). *Science and success: Sex education and other programs that work to prevent teen pregnancy, HIV and sexually transmitted infections* (3rd ed.). Washington, DC: Author. Retrieved from http://www.advocatesforyouth.org/programs-that-work-publications

Anderson, L. M., Scrimshaw, S. C., Fullilove, M. T., & Fielding, J. E. (2003). The Community Guide's model for linking the social environment to health. *American Journal of Preventive Medicine, 24*(S3), 12–20.

Bandura, A. (1977). Self-efficacy: Toward a unifying theory of behavioral change. *Psychological Review, 84*(2), 191–215.

Bandura, A. (1986). *Social foundations of thought and action.* Englewood Cliffs, NJ: Prentice Hall.

Bandura, A. (1989). Human agency in social cognitive theory. *American Psychologist, 44*(9), 1175–1184.

Bandura A. (1994). Social cognitive theory and exercise of control over HIV infection. In R. J. DiClemente & J. L. Peterson (Eds.), *Preventing AIDS: Theories and methods of behavioral interventions.* New York: Plenum.

Bandura, A. (1997). *Self-efficacy: The exercise of control.* New York: WH Freeman.

Bandura, A. (2000). Exercise of human agency through collective efficacy. *Current Directions in Psychological Science, 9*(3), 75–78.

Bandura, A. (2004). Health promotion by social cognitive means. *Health Education & Behavior, 31*(2), 143–164.

Bandura, A., Ross, D., & Ross, S. A. (1961). Transmission of aggression through imitation of aggressive models. *Journal of Abnormal and Social Psychology, 63,* 575–582.

Bandura, A., Ross, D., & Ross, S. A. (1963). Imitation of film-mediated aggressive models. *Journal of Abnormal and Social Psychology, 66*(1), 3–11.

Bandura, A., & Wood, R. E. (1989). Effect of perceived controllability and performance standards on self-regulation of complex decision-making. *Journal of Personality and Social Psychology, 56,* 805–814.

Barrera, M. (2000). Social support research in community psychology. In J. Rappaport and E. Seidman (Eds.), *Handbook of community psychology* (pp. 215–245). New York: Kluwer Academic/Plenum.

Bauman, A. E., Reis, R. S., Sallis, J. F., Wells, J. C., Loos, R. J., & Martin, B. W. (2012). Correlates of physical activity: Why are some people physically active and others not? *Lancet, 38,* 258–271.

Berkman, L. (1984). Assessing the physical health effects of social networks and social support. *Annual Review of Public Health, 5,* 413–432.

Berkman, L. F., Glass, T., Brissette, I., & Seeman, T. E. (2000). From social integration to health: Durkheim in the new millennium. *Social Science and Medicine, 51,* 843–857.

Berkman, L. F., & Syme, S. L. (1979). Social networks, host resistance, and mortality: A nine-year follow-up study of Alameda County residents. *American Journal of Epidemiology, 109*(2), 186–204.

Bilukha, O., Hahn, R. A., Crosby, A., Fullilove, M. T., Liberman, A., Moscicki, E., et al. (2005). The effectiveness of early childhood home visitation in preventing violence: A systematic review. *American Journal of Preventive Medicine, 28*(2 Supple 1), 11–39.

Burke, L. E., Wang, J., & Sevick, M. A. (2011). Self-monitoring in weight loss: A systematic review of the literature. *Journal of the American Dietetic Association, 111*(1), 92–102.

Centers for Disease Control and Prevention (CDC). (2013). *Strategies to prevent obesity and other chronic diseases: The CDC guide to strategies to support breastfeeding mothers and babies.* Atlanta: U.S. Department of Health and Human Services.

Civljak, M., Sheikh, A., Stead, L. F., & Car, J. (2010). Internet-based interventions for smoking cessation. *Cochrane Database of Systematic Reviews, 9*(2), CD007078.

Cohen, S. (2004). Social relationships and health. *American Psychologist, 59*(8), 676–684.

Cohen, S., Mermelstein, R., Kamarck, T., & Hoberman, H. M. (1985). Measuring the functional components of social support. In I. G. Sarason & B. R. Sarason (Eds.), *Social support: Theory, research, and applications.* The Hague, Netherlands: Martinus Niijhoff.

Cohen, S., & Wills, T. A. (1985). Stress, social support, and the buffering hypothesis. *Psychological Bulletin, 98*(2), 310–357.

Committee on Public Education (2001). Media violence: Report of the Committee on Public Education. *Pediatrics, 108*(5), 1222–1226.

Community Preventive Services Task Force. (2012). 2012 Annual Report to Congress and to agencies related to the work of the task force. Retrieved from http://www.thecommunityguide.org/annualreport/index.html

Cotter, A. P., Durant, N., Agne, A. A., & Cherrington, A. L. (2014). Internet interventions to support lifestyle medication for diabetes management: A systematic review of the evidence. *Journal of Diabetes Complications, 28*(2), 243–251.

Coyle, K., Basen-Engquist, K., Kirby, D., Parcel, G., Banspach, S., Collins, J., et al. (2001). Safer Choices: Reducing teen pregnancy, HIV, and STDs. *Public Health Reports, 116*(Suppl. 1), 82–93.

Coyle, K., Basen-Engquist, K., Kirby, D., Parcel, G., Banspach, S., Harrist, R., et al. (1999). Short-term impact of Safer Choices: A multicomponent, school-based HIV, other STD, and pregnancy prevention program. *Journal of School Health, 69*(5), 181–188.

DiMatteo, M. R. (2004). Social support and patient adherence to medical treatment: A meta-analysis. *Health Psychology, 23*(2), 207–218.

Tobacco Use and Dependence Guideline Panel (2008). *Treating tobacco use and dependence, 2008 update: Clinical practice guideline.* Rockville, MD: U.S. Department of Health and Human Services, Public Health Service.

Glanz, K., & Bishop, D. B. (2010). The role of behavioral science theory in development and implementation of public health interventions. *Annual Review of Public Health, 31*(1), 399–418.

Governors Highway Safety Association. (February 2014). *Graduated driver licensing (GDL) laws.* Retrieved from http://www.ghsa.org/html/stateinfo/laws/license_laws.html

Guide to Community Preventive Services. (2014). *All findings of the Community Preventive Services Task Force.* Retrieved from http://www.thecommunityguide.org/about/conclusionreport.html

Gwaltney, C. J., Metrik, J., Kahler, C. W. & Shiffman, S. (2009). Self-efficacy and smoking cessation: A meta-analysis. *Psychology of Addictive Behavior, 23*(1), 56–66.

Hogan, B. E., Linden, W., & Najarian, B. (2002). Social support interventions: Do they work? *Clinical Psychology Review, 22,* 381–440.

House, J. S. (1981). *Work stress and social support.* Reading, MA: Addison-Wesley.

House, J. S., Kahn, R. L., McLeod, J. D., & Williams, D. (1985). Measures and concepts of social support. In S. Cohen & L. S. Syme (Eds.), *Social support and health* (pp. 83–108). San Diego: Academic Press.

House, J. S., Umberson, D., & Landis, K. R. (1988). Structures and processes of social support. *Annual Review of Sociology, 14,* 293–318.

Kirby, D. B., Baumler, E., Coyle, K. K., Basen-Engquist, K., Parcel, G. S., Harrist, R., & Banspach, S. W. (2004). The Safer Choices intervention: Its impact on the sexual behaviors of different subgroups of high school students. *Journal of Adolescent Health, 35*(6), 442–452.

Kirby, D. B., Laris, B. A., & Rolleri, L. A. (2007). Sex and HIV education programs: Their impact on sexual behaviors of young people throughout the world. *Journal of Adolescent Health, 40*(3), 206–217.

Lin, J. S., O'Connor, E., Whitlock, E. P., & Beil, T. L. (2010). *Behavioral counseling to promote physical activity and a healthful diet to prevent cardiovascular disease in adults: A systematic review for the U.S. Preventive Services Task Force* (AHRQ Publication No. 11-05149-EF-3). Retrieved from http://www.uspreventiveservicestaskforce.org/uspstf11/physactivity/physart.htm

Lopez, L. M., Tolley, E. E., Grimes, D. A., Chen, M., & Stockton, L. L. (2013). Theory-based interventions for contraception. *Cochrane Database System Reviews,* CD007249.

Mann, T., de Ridder, D., & Fujita, K. (2013). Self-regulation of health behavior: Social psychological approaches to goal setting and goal striving. *Health Psychology, 32*(5), 487–498.

Merson, M. H., O'Malley, J., Serwadda, D., & Apisuk, C. (2008). The history and challenge of HIV prevention. *Lancet, 372,* 475–488.

Nokes, K., Johnson, M. O., Webel, A., Rose, C. D., Phillips, J. C., Sullivan, K., . . . Holzemer, W. L. (2012). Focus on increasing treatment self-efficacy to improve human immunodeficiency virus treatment adherence. *Journal of Nursing Scholarship, 44*(4), 403–410.

Plotnikoff, R. (2013). Social cognitive theories used to explain physical activity behavior in adolescents: A systematic review and meta-analysis. *Preventive Medicine, 56*(5), 245–253.

Prati, G. (2012). A social cognitive learning theory of homophobic aggression among adolescents. *School Psychology Review, 41*(4), 413–428.

Renfrew M. J., McCormick, F. M., Wade, A., Quinn, B., & Dowswell, T. (2012). Support for healthy breastfeeding mothers with healthy term babies. *Cochrane Database of Systematic Reviews 5*, CD001141.

Rinderknecht, K., & Smith, C. (2004). Social cognitive theory in an after-school nutrition intervention for urban Native American youth. *Journal of Nutrition Education & Behavior, 36*(6), 298–304.

Smith, K. P., & Christakis N. A. (2008). Social networks and health. *Annual Review of Sociology, 34*, 405–409.

Stansfeld, S. (2006). Social support and social cohesion. In M. Marmot & R. G. Wilkinson (Eds.), *Social determinants of health* (2nd ed., pp. 149–170). Oxford: Oxford, University Press.

Stead, L. F., Hartmann-Boyce, J., Perera, R., & Lancaster, T. (2013). Telephone counseling for smoking cessation. *Cochrane Database of Systematic Reviews, 8*, CD002850.

Task Force on Community Preventive Services. (2002). Recommendations to increase physical activity in communities. *American Journal of Preventive Medicine, 22*(4S), 67–72.

Thoits, P. A. (2011). Mechanisms linking social ties and support to physical and mental health. *Journal of Health and Social Behavior, 52*(2), 145–161.

Uchino, B. N. (2009). Understanding the links between social support and physical health: A life-span perspective with emphasis on separability of perceived and received support. *Perspectives on Psychological Science, 4*(3), 236–255.

Umberson, D., Crosnoe, R., & Reczek, C. (2010). Social relationships and health behaviors across the life course. *Annual Review of Sociology, 36*, 139–157.

U.S. Department of Health and Human Services (USDHHS), National Health Lung and Blood Institute (NHLBI). (1998). *Clinical guidelines for the identification, evaluation and assessment treatment of overweight and obesity in adults.* Retrieved from www.nhlbi.nih.gov/guidelines/obesity

U.S. Department of Health and Human Services (USDHHS), National Health Lung and Blood Institute (NHLBI). (2004). *The seventh report of the Joint National Committee on Prevention, Detection, Evaluation, and Treatment of High Blood Pressure: Complete report.* Retrieved from www.nhlbi.nih.gov/guidelines/asthma

U.S. Department of Health and Human Services (USDHHS), National Health Lung and Blood Institute (NHLBI). (July 2007). *Guidelines for the diagnosis and management of asthma (EPR-3).* Retrieved from www.nhlbi.nih.gov/guidelines/hypertension.

Wethington, E., & Kessler, R. C. (1986). Perceived support, received support, and adjustment to stressful life events. *Journal of Health and Social Behavior, 27*(1), 78–89.

Wortman, C. B., Loftus, E. F., & Weaver, C. A. (1998). *Psychology* (5th ed.). New York: McGraw-Hill.

CHAPTER 7

Theories of Networks and Communities

KEY TERMS

actor	dissemination	isolate	social cohesion
centrality	distance	laggards	social networks
cluster	early adopters	late majority	system
community	early majority	node	ties
community readiness	homophily	policy	
density	innovation	reciprocity	
diffusion	innovators	social capital	

LEARNING OBJECTIVES

1. Describe properties of social networks.
2. Explain how relationship ties influence the spread of information, resources, and health behaviors.
3. Identify properties of groups that influence community action.
4. Categorize stage of community readiness in a population.
5. Classify network members by the extent of innovativeness and explain how membership influences the movement of ideas and behaviors.
6. Compare a system approach to interpersonal approaches to behavioral change.

IN THE NEWS ...

Are you in or out? This question was a hot topic on news shows and on current events websites for much of 2013. More specifically, the question was, "Will your state expand their Medicaid coverage?"

Medicaid was created in 1965 to provide health care and long-term care coverage for low-income individuals (KFF, 2013). Medicaid is a state-federal partnership to improve access to health insurance and preventive primary care to individuals with a disability and those who are living at or below a poverty threshold. It also provides a safety net in the event of job loss or economic downturn. While this program provides coverage to millions of people, many are still left without access to health coverage, including adults without children and many people who make just a bit too much money but still struggle to make ends meet. States define and manage their own Medicaid programs, yet at least 50% of the funding comes from the federal government. Because a state's Medicaid population depends on its socioeconomic and demographic characteristics, no two states are alike in their Medicaid makeup and funding situations.

On June 28, 2012, the U.S. Supreme Court upheld the constitutionality of the Affordable Care Act (ACA), which includes legislation to expand Medicaid coverage to everyone under the age of 65 who earns at or below 133% of the federal poverty level (National Association of States United for Aging and Disability, 2013). One significant part of the ruling, however, was that the federal government could not require states to expand Medicaid enrollments, that is, states are able to opt in or opt out. Some states were early adopters of the expansion, while a greater number of states waited for the Supreme Court ruling. At the time of this writing, 26 states are participating in the Medicaid expansion, and three other states are leaning toward participation (Advisory Board Company, 2014). Most states not participating in the expansion cite concerns about their state's long-term financial obligations, while other states noted bipartisan support and dissent (Advisory Board Company, 2014). Access the State Medicaid Expansion Tracker online for more information on the status of the expansion.

Introduction

Health behaviors both shape and are shaped by the social and built environment. Community, organization, and policy factors represent the outer levels of influence and are the topic of this chapter. The previous chapters discussed intrapersonal and interpersonal levels of influence. Health behavior theory provided a useful framework of detailed information and hypothesized relationships for understanding intrapersonal and interpersonal factors. This chapter will discuss common properties of factors on the outer levels of influence—those of institutions, organizations, and policy (Figure 7-1). Health behavior theory provides a guide for the chapter; however, theoretical constructs and understanding for communities and organizations are not as clearly defined as constructs in the previous chapters (Green, 2006; Luke & Stamatakis, 2012).

Social network theory, community readiness, and diffusion of innovations are health behavior theories currently used to describe community-level factors of influence. Social network theory explores how people are connected and has been useful in describing chronic disease, the spread of infectious disease, preventive actions such as influenza vaccinations, and adolescent risk behaviors such as tobacco use. Community readiness describes stages of readiness to change in groups of people and is similar to the constructs of individual stages of change. When communities demonstrate a readiness to act, health-promoting strategies are more successful. A community's adoption of a new health behavior or social norm, or its acceptance of a public health intervention can also be discussed in the context of diffusion. Diffusion is the movement and adoption of a product, idea, or practice through different social systems (Rogers, 2003). Innovation is the new idea, product, or practice.

Collectively, the levels of influence along with the numerous factors on each level of influence form a system. A **system** is the set elements organized and interconnected into a structure that produces a set of behaviors (IOM, 2013). Systems contain elements of social and physical environments, along with the practices and policies of communities (see Figure 7-1). Systems organize to fulfill a function or purpose. A health care system and a food system are two examples of purposeful systems. Policy, along with systems, often gets mentioned in the title of the outer level of influence in a social ecological model. Policy is a type of health promotion intervention that influences the availability of resources and networks across all levels of influence. Policy is included in the system category as a factor of influence on a health behavior because of its relationship with creating the factors on the earlier levels of influence.

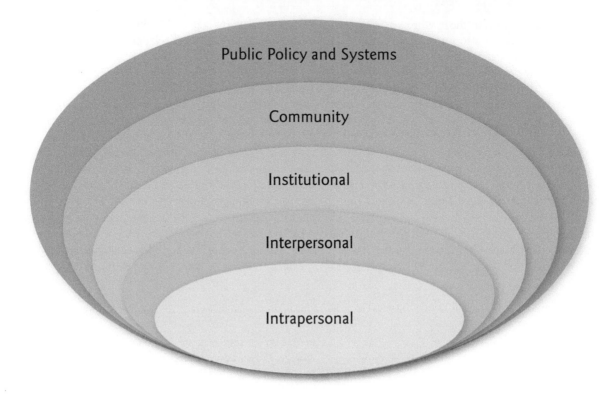

Figure 7-1 Social Ecological Model

Concepts Of Community

A **community** is a group of people who have something in common, whether it is a trait, an interest, geographical proximity, or a common goal. A neighborhood, a student community, a religious group, a professional organization, and an informal recreational group are a few examples. People can come together for functions, interests, and/or support. Individuals can belong to many communities, and their membership can change over time as their identities, locations, and interests change or evolve.

Community membership can be intentional or unintentional. People can choose to join a group or a cause such as breast cancer advocacy group or a parent teacher association (PTA). Other group memberships are more automatic and are based on where a person lives, where a person works, and/or their families. These groups include co-workers and professional colleagues, neighbors, extended families, and other connected contacts. Membership in these groups is not always a conscious decision, and individuals may move in or out of these communities as their lives change.

Communities exist because of the relationships of their members; therefore, social networks are created within communities. The characteristics and demographics of a community can help identify factors influencing health behavior and community-based health promotion strategies of change within its social networks. Information and resources flow through networks and significantly influence health behavior. Collective properties also emerge within communities, that is, the group develops attributes that are not observed in the individual members. An attribute exists because of the collective beliefs, resources, or behaviors of the group. Collective efficacy, discussed in the previous chapter, is one network-based attribute. Collective efficacy is a group's shared belief in the combined abilities to accomplish tasks. Similar to individual self-efficacy, collective efficacy influences task effort and expectations for success. Other collective-based attributes that will be discussed in this chapter are network structures, social capital, cohesion, and readiness.

Social Networks

Social networks refer to the structure of people's connections to one another. **Social networks** are the structure, or the frame, of the social relationships. Networks have been described as webs, where the dots represent people and the lines represent relationships (Berkman, 1984; Smith & Christakis, 2008). Social network analysis is the study of the properties of those dots and lines, *as well as* the larger web (see Figure 7-2). Networks can be large, small, and every size in between. Networks vary in density, in member likeness, and in cohesion. Network analysis is interested in those structures, the composition and the specific resources that flow through the network (Berkman & Glass, 2000; Christakis & Fowler, 2009; Hawe, Webster, & Shiell, 2004). Network analysis differs from the interpersonal focus of social cognitive theory and social support. In the latter, the properties of people are of interest. Social network theory asserts that the social structure of the network itself is largely responsible for determining individual behavior and attitudes by shaping context and influencing the flow of resources (Berkman & Glass, 2000).

People are a fundamental unit of a network, and the term **actors** is assigned to participants in a social network. Actors can be any entity that can have a relationship with people. Actors can also have relationships through groups, organizations, informational websites, and online forums (Luke & Stamatakis, 2012). Alter and ego are two specific actor roles. An ego is the person whose behaviors is being analyzed, and alters are the persons connected to the ego. In the sample network of Figure 7-2, Mary is the ego. George, Joe, Lucy, and Nick are alters. Networks are important because of the resources and contexts they create. The linkages between people influence the flow of information and social norms, and they provide social capital and create cohesion. Social networks can exist in a variety of formats and mediums, but they tend to share many of the same structural characteristics.

Properties of Social Ties and Networks

The connections between two people in a network are called ties. Social **ties** represent the relationships between people: Joe is tied to George, George is tied to Mary, and Lucy is tied to Joe and Mary. As would be expected, whom people are linked to, how people are linked, and the influence of those relationships differ. Persons can belong to multiple social networks, within both formal structures (e.g., work and places of worship) and informal structures (e.g., family and friends). Social ties also vary across a life span. As members age, couple, uncouple, build families, work, and relocate, so does their network. Location of the actors and the ties that indicate their relationships are the framework of study in social network theory. Table 7-1 summarizes terms used in describing properties of social network.

Within a network, actors hold different positions and locations. An individual's location in the network and his or her ties with others affect his or her behaviors, perceptions, and attitudes (Kobus, 2003). **Centrality** is the degree to which a person is centrally located in a network (Hawe et al., 2004; Valente, Gallaher, & Mouttapa, 2004). There is often a person or persons at the middle of the network around whom much of the network's activities occur. Visually, centrality is a central **cluster** of "key players" in a network. Central actors have ties to one another. This focal individual or cluster may be the person(s) trying to make a behavior change, or it may simply be a person with a number of connections to others in the network. This central individual likely influences the behavior, knowledge, resources, and reinforcements in the network due to his or her central role. The other actors in the social network are often connected through this central individual or cluster and provide some sort of support, influence, emotional relationship, or resources to the focal individual and other individuals in the network.

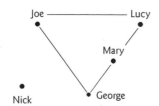

Figure 7-2 Sample Social Network

TABLE 7-1 Terms Related to Social Networks Structure

Term	Definition
Ego	The person whose behavior is being analyzed.
Alter	A person connected to the ego that may influence the behavior of the ego.
Node	A person that may or may not be connected to other objects in a network.
Ties	A connection or relationship between two nodes.
Directionality	The direction in which members exchange information and resources. This concept is also referred to as reciprocity.
Centrality	The degree to which a person or small group is located in the center of network. Isolates and bridges refer to individuals not centrally located, that is, they are on the periphery of the network.
Cohesion	The interconnectedness and solidarity of the network actors; a function of the strength of ties, distance, and density.
Density	The number of connections in the network as a proportion of those possible.
Distance	The number of steps connecting two people. Social distance is the number of steps, or degrees of separation, between two people in the network. Geographic distance is the physical dispersion of members.
Homophily	The tendency for people to have relationships with others who have similar attributes.
Induction	The spread of a behavior or trait from one person to another.
Cluster	A group of nodes. Each node is connected to at least one other node in the group.

Source: Adapted from Christakis & Fowler, 2007; Valente et al., 2004

By contrast, isolates and bridges are actors whose place is on the periphery of a network. **Isolates** are persons not connected to any one in the group (Valente et al., 2004). In Figure 7-2, Nick is an isolate. Isolates tend to experience less social pressure because of limited ties to others. In studies of adolescent tobacco use, isolates were less likely to conform to the network norm on tobacco use. In instances where isolates were more likely to smoke, smoking was prevalent, and central members had higher smoking rates (Kobus, 2003; Valente et al., 2004). If the group norm is positive toward smoking, the isolate is protected from the perceived pressure, whereas the central members are influenced by group norm. Bridges have ties in the network, as well as ties to other networks. Bridges serve as liaisons between two or more otherwise unlinked groups; they bridge the gap between the two groups. Their location on the periphery allows them to move between two or more groups, which can be important for the diffusion of ideas, norms, and behaviors. Bridges between multiple networks also expose members to the norms, resources, and opportunities of the different networks. The impact of the increased network exposure can be positive or not, depending on the network properties (Kobus, 2003; Valente et al., 2004).

Directionally refers to the flow of exchange between two or more members. This property is also called reciprocity (Berkman & Glass, 2000; Hawe et al., 2004; Valente et al., 2004). **Reciprocity** refers to whether social support and resources move both ways between actors in a network. In a network that has a focal individual who requires the support and resources of the others, it is possible that the majority of actors will be giving rather than receiving aid.

Two-way exchanges are mutual relationships (Christaskis & Fowler, 2007). Mary is friends with Joe, *and* Joe reports that he is Mary's friend. The relationship is reciprocated between Mary and Joe. One-way ties are not mutual relationships. One of the actors reports a relationship that the other person does not perceive. Mary reports a friendship with Joe, but Joe does *not* report a relationship with Mary—their relationship is directional. Family relationships are most often bilateral or two-way ties because members support one another. One-way relationships do not have this reciprocal flow. One person in the network is more responsible (and sometimes more powerful) than another person. Networks—including friendships and occupational, school, and community organizations—can have a surprising number of directional ties. The directionality between two nodes is important because the information, resources, and behavioral norms flow in these directions. For example, in a longitudinal study of obesity, mutual friends had a much greater impact on each other's weight status than did people in one-way nonreciprocal relationships (Christakis & Fowler, 2007).

Ties are also described in terms of strength. Persons have a number of ties, and they vary in strength from strong to weak relationships. Strength is a product, "a combination of the amount of time, the emotional intensity, the intimacy, and the reciprocal services which characterize the tie" (Granovetter, 1973, p. 1361). Strong ties occur through close-knit, dense linkages, like those between close friends. Weaker ties come from less dense, casual linkages, such as between co-workers and acquaintances. Despite their lower strength, weaker ties have important functions in social networks and health promotion.

The strength of weak ties was a groundbreaking position introduced by American sociologist Mark Granovetter (1973). Granovetter suggests that weak ties between individuals are crucial for creating new opportunities, enabling resource and information diffusion, and successfully integrating different social groups. Strong ties create local cohesion but will ultimately lead to social fragmentation. Weak ties strengthen wider cohesion through the integration of subgroups or fragmented members of a network (Kadushin, 2012). Not all weak ties are equally important, however. Those that act as bridging ties between two different networks of strong ties— along which ideas, innovations, information, and resources flow—tend to be the most important. Weak ties expedite the spread of norms, fads, and opportunities (e.g., locating a job) (Granovetter, 1973, 1983). The idea of ties will be revisited later in this chapter in the section about diffusion of innovations.

Network Properties

"Centrality," "direction," and "strength" are terms often used to describe ties between nodes. The study of networks is also interested in characteristics of the whole. Groups take on properties of their own that can influence information, norms, and behavior. Likeness, distance, density, and cohesion are central properties of networks that influence health behaviors.

Characteristics shared by the whole group can be used to describe a social network's cohesiveness. Homogeneity refers to how similar the group members are in terms of demographics such as age, race/ethnicity, income, and education level. Social networks tend to have **homophily**, meaning members share similar attributes (Christakis & Fowler, 2007; Kobus, 2003; Smith & Christakis, 2008). The more similar the members are, the more homogeneous the social network is said to be. As mentioned previously, communities are formed around a similar trait, such as a neighborhood or an interest. Homophily extends beyond the common characteristic. Some attribute brought members together; however, networks tend to have likeness of the members beyond the community-forming trait.

Do individuals choose to be in groups with members of similar behaviors, or does the group relationship exert an influence on the person and the behavior? The answer is both—there is a group selection process as well as a group influence process at work in social networks. The type of influence can be associated with the type of relationship. For example, nonsmoking adolescents in stable friendships with smokers are more likely to become smokers. However, when adolescents change friends over the course of a year, they are much more likely to select friends of similar smoking status (Bearman, Moody, & Stovel, 2004; Kobus, 2003; Simons-Morton & Farhat, 2010). Similarly, individuals tend to select partners and friends of similar weights as well as be strongly influenced by changes in the weight status of family, friends, and spouse (Christakis & Fowler, 2007; Cunningham et al., 2012; Smith & Christakis, 2008). Overall, a person's current relationships exert indirect pressure to conform to behaviors; however, when given a choice, individuals more often choose to be connected with others who have likeminded behaviors.

Distance is another characteristic of a network. **Distance** refers to the space between actors in the network. Persons can be social and physically separated. Social distance is the number of steps between an ego (person of interest) and other persons in the network. In the plot of the network, social distance is measured as the length of shortest distance between nodes (persons) (Kadushin, 2012). Direct ties, formally called first-order ties, reflect a person's interpersonal social environment (Kadushin, 2012). In Figure 7-2, George is 2 degrees separated from Lucy and 1 degree separated from Mary and Joe. Social distance can have a powerful impact on health and behaviors. It is through the ties that information, influence, and resources flow. Conceptually, persons closer to us exert stronger influence (Kincaid, 2004; Smith & Christakis, 2008).

Geographical distance is the actual space between members. Geographical distance can be a measure of space, like miles, between friends and family, but also a measure of the sharing of common space. Co-location includes living in the same dorm, attending the same classes, or eating lunch in the cafeteria at the same time. Members share a common space together. Geographical distance has an interesting relationship with social distance. Nodes are more likely to have social relationships with people with whom they share physical space (Kadushin, 2012). Social relationships develop between neighbors and co-workers because of the opportunity of interaction *and* the likelihood of homophily (Kadushin, 2012). Being in the same place as others may occur because of shared interests or attributes. For example, students who live in the same dorm are likely of similar age, interests, and aspirations. Geographic dispersion can create challenges in a social network. When members are separated by distance, they may not know each other well or at all. With other conditions being equal, when members are spread out geographically, network cohesiveness is impacted. In the spread of unhealthy practices, distance may be good.

Density refers to the compactness of the ties in the network. The more direct relationship ties in a cluster, the denser the network. **Density** influences the extent to which actors are acquainted and interact. Density facilitates the dissemination of information, behaviors, and activity. "Density is at the heart of community, social support, and high visibility" (Kadushin, 2012, p. 29). With density, people in a network can see what others are doing and monitor the network.

Through the visibility of members, many other community attributes are communicated and shared. Dense networks also tend to have well-established and stable value systems and norms. Other things being equal, the greater the density, the more likely a network is to be considered a cohesive community, a source of support, and an effective transmitter of ideas and resources (Kadushin, 2012).

Social cohesion represents a network's collective characteristic. **Social cohesion** refers to the extent of connectedness and solidarity among members of the population (Kawachi & Berkman, 2000). One or two members do not create cohesion, nor does one individual member possess the trait. Cohesion is a quality of the whole network. It is the glue of the group. Cohesion is twofold: it occurs through the absence of social conflict and through the presence of strong social bonds. Strong social bonds are characterized by trust, reciprocity, and often density. Cohesive networks also have an abundance of social bridges. In large networks or populations, bridges can be organizations as well as members (Kawachi & Berkman, 2000). A nonprofit organization can bridge a gap between a health care system and subgroup of the network, much like a person, can bridge a gap between two clusters in a network. Cohesive groups have more social capital.

Social capital

One of the interesting and powerful features of networks is the development of collective properties through the structure of the group. Social capital is one of those collective characteristics of a network. **Social capital** refers to the social resources and benefits that emerge from strong social ties or social cohesion and facilitate collective action (Kawachi & Berkman, 2000). It is similar to social support, but it extends well beyond what one member can offer another member. It is the available resources (capital) that accrue through the mutual acquaintance of members (social) (Bourdieu, 1986; Macinko & Starfield, 2001). Social capital is very much a collective and social process. Both types of support and influence are important—social support operates at the interpersonal level; social capital extends to the community, organization, and system levels (see Table 7-2).

Social capital encompasses the positive benefits of belonging to a social network, including bonding, information,

TABLE 7-2 Functions of Social Networks

Function	Definition
Social support	Emotional, informational, and instrumental resources offered between persons
Social capital	Social resources and benefits that emerge from strong social ties or social cohesion and facilitate collective action
Social influence	The normative guidance, from direct and indirect interactions, of a group
Social engagement	Participation with members for companionship, activity, and completion of life tasks

Source: Berkman et al., 2000

encouragement, and anything else an individual believes he or she gains from membership in the network. Social capital is both structural and operational. First, capital is built through a network or structure; it is an ecological characteristic (Kawachi & Berkman, 2000). Without members and ties, there is no social capital. Second, social capital is an accrual of resources. These resources differ from those of social support. The collective resources are a "public good" whose benefits are available to all members of the social structure (Kawachi & Berkman, 2000). In addition to tangible resources such as money and goods, trust, compassion, and civic action are commonly considered to be part of social capital.

"Social capital" is a bit of an abstract term with an evolving definition and measurement. Typically, social capital is estimated by a network's level of trust, reciprocity, and safety. In cohesive networks with corresponding levels of social capital, members have high levels of trust in other members. As noted earlier in this discussion, there is more social capital in cohesive groups and as a result, there can be some overlap in the measurement of concepts. Some researchers have looked at levels of community involvement and links between organizations both within and outside of a community (Kawachi & Berkman, 2000; Lantz & Pritchard, 2010). Population indicators of social capital that can be compared across socioeconomic environments include the number and density of community organizations, volunteerism or per capita participation in voluntary organizations, voter registration, and voter turnout (Lantz & Pritchard, 2010).

Social capital influences health behavior by allowing strongly connected communities or networks to use shared resources to facilitate collective action that benefits the health of members (Lantz & Pritchard, 2010). Social capital allows for achievements that would not be attainable in its absence. Social capital has been linked to decreased mortality and improved self-perceived health (Ferlander, 2007). It is also possible that social capital improves the health and chances of survival of those who are already ill (Berkman, Summers, & Horwots, 1992). Additionally, solidarity, trust, and other positive forms of social capital may allow healthy individuals to maintain or improve their health and further strengthen the network or community.

A lack of social capital can disadvantage populations. Low-resource communities, particularly communities with members living in poverty and/or segregation, have fewer resources to pool. Less obvious, though, is that disadvantaged communities tend to have fewer of the qualities that make communities cohesive. Low interpersonal trust and minimal reciprocity create low cohesiveness, which makes for low social capital. Disadvantage, cohesion, and social capital then become cyclic. Living in poverty or isolation does not ensure lack of community cohesion. Linking members, building trust, and bridging clusters of members can build cohesion and capital. Communities with strong bridging organizations, such as civic groups, schools, and places of worship, can successfully foster social capital. Coalition building also builds a network that can harness existing resources, build trust, *and* build bridges to other networks. Bridges outside the immediate community create a wider base of cohesion and expand the information and resources made available for the common good.

Check for Understanding List five communities of which you are a member. What is the unifying trait of each community? Pick one community and map membership of at least 10 of the actors. Use arrows to indicate directional ties. Describe the network in terms of centrality, density, and distance. Is there homophily in the network? Refer to Table 7-1 as needed.

Obesity in a Social Network

Understanding the spread of infectious diseases through social ties seems plausible; germs spread through people. Strong evidence is also emerging on the relationships of network structure with noninfectious health behavior outcomes. Researchers have tapped into the Framingham Heart Study (FHS), the landmark epidemiological study initiated in 1948 about cardiovascular risk factors, to study the impact of social networks on smoking, obesity-related behaviors, and happiness (Christakis & Fowler, 2007, 2008, 2009, 2012). When the FHS study was initiated in 1948, there were 5209 people in Framingham, Massachusetts, enrolled into the original cohort.

The offspring cohort, composed of children of the original cohort and their spouses, was enrolled in 1971 and consisted of 5124 people. In 2002, enrollment of the third-generation cohort began, and it consisted of 4095 of the children of the offspring cohort. The origins and seminal findings of the FHS were discussed in the Behavioral Science in Action feature in Chapter 1.

Researchers were able to identify relatives, close friends, place of residence, and place of work of cohort members *and* the changes in these variables over 32 years. This information was captured as a person's family changed due to birth, death, marriage, or divorce, and as their contacts changed due to residential moves, new places of employment, and new friendships. Overall, there were 53,228 observed social ties between the 5124 egos and alters in the FHS cohorts, yielding an average of 10.4 ties to family, friends, and co-workers over the course of follow-up (Christakis & Fowler, 2007).

Figure 7-3 illustrates the largest connected subcomponent social network in a study of the spread of obesity. There are 2200 persons, family, and friends represented in this cluster. Nodes and ties are color-coded by weight status, gender,

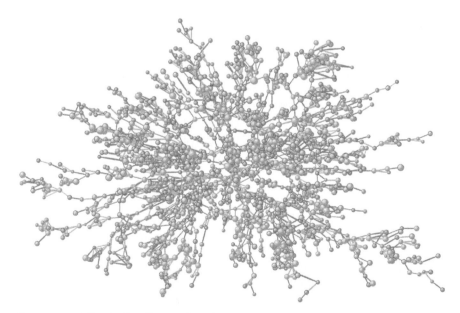

Figure 7-3 Obesity in a Face to Face Network
Source: Christakis and Fowler, www.nicholaschristakis.net/pages/research/r-images.html

and type of relationship. In this study, a person's likelihood of becoming obese was partially determined by whether his or her social contacts became obese. In some relationships, the impact was large, and the type of relationship was important to the magnitude of risk. In mutual friendships, a person's risk for obesity was 171% higher if the friend became obese (Christakis & Fowler, 2007). If the friendship was directional (one-sided), a person's risk for obesity depended on the direction of the relationship. If an ego reported that a friend became obese, it increased the likelihood that he or she would become obese by 57%. The opposite, however, was not true. In an "alter-perceived friend," in which an alter identifies an ego as a friend, there was no increased risk of weight gain. In general terms, if a person who an individual perceives to be a friend becomes obese, he or she is more likely to become obese.

Adult sibling relationships had similar risks, but of lesser magnitude. If an adult sibling became obese, the other siblings' chance of becoming obese increased by 40% (Christakis & Fowler, 2007). For a sibling of the same sex, the risk increased by 55%. There was no such association between neighbors. A person who experienced weight changes had no impact on the weight status of his or her neighbors. This finding is interesting given that neighbors share common community physical environments. Neighbors have similar sidewalks, fitness facilities, grocery stores, and fast-food restaurants. Social distance—not geographical distance—had the greatest impact on obesity. Overall, changes in weight status were explained through social relationships (spouse, sibling, or friend) and were not modified by distance.

Other interesting studies of the spread of behaviors through social network structures include influenza vaccinations, chronic disease treatment compliance, adolescent tobacco use, healthy aging, and sexual behaviors. The studies focus on defining the structure of networks and identifying the ties within the structure. In some studies, like that of the spread of obesity, researchers measured members' actions (or health outcome) and corresponding influences by the structure and ties. Brunson (2013) found that parents' vaccination decisions for their children were significantly influenced by the people in their network. The strongest predictor of a vaccination decision was the percentage of people in the network recommending nonconformity to vaccination recommendations. Bearman, Moody, and Stovel (2004) mapped a Midwest high school social network and the corresponding dating patterns of the members to later predict the transfer of sexually transmitted infections (STIs). In this unique study, 52% of all romantically involved students were tied in one large cluster, which the researchers called a spanning tree. Unlike the large round cluster in Figure 7-3, the social ties formed by these high school students formed a long chain of interconnected nodes (Figure 7-4). Previous models of STI transmission assumed a central cluster of high sexual activity; treat the central core, protect the network. The spanning tree, with the small number of redundant ties, does not have a central core with high density.

Community Readiness

Community readiness is another characteristic of a connected group that influences behavioral action. **Community readiness** is the degree to which a community is prepared to take action on a specific issue (Plested, Edwards, & Jumper-Thurman, 2006). Like people and their stages of change, communities can also be at different stages of motivation and/or action. Intervention strategies should match a group's stage of readiness. If a community is unaware of a health issue, strategies should seek to build awareness. If a community is aware and prepared to take action, strategies should support the community's actions of change. The ability to evaluate readiness is central to determining whether a community can successfully execute a given intervention and to identifying a starting place for researchers and practitioners who are designing programs or interventions. Successful health promotion programs help communities progress to future stages.

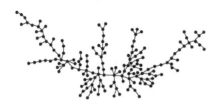

Figure 7-4 Example of Spanning Tree Network

Model for Understanding: Violence   Violence, particularly gang and intentional shootings, has reached epidemic levels in some communities. In one Chicago community, for example, the annual rate of homicide between 2006 and 2011 was 55.2 per 100,000 residents. By contrast, the same rate in the general Chicago population was 14.7 per 100,000. The difference is huge (Papachristos & Wildeman, 2014). For residents and others that followed the news, the difference in the homicide rates was not surprising, though. Researchers' study of the phenomena was a new approach, though. In an article in the *Washington Post*, sociologist and lead researcher Andrew Papachristos reflected that social network theory could help provide a deeper and more practical understanding than comparisons of epidemiological rates could.

> Epidemics of any kind are not random. HIV is a blood-borne pathogen transmitted primarily through sex or intravenous drug use. Once its patterns of transmission and the communities most affected were identified in the United States, extensive public health campaigns helped transform AIDS from an always-fatal disease into one that is chronic and manageable for many of those infected. ... So it is with gun violence. There are patterns of transmission in the United States that go beyond aggregate factors such as race, age, gender and income. On an individual level, social networks—the people one hangs out with—can predict a given person's likelihood of being shot and killed. (Papachristos, 2013)

Early findings from Chicago indicate that mapping social network structures and the pathways of influence can improve understanding of fatal and nonfatal shootings. In the initial study of Chicago shootings, 41% of all gun homicides occurred within a network component containing less than 4% of the neighborhood's population. For each social tie removed from a homicide victim, a person's likelihood of becoming a homicide victim dropped by 57% (Papachristos & Wildeman, 2014). In a follow-up study that examined nonfatal injuries, most of the shootings (70%) were confided to specific networks. A majority of those shootings (89%) occurred in a network cluster (Papachristos, Wildeman, & Roberto, 2014). Another study showed similar location-specific shooting risk patterns in a Boston community. A high percentage (85%) of all the shooting victims were within a single social network, and the risk of getting shot dropped 25% each step an individual was removed from a victim (Papachristos & Wildeman, 2014). Overall, the closer one's tie to a gunshot victim, the greater the probability of one's own victimization.

At first glance, these findings may seem obvious. We have long heard that few acts of violence are truly random. These initial examinations are significant for practice and future research. First, they confirm that network analysis is a viable and useful methodology for exploring acts of violence. These studies confirm general hypotheses that violence is not random; the measures of association and the bounded clusters in which it takes place add to the body of understanding about gun violence. Second, the findings suggest significant implications for *targeted* interventions. As Papachristos notes, "Prevention efforts can be directed toward those individuals and communities most susceptible to the infection. The solution is not broad, sweeping policies, such as New York's 'stop and frisk' or mass arrests, but the opposite: highly targeted efforts to reach specific people in specific places" (2013). The application of social network theory to the public health problem of gun violence is in its infancy. Future studies will build understanding by exploring additional network structures such as directionality, density, and the role of bridges.

Readiness is specific to a particular health behavior or problem. Readiness for tackling secondhand smoke in the community may differ from other issues like prescription drug overdoses or unplanned pregnancies. Communities, like people, must be at certain stages of readiness before they can take action. The resources needed vary by the level of community readiness. Building interest in or motivation toward a topic requires completely different resources than taking specific action. Building community interest involves information sharing and campaigns, whereas taking action requires developing action plans and aligning tangible and service resources.

Building capacity in a community requires a clear understanding of the current readiness. To build more capacity, communities grow to the future stages of readiness (Jumper-Thurman, Vernon, & Plested, 2007). There are six dimensions of readiness: community efforts, knowledge of the efforts, leadership, community climate, knowledge about the issue, and resources related to the issue (Plested et al., 2006). Community effort is the current state of strategies, programs and policies in place to address the issue at hand. Simply, what is happening right now to try and change the issue? The second dimension is the community's knowledge of the local efforts to address the issue. Members can be completely unaware of strategies, which reflects a disconnect between practice and community. Leadership is the third dimension and reflects the extent to which appointed leaders and influential members of the community support the issue. Leaders can come from across the community: city government, law enforcement, medical and other health professionals, clergy, youth, and community activists are segments to consider.

Community climate is the overarching attitude of the community toward the selected issue. Like individuals, communities may feel varying degrees of responsibility, empowerment, and/or helplessness related to the issue (Plested et al., 2006; York & Hahn, 2007). Community knowledge about the issue is the extent to which members understand the problem, its consequences, and how it impacts the community. This type of knowledge differs from knowledge of the activities related to the issue (dimension 2). Knowledge about the issue is a higher level of understanding of the issue and its connected pieces. The sixth dimension of a community's ability to take action is the resources related to the issue. Communities often need a range of resources—people, money, space, and time—to improve efforts. Variations across these six dimensions form the stages of community readiness.

Stages of Community Readiness

The community readiness model (CRM) consists of nine stages that reflect a community's readiness to address a social issue. The higher the stage of development, the greater the degree of readiness. Broadly, communities range from little to no awareness of a community health issue to sustaining ongoing efforts related to a community health issue. Determining a community's stage of readiness to act helps in the development of a community's resource- and strategy-specific plan. See Table 7-3 for more information about the stages of community readiness.

Check for Understanding College campuses are communities that also vary in readiness. If you were to measure community readiness for a selected topic related to your campus, what measurement strategies might you employ?

Assessing Readiness

Once a community and issue are defined, community readiness can be assessed. Key informant interviews are the primary means of measuring readiness. A key informant is a community member who is knowledgeable about the issue; existing programs, or efforts aimed at the problem; and community leadership. A key informant is not necessarily a community leader or decision maker, but rather someone who can provide detailed information about the specific community issue (Plested et al., 2006; York & Hahn, 2007). Four to six members of a community participate in a semistructured interview. The scope of the interview includes knowledge/acceptance of an issue and the community's capacity to address the issue. A community can be made up of many groups, so it is important to select key informants from different subpopulations (Plested et al., 2006). The health problem to be addressed likely affects most, if not all, of the subgroups but perhaps in different ways, so having input from these groups can yield vital information that is relevant to the future intervention.

Semistructured interviews with key informants are conducted via telephone or in person. Interview questions are specific to the problem and are modified to reflect the language of the community (Plested et al., 2006). Questions assess the six readiness dimensions and lead to identification of the stage of readiness for change. For example, readiness for tobacco control differs from other health issues. Thus, questions should specifically ask about efforts, awareness, climate, and resources related to the health issue. Informant responses are scored on a rating scale.

TABLE 7-3 Stages of Community Readiness

Stage of Readiness	Description	Intervention Goal
No awareness (also called community tolerance)	Health behavior is typically accepted or not viewed as a problem in the community	Raise awareness of health issue in general
Denial/resistance	Some community members acknowledge health issue, but it is not viewed as a concern in the local community	Raise awareness that health issue exists in the community
Vague awareness	Many community members agree that there is a problem related to the health issue, but there is little motivation to make a change	Develop and encourage the idea that the community can do something to impact the health issue
Preplanning	People realize the health issue must be addressed in the community, but efforts are not well planned or executed	Develop and promote concrete ways to address the health problem
Preparation	Leaders undertake planning and offer support	Collect information in order to plan, implement, and improve programs
Initiation	There is sufficient information to justify intervention efforts, and activities begin to address the health issue	Provide information on the health issue and interventions that is tailored to the community
Stabilization (also called institutionalization)	Community leaders and administrators support activities, and program staff is trained and experienced	Stabilize intervention efforts and programs in the community
Confirmation/Expansion	Program is in place, and community members use and approve of services offered; data are continually collected	Increase services and broaden reach in the community
High level of community ownership (also called professionalization)	The program has detailed data about prevalence and local causes and risk factors; staff is highly trained, and program is regularly evaluated	Continue to maintain and expand the program

Source: Adapted from Kelly et al., 2003; Plested et al., 2006

Anchored rating scales include descriptive statements that best describe a community's position within each of the six dimensions.

Application of the Community Readiness Model

Children in Balance staff from Tufts University used the community readiness model (CRM) as they worked to select communities for a funded community-wide prevention project: The Balance Project: Bringing Healthy Eating and Active Living to Children's Environments (Sliwa et al., 2011). The 2-year funded project was a replication (or dissemination) project, meaning the program intervention was developed and the funded project aims were to diffuse and evaluate the Balance Project in additional real-world settings. The CRM was used to measure community readiness for action and supplemented applicant-supplied information.

Four stakeholder interviews were conducted in communities interested in participating in the Balance Project. The stakeholders were the mayor or city manager, the school superintendent, the school food service director, and a community coalition representative. The community members selected for the interviews were in leadership positions, and their support and collaboration seemed integral to achieving the project's objectives. Each interview included 23 questions to assess six dimensions of readiness: existing community efforts to prevent childhood obesity, community knowledge about the efforts, leadership, community climate, knowledge of the issue, and resources.

The overall CRM scores demonstrated that the communities ranged from vague awareness to preparation stages of change, ranging from 2.97 to 5.36 on a 9-point readiness scale. Communities scored highest in resources and current efforts, that is, the stages of preplanning and preparation. Community climate scores were lowest (Sliwa et al., 2011). Communities with a high overall score appeared to have sufficient motivation and momentum to initiate and sustain the set intervention components. Scores of leadership supported varied the most across the applicants. The selection committee noted that leadership support would be necessary for project implementation and sustainability, and therefore, they considered low leadership scores "a red flag" (p. 5). One community had a readiness score of 2.97, indicating vague awareness of the problem of childhood obesity, and it was removed from consideration.

Community readiness scores, along with applicant materials, were used to rank the 10 finalists. Six communities were selected for a site visit and then for participation in the project. The communities were selected because their stage of readiness indicated they were prepared for but did not yet have a comprehensive obesity prevention program. The CRM information supplemented other applicant materials and was an important, but not the sole, tool for selection.

Diffusion of Innovations

Another theoretical framework for understanding health behavior in networks and organizations is diffusion of innovations. Earlier in the chapter, the concept of weak ties was introduced. It was explained that members outside the centralized cluster of a network play a pivotal role in bringing new ideas, behaviors, and opportunities into the network. Members located outside the central cluster, or members with ties to other networks, tend to be exposed to ideas and opportunities from other networks or clusters. After exposure, these bridges or weaker ties can bring new ideas to the centralized group. The process of the idea or resource moving from one group of members to another group is called diffusion. **Diffusion** is the process by which an innovation moves through channels of a social system (Rogers, 2003).

In health promotion, an innovation is a new health behavior, a social norm, or an intervention. **Innovations** are defined as ideas, practices, or objects that are perceived as new by an individual or other unit of adoption (Rogers, 2003). Innovations can be designed interventions, such as a health promotion program or a technology product, or they can represent new ideas emerging or transferring from other groups. Adoptions of innovations can enhance population health or represent a source of potential harm for adopting members (Haider & Kreps, 2004). The widespread adoption of seat belt use has improved the health status of groups, whereas the current spread of e-cigarette use is not as beneficial.

Change occurs through diffusion. A new idea, product, or behavior is adopted by one member and then spreads to another member and so forth. Diffusion occurs through both planned and spontaneous processes. Spontaneous diffusion is a natural spread of information that occurs without the implementation of planned strategies. By contrast, companies, community-based organizations, and public health practitioners can design information campaigns and strategies of change that promote diffusion and adoption. **Dissemination** is the active process of using planned strategies to spread information to promote adoption (Brownson et al., 2013). Dissemination leads to diffusion.

Members of a group do not adopt all new ideas. Some ideas "take off," whereas others "die on the vine." In diffusion of innovation theory, the rate and scope of adoption is explained by attributes of the innovation, the social environmental context (or network properties of the community), and the characteristics of adopters (Green et al., 2009; Haider & Kreps, 2004; Kincaid, 2004; Rogers, 2003).

Categories of Adopters

Individuals in a community play different roles in the adoption of new norms and health behaviors. In social network theory, individuals are mapped by their location in the community and their relational ties to others. These interpersonal ties influence the flow of information and resources. With the introduction of new ideas and behaviors, individuals, and therefore organizations and networks, do not accept an idea or adopt an innovation at the same time. Adoption occurs over time and follows a pattern in which select members of a community participate at predictable moments in a community's adoption of the behavior or program.

Innovativeness is a key attribute by which members of a system vary. Innovativeness is the degree to which an individual or unit of adoption is earlier in adopting new ideas than other members of a system (Rogers, 2002, 2003). Adopters can be divided into subgroups by their innovativeness and described by similarities in personal characteristics and communication style. **Innovators** are the initial users of an innovation and tend to be described as adventurous and comfortable with risk (Rogers, 2003). Innovators find "newness" and "cutting edge" to be appealing product attributes. Subsequent groups of adopters are less innovative and have a greater aversion to risk. Table 7-4 describes the remaining categories of adopters: early adopters, early majority, late majority, and laggards.

The predictable sequence of participation by these five groups of adopters follows a bell-shaped curve known as the curve of adoption, which is illustrated in Figure 7-5. Innovators are the first 2.5% of individuals in a system to adopt an innovation. Their interest in new ideas and their location on

TABLE 7-4 Categories of Adopters

Category of Adopter	Innovative Descriptors	Personal Characteristics	Social and Communication Systems
Innovators	Adventurous, cosmopolitan, daring, comfortable with uncertainty	Have financial resources, higher than average education	Peer group of fellow innovators, peer group not geographically bound, communicate with fellow innovators, not tied to local audience or system
Early adopters	Local trendsetters, comfortable with uncertainty	Respected by peers, higher than average education	Integrated in local social system, high proportion of opinion leaders, perceived as role models for other adopters, information source for future local adopters, central position in communication network
Early majority	Deliberate when making decisions, longer decision-making period than for earlier adopters	Willingness to adopt, average to above average education	Interact frequently with peers (but not as opinion leadership), link between early and late adopters
Late majority	Skeptical, cautious, most uncertainty must be removed	May be responding to economic necessity	Peer pressure or norm necessary for adoption, less social participation than earlier groups
Laggards	Traditional, last to adopt, suspicious, lengthy decision-making process	Have limited resources, less than average education level	Near isolates, almost no opinion leaders in group, minimal contact with change agents, decision making is based on past experiences

Source: Adapted from Rogers, 2003

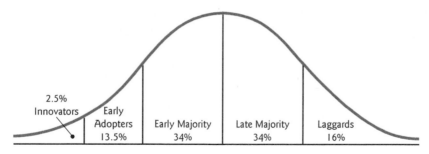

Figure 7-5 Adoption Curve
Source: Adapted from Rogers, 2003

the periphery of a network leads to exposure and fostering of new ideas, products, and behaviors. The **early adopters** are the next 13.5% of individuals in a system to adopt an innovation (Rogers, 2002, 2003). Early adopters are more integrated into the social system, that is, they are more centrally located with dense ties. This category of adopters has the highest proportion of opinion leaders. Early adopters play an important role in the spread of information. Their dense ties to others facilitate the spread of information, interest, and influence.

The **early majority** are the next 34% of individuals in a system to adopt an innovation. Their decision process is described as deliberate; they take time to evaluate the innovation's attributes. Members of the early majority are likely to adopt the innovation just before the average person (Rogers, 2002, 2003). At this point in the adoption process, the innovation reaches a 50% threshold, and it is not the new social norm. Late majorities, another 34% of the social system, follow the early majority. **Late majorities** participate as a result of peer pressure and/or sheer need. The innovation is now the new norm; late majorities merely conform. Conformity may provide economic advantage because the new norm is cheaper, or conformity may provide emotional relief. **Laggards** are the last 16% of individuals in a system to adopt the innovation. Laggards tend to have fewer resources than other members of the system as well fewer social ties. The decision to adopt can be lengthy and/or never occur.

Check for Understanding   List examples of innovations in the following categories: technology, social policy, and health behaviors. In general, into which category of adopter do you fall? Why?

Social Systems and Communication Channels

Social systems and communication channels are two other important concepts related to diffusion. Together, they form an environmental context for diffusion. Social systems are groups of people defined by a common goal, characteristic, or boundary. *Innovations move through social systems.* Communication channels are the routes, related to both distance and direction, through which information is shared. Adoption of healthy behaviors by populations, not by singular neighborhoods or classrooms, produces substitutive changes in health status. To achieve higher rates of adoption, the innovation needs to spread through multiple network clusters and social systems. Further, the higher the rates of adoption, the more likely individual behaviors are to be maintained. There comes a point at which so many people have adopted the behavior (a critical mass) that future behavior adoption is self-sustaining. In the popular book *The Tipping Point* (2002), author Malcolm Gladwell refers to this point of critical mass as the tipping point.

Wide adoption of a new belief or behavior by groups of people creates a new social norm. Yet, "every innovation begins as a deviation from existing social norms" (Kincaid, 2004, p. 37). This is a powerful idea—social norms, the normative beliefs and practices of a group, often begin as a minority position or as a "deviant" group act. So how does an uncommon belief or practice move to the majority? In the previous section, the role of social network bridges was introduced. Innovations initiate on the periphery of a network, not in a central dense cluster. Singular bridges or members do not create a norm, though. They do not walk over to the central cluster and introduce a new idea, product, or practice. Rather, a subcomponent of members in a network starts to develop around the innovator or innovation (Kincaid, 2004). The innovator influences those closer to him or her (likely socially closer), and a bounded cluster with a similar practice develops. As that density of the subcluster grows, so does the norm.

Opinion leaders play a pivotal role in the spread of ideas and behaviors in social networks. Opinion leaders influence the opinions, attitudes, and behaviors of others. They are centrally located in the network and are held in esteem by others. Opinion leaders are traditionally early adopters but not innovators (Valente & Pumpuang, 2007). Innovators are few and are less centrally located; opinion leaders adopt early in the process and influence others. Opinion leaders are crucial to widespread diffusion because of their location in regard to many others.

In dissemination projects, locating and engaging the opinion leaders can greatly influence program or product adoption. Two of the most common methods for identifying opinion leaders in a network are self-report techniques and sociometric mapping (Valente & Pumpuang, 2007). Self-identification methods tend to be cost efficient and easy to implement; however, there can be selection bias. Asking an individual if she is an opinion leader in her network may not identify the most influential opinion leaders of the group. In an interesting study of physician adoption of new pharmaceutical medications, this selection bias was confirmed. Self-reported opinion leaders were not actually centrally located in the network. Researchers concluded that self-identification captured a person's self-confidence, not their position of influence in the network (Ivengar et al., 2011). By contrast, mapping a network of who is linked to whom is a much more accurate way of identifying opinion leaders and key network bridges (Ivengar et al., 2011; Valente & Pumpuang, 2007). To map a network, members are interviewed and asked a series of questions about whom they consider friends, who their colleagues are, and where they get their information. **Nodes** (members) and ties (relationships) are then mapped. Influential members and cluster bridges are subsequently identified (Christakis & Fowler, 2007; Ivengar et al., 2011; Valente & Pumpuang, 2007). This sociometric method, along with its variations, is a more accurate means than self-identification, yet it can be time consuming and expensive.

Organizations should also be considered as intended audiences for adoption. The properties of the innovation and

the pattern of adoption described earlier with individuals also apply to organizations. Organizations are more likely to adopt when the innovation offers *advantages* to the current practice or belief, it is *compatible* with the current system, adopters can *trial* aspects of the innovation, and the use of the innovation by the organization or other systems is *observable* (Rogers, 2003). Organizational behaviors of adoption tend to be different from individually targeted behaviors. For example, smoking cessation is an intrapersonal behavior with strong interpersonal influences; individuals quit smoking and are more likely to be successful with the support of family and friends. By contrast, the adoption of smoke-free laws is an organization behavior. Groups of individuals, in an organization or larger system, pass legislation or organizational policy that restricts smoking in select places. The creation and adoption of the smoke-free policy is the behavior of the organization. For example, individual states are in the process of banning smoking in public spaces. As of 2014, there were 36 states with statewide bans on smoking in select public spaces (ALA, 2014; Americans for Nonsmokers' Rights Foundation, 2014).

Diffusion of Smoke-Free Policies

The movement of smoke-free policies across and between states is an example of an innovation, in this case a new practice, moving through different social systems. The widespread adoption through various social structures creates and reflects a new social norm. California is typically credited with being the true innovator of statewide smoke-free policy adoption. In 1994, California passed a statewide ban on smoking in select public places. The California policy restricted smoking in public places, most workplaces, and restaurants without bar areas. It did allow for smoking in designated indoor areas with proper ventilation and gave several workplace exemptions. In 1998, smoking restrictions in all bars and restaurants were added. Eight years later, in 2002, Delaware became the first state to implement a *comprehensive* smoke-free law, followed by New York in 2003, Massachusetts in 2004, and Rhode Island and Washington in 2005 (CDC, 2011). It is important to note that the designated space exemption is still in place in the California policy, making it fall outside the definition of a comprehensive policy.

In the span of a decade, smoke-free workplaces, restaurants, and bars went from being relatively rare to being the norm in half of the states and the District of Columbia. The number of states that implemented comprehensive statewide smoke-free laws that prohibit smoking in private workplaces, restaurants, and bars increased sharply, from zero states in 2000 to 27 states in 2014, including Washington, DC (CDC, 2011; 2014).

Figure 7-6 illustrates the movement of comprehensive smoke-free policies over the past 14 years. More than 50% of states have adopted comprehensive indoor smoke-free policies. Seven states are potential late adopters and/or laggards for indoor smoking policy adoption. Indiana, Kentucky, Mississippi, South Carolina, Texas, West Virginia, and Wyoming have no statewide laws restricting smoking in worksites, restaurants, and/or bars (Americans for Nonsmokers' Rights Foundation, 2014; CDC, 2014).

Early in the statewide adopt process, hospitals began to explore smoke-free campus policies. Ideas and practices in municipality and worksite networks were influencing other social systems. Similarly, the success and acceptance of the restrictions was visible to members of these other systems. No state experienced a revolt or significant drops in restaurant/bar revenue. To date, approximately four national health systems (Kaiser Permanente, Mayo Clinic, SSM Health Care, and Cigna Corporation) have 100% smoke-free grounds. The number of smoke-free local and state hospitals is a bit more difficult to count. Over 3500 local, state, and territorial hospitals and health care systems are estimated to have smoke-free grounds (Americans for Nonsmokers' Rights Foundation, 2014). Other social systems in earlier stages of adopting smoke-free policies include college campuses, parks and

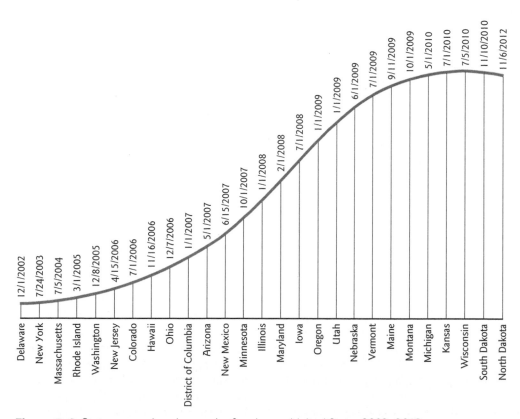

Figure 7-6 State comprehensive smoke-free laws – United States 2002–2013

recreation spaces, and public housing. As of January 2014, at least 1182 college or university campuses in the United States had adopted 100% smoke-free campus policies that eliminate smoking in indoor and outdoor areas across the entire campus, including residences (Americans for Nonsmokers' Rights Foundation, 2014). This number grew from the 586 campuses two years earlier (October 2011) and 446 campuses three years before (October 2010).

Community readiness is an important factor for statewide adoption of policies. Readiness grows as information about, advantages of, and trial use related to the innovation spread through network clusters or subcomponents. Strong smoking restrictions have traditionally started at the local level and then spread into larger parts of the state (USDHHS, 2006; York & Hahn, 2007). In 1990, the community of San Luis Obispo, California, adopted the first law in the country eliminating smoking in bars (CDC, 2012). The first local *comprehensive* smoking law was implemented by Shasta County, California (NCI, 2000). During the decade of incredible progress, more states enacted comprehensive indoor smoking laws, often after a number of local jurisdictions in the state had implemented such laws (CDC, 2011; USDHHS, 2006). Currently, six of the seven states without statewide smoke-free polices have local comprehensive policies restricting smoking in public places (Americans for Nonsmokers' Rights Foundation 2014; CDC, 2012). Only Mississippi does not have any comprehensive local smoking bans. The number of local policies can be high: South Carolina has 38 municipalities with comprehensive bans, and the other states without statewide bans are not far behind: Texas has 35 municipalities with comprehensive bans, West Virginia has 27, Kentucky has 21, Indiana has 18, and Wyoming has 2. In the linking language of the social network theory, cities and their influences can serve as bridges of support for greater adoption of comprehensive policy into the statewide network.

Properties of Innovations

The rate and scope of adoption is largely influenced by the properties of the innovation. Rogers (2003), the original author of diffusion theory, estimates that 49–87% of adoption can be explained by the *advantages, compatibility, complexity, trialability,* and *observability* of the innovation (see Table 7-5). First, the introduced method or product should offer advantages over the older method or product. Across studies, relative advantage appears as the most influential set of attributes in the rate and scope of innovation adoption (Rogers, 2003). There must be some perceived advantages for individuals and organizations to "change their ways." Advantages can include economic benefits, physiological or emotional outcomes, recognition by others, and convenience. In health promotion, financial incentives can also increase adoption by providing an economic advantage, which serves as a cue to act (Rogers, 2003).

Second, compatibility is the degree to which the innovation fits within the individual or organization's system. Ideas and products that fit within the current lifestyle or environment are more readily adopted and sustained. Compatibility, or fit, of health promotion interventions and behaviors also needs to be considered when they are being introduced to audiences. The easier it will be to integrate a particular intervention with current structures, the more likely the intervention or behavior will be trialed. Specific fit issues include amount of proposed time, amount of space needed, amount and type of equipment, and flexibility within the schedule. Compatibility issues can also be related to the individual, including beliefs about the behavior, interest, comfort, and abilities.

In health promotion, Rogers (2003) notes that communicating issues of compatibility to an intended audience begins with the name of the introduced behavior and program. For example, Brain Gym® and Energizers are names of two programs for structured classroom physical activity breaks. The names are designed to appeal to teachers by communicating the perceived advantages of these activities: students will be more energized, and it is a workout for their brain. In practice, Rogers recommends the use of receiver-oriented names, where the name is associated with a desired meaning for the audience. Finally, encouraging audiences to personalize the innovation increases perceived degrees of compatibility. With technology products, personalization occurs via colors, size, logos, and noises, such as ringtones.

Complexity, or ease of use, is negatively related to rate of adoption. The higher the perceived complexity, the lower the rate of adoption. By definition, innovations are new to the intended audience, and therefore persons will process new information for all innovations. However, certain innovations may be perceived as having higher degrees of complexity. These products, ideas, and behaviors that are considered harder to process and adopt are less likely to be trialed and adopted.

TABLE 7-5 Attributes of Innovations That Influence Diffusion

Attribute	Definition	Considerations for Health Behavior Interventions
Relative advantage	Degree to which an innovation is perceived as better than the current product, idea, or method	• Limit costs and provide incentives • Promote prestige, innovation, and social outcomes • Make strategies convenient • Understand the desired benefits to different user groups
Compatibility	Degree to which an innovation is perceived as consistent with beliefs, past experiences, and current lifestyle	• Appeal to interest • Address a need • Fit within structures of audience environment • Encourage customization • Use a receiver-oriented name
Complexity	Degree to which an innovation is perceived as difficult to use or adopt	• Provide ready-made materials • Gear materials to abilities of intended audience • Build on previous learning and experiences
Trialability	Degree to which an innovation can be experimented with prior to adoption	• Offer trial events • Divide intervention for trial • Offer incentives or free product
Observability	Degree to which the advantages and results of an innovation are visible to others	• Measure and communicate successes • Showcase adopters • Implement select strategies in visible ways • Brand strategies to program

Source: Adapted from Rogers, 2003

Level of knowledge, scope of skills, and product or collaborative requirements can influence the degrees of complexity. Past experiences with a similar product or process can also influence perceived complexity. The ability to use previously acquired skills and knowledge with the new intervention makes an innovation appear less complex (Rogers, 2003). Overall, degree of complexity appears less influential than relative advantages and compatibility. If use of a behavior or product is within a person's abilities and resources, trial and adoption are probable.

Practices and products that can be easily trialed also diffuse more quickly and at higher rates. Trialing allows an individual or organization to readily experiment with the new product or process without making large financial, time, or other commitments. Finally, other adopters or social systems are more likely to try the innovation if the innovation and its advantages are observable by others. Observability promotes member discussion of the new idea, product, or practice.

A nonadopter sees the advantages of innovations and asks the adopter about the innovation. Other attributes being equal, observable innovations diffuse more quickly. Observability of the innovation becomes more important in the later stages of the adoption curve (Rogers, 2003). Early majority and late majority adopters require more information and are influenced by the actions of others; therefore, visibility of the innovation facilitates the spread of information and creates perceived peer pressure.

Dissemination

Dissemination is planned systematic efforts designed to make a program or innovation more widely available. Diffusion is the outcome of these efforts. Health behavior programs should be designed and modified for diffusion. First and foremost, the advantages of the health promotion program or new practice should be communicated to the members of the target audience (Rogers, 2002). Next, the fit of the intervention or behavior within existing structures and routines of the current lifestyle of the intended audiences should be maximized. The easier it is to be integrated into the current structures, the likelier the intervention or behavior will be trialed and maintained. The innovation should be as simple as possible because the higher the perceived complexity, the lower the rate of adoption. Finally, other adopters or social systems are more likely to try the innovation if it and its advantages are observable by others. If the desired change is not easily visible, what can be done to draw attention to early adopters' successes? Potential late adopters will be watching.

In addition to the structure of the innovation, planned strategies for how and where the innovation is introduced into the social system are equally important. Opinion leaders, or change agents, are crucial to diffusion (Rogers, 2002). Opinion leader recruitment early in the process increases the rate and speed of adoption by the network. Large networks can have multiple change agents that bridge groups. Recruit opinion leaders across clusters of the network. Early adopters willingly try and experiment with the innovation, and their experiences create visibility for late adopters.

Late adopters will be enticed or drawn in by the successes and progress of the innovation. It may not be a good use of early project resources to aggressively recruit late adopters. Late adopters experience trialability vicariously through observing and interacting with the early adopters (Rogers, 2003). Trial and awareness strategies are more important to early adopters. Peer pressure and conformity are more important to late adopters. With late adopters, peer recruitment via buddy-type programs may be more efficacious than trial events. Similarly, the methods by which select objectives are approached may be customized to adopter characteristics. Innovators may appreciate minimally guided and electronic strategies for skill development, while late adopters may require traditional face-to-face coaching and feedback.

Systems

A system is a combination of factors operating across multiple levels of influence that work toward a common goal (IOM, 2013; Meadows & Wright, 2008). In population health, the social ecological model is the conceptual framework for a system. Factors of the individual, groups of people, and

environments interact to influence health behavior and status. Other disciplines use different models to understand systems such as socio-technical modeling (human factors engineering), protein modeling (bioinformatics), and solid modeling (computer-aided engineering). Educating children, reducing tobacco use, providing health care, and advancing a political cause are various types of system goals. Public health successes such as tobacco control and immunizations are often attributed to a systems approach. Future interventions call for a more all-encompassing approach that will work with existing systems to impact more individuals (NCI, 2007).

Systems, like communities, operate around a purpose or goal. Unlike communities, though, systems operate across multiple levels of influence, operate in nonlinear fashions, and contain heterogeneous elements (Luke & Stamatakis, 2012; Meadows & Wright, 2008). Differing elements interacting together over various levels of influence produce an outcome that is collectively larger than that of the individual elements (Luke & Stamatakis, 2012). The resulting effect is usually enduring and able to adapt to a changing system (Luke & Stamatakis, 2012).

A system is the context for health behavior action or inaction. To improve community health, an understanding of the system elements, connections, and purpose is critical. The health behavior theories and the constructs within the theories describe the interconnected factors of influence at work in systems (Gillen et al., 2014). Attributes of people, their relationships, and organizational properties have been discussed; the next section briefly explains the role of policy in a system. Chapter 8 then provides a useful tool for pulling the multilevel information from different health behavior theories into one framework, representing the system of factors influencing behavior.

Policies

The outer level of influence in the social ecological model includes policy. **Policies** are defined as local, state, and national laws, decisions, and plans that create built and social environments and systems. They tend to create and/or influence the structures, resources, reinforcements, and norms in multiple levels of influence in the social ecological map. A health policy in particular is some form of action, whether it is a law or a less formal plan that seeks to achieve certain health-related goals within a certain population. Recall the discussion of Medicaid in this chapter's In the News feature. States spent 2013 debating whether to expand Medicaid, the health insurance program for persons of low income and/or with a disability. Expanding the Medicaid program increases the number of people with health insurance, and policies such as Medicaid expansion are powerful determinants for social and physical environments. Policies change environments. They can mandate conditions, which in turn change variables of influence across most, of not all, levels of influence. Medicaid expansion gives individuals health insurance, which in turn improves access to health care providers, treatments and medications, and education.

Policies exist on all levels of influences and influence behavior of the individual and of organizations. Some policies, like seat belt and helmet laws, have an impact mainly on the intrapersonal level. Policies that influence population-level health tend to target organizations, institutions, and governments to reach the greatest number of individuals. Numerous public health policies have altered the context for health behaviors. On a federal level, the Breast and Cervical Cancer Mortality Prevention Act of 1990 and the Affordable Care Act, passed in March 2010, increased access to preventive cancer screenings by removing financial barriers for individuals, and mandating

community health care services. On a state level, tobacco-free policies and excise taxes reduce exposure to smoking and create penalties for tobacco use. As highlighted within in this chapter's discussion of dissemination of innovations, tobacco-free policies have also been implemented on institutional levels in hospitals, schools, and places of employment. In the physical activity model discussed in Chapter 4, city policies and regulations were also identified as being instrumental for creating access to connected pathways, sidewalks, and mixed land use that promote walking and biking for transportation.

Policies are a category of health promotion intervention, and they are a strategy that can be used within health promotion to facilitate change. Later in Chapter 10, policies will be discussed with other types of health promotion programming. Policies are often seen as a determinant of health behavior because of the strong influence they can have on factors across the social and environmental levels of influence.

Check for Understanding List 10 to 20 components of the U.S. health care system. Can you place the components in the corresponding level of the social ecological model?

SUMMARY

Groups take on properties, and these properties influence the actions of the groups' members. As with an individual, group properties can be beliefs, abilities, or resources of the group. Also, like the individual, communities need to be motivated, able, and reminded to act. The properties of networks and organizations reflect the properties of the members but can take on stronger influence or magnitude in their collective nature. Social capital refers to the social resources and benefits that emerge from strong social ties or social cohesion and facilitate collective action. Social capital is very much a collective and social process. Similarly, community readiness reflects the degree to which a community is prepared to take action on a specific issue. Like capital, readiness reflects the awareness, efforts, and

resources of a community. Communities with higher degrees of social capital and readiness have higher capacity for change.

Network properties can also influence the manner in which ideas, behaviors, and products move through a community. New ideas and practices tend to come from members on the periphery, yet adoption by centralized members is required for greater network adoption. Systems, a social ecological model, operate in a manner that produces long-term outcomes greater than those of the smaller pieces and is able to adapt to changes in individual components of the system. Individuals take action, but action is more likely in social and physical environments that support the action.

BEHAVIORAL SCIENCE IN ACTION

Snowballing and Other Sampling of a Social Network

Social network analysis (SNA) is the mapping of actors and their relationships. As in much of research, there are a variety of methods available to study this issue. In the spread of obesity study by Christakis and Fowler (2007, 2012), the researchers were able to use existing interview notes from within the Framingham Heart Study. For many decades, handwritten interview notes documented relatives, friends, and co-workers. Addresses were recorded, and therefore, neighbors could also be identified. The researchers note that given the completeness and the length of time covered, it really is a unique data set for studying social networks and health (Christakis & Fowler, 2012). In the gun violence studies by Papachristos and colleagues, researchers used existing data sources, but in this instance, the sources were police records. Data were derived from two sources: (1) homicide records with details of incidents and participants involved and (2) records of all arrests among residents in the community of study. Arrest records allowed researchers to map nodes and ties into what that they called co-offending networks (Papachristos & Wildeman, 2014).

All methods measure ties to other actors. In the most basic format, social network analysis measures existing relationships. Two people have a relationship—a tie. In the gun violence study, the data source identified people in the same place and the same time, and being in the same place and the same time implied a relationship. Methods for quantifying relationships can become more complex than just establishing co-existence. Some methods for data collection measure reciprocity and the degrees of separation. When examining the spread of obesity, the researchers were able to quantify whether relationships were mutual or directional friendships. Similarly, because of the wide scope of the sample, degrees of separation were also

measured. Sampling, whether of available data or of researcher-collected data, is an important measurement decision. Full network sampling, snowball sampling methods, and egocentric methods are common sampling methods in social network analysis (Hanneman & Riddle, 2005).

Full network methods require information to be collected about each actor's ties with all other actors. In essence, this approach takes a census—rather than a sample—of ties in a population of actors. Information from the Framingham Heart Study was largely census data. The original cohort had almost no loss other than because of death (Christakis & Fowler, 2012). Similarly, a study at a Midwest high school was largely census data—all students in the high school were interviewed (Bearman et al., 2004). Full network data give a complete picture of relations in the population. Full network data is necessary to properly define and measure many of the structural concepts of network analysis (e.g., between-ness). Full network data allow for powerful descriptions and analyses of social structures. Obtaining data from every member of a population, and having every member rank or rate every other member, can be very expensive and difficult to collect.

Snowball methods begin with an initial actor or set of actors. Each of these actors is asked to name some or all of his or her ties to other actors (the process is called name generation). Then all the actors who were named (and who were not part of the original list) are tracked down and asked for some or all of their ties. The process continues until no new actors are identified, names start to repeat, or the researcher decides to stop. Name generation can identify individuals that the researchers were unaware of and locate subjects when there is not a defined list. One concern with the snowball method of sampling is that the sample is influenced by where the researcher initially starts the collection. Mapping of the network is likely biased by where the snowball started. In some instances, there may be a natural starting point: a power position, a community or organization leader, or a person of interest. In other instances, the question is where should the researcher start? Finally, actors who are not connected (isolates) are not located by this method. The presence and numbers of isolates can be an important feature of populations for some analytic purposes.

A third method of sampling actors within a network is related to *egocentric networks*. As the name implies, sampling begins selection of focal nodes (egos). The sampling then moves from the focal point, ego, outward. The egos identify the nodes to which they are connected. Contacting each of the actors can identify ties to other actors. This kind of approach can be effective for collecting a form of relational data from very large populations and can be combined with attribute-based approaches. For example, one might take a simple random sample of male college students and ask them to report who their close friends are and which of these friends know one another (Hanneman & Riddle, 2005). This kind of approach can give a reliable picture of the kinds of local networks in which individuals are embedded, as well as how many connections nodes they have and the extent to which these nodes are close-knit groups. Many network properties—distance, centrality, and density—cannot be assessed with egocentric data. Some properties, such as overall network density, can be reasonably estimated with egocentric data. Some properties—prevalence of reciprocal ties and cliques—can be estimated from egocentric sampling.

IN THE CLASSROOM ACTIVITIES

1) Think about a work, class, or club project. Create a list of all the people or organizations involved in the work. Map the network. Write the names of people and organizations on sticky notes, place the sticky notes on a sheet of paper, and then draw arrows of relationships. Use one-way and two-way arrows to depict directionality. Describe the network in terms of density and other structure terms from Table 7-1. Do some actors have few or no arrows or relationships and should be moved further away from other sticky notes to indicate their lack of connections?

2) Take the project from number 1. Use the snowball sampling technique and the prompt "Who do you work with on this project?" to map the project.

3) As a class, pick a campus or other community public health issue. Using the resources from the Tri-Ethnic Center, develop an interview guide. Create a list of interviewees and conduct four interviews. What is the community's stage of readiness for the issue? How does the community's readiness relate to social cohesion and social capital?

4) In the social network map from number 1 or number 2, where are new ideas most likely to come from in the network? Why? How might innovations move through the group? What factors would influence diffusion?

5) For the community public health issue in number 3, can you identify campus groups or individuals in early stages of adoption? How do the attributes of adopters and the adopters vary?

WEB LINKS

Connected: The Surprising Power of Social Networks: http://connectedthebook.com/

Tri-Ethnic Center: www.Triethniccenter.colostate.edu/communityReadiness.htm

REFERENCES

Advisory Board Company. (2014). *Where each state stands on ACA's Medicaid expansion.* Retrieved from http://www.advisory.com/daily-briefing/resources/primers/medicaidmap

American Lung Association (ALA). (2014). *Smokefree air laws.* Retrieved from http://www.stateoftobaccocontrol.org/state-grades/state-rankings/

Americans for Nonsmokers' Rights Foundation. (2014). *U.S. tobacco control laws database.* Retrieved from http://www.no-smoke.org/goingsmokefree.php

Bearman, P. S., Moody, J., & Stovel, K. (2004). Chains of affection: The structure of adolescent romantic and sexual networks. *American Journal of Sociology, 110*(1), 44–91.

Berkman, L. (1984). Assessing the physical health effects of social networks and social support. *Annual Review of Public Health, 5,* 413–432.

Berkman, L., & Glass, T. (2000). Social integration, social networks, and health. In L. F. Berkman & I. Kawachi (Eds.), *Social epidemiology* (pp. 137–174). Oxford: Oxford University Press.

Berkman, L., Summers, L., & Horwots, R. I. (1992). Emotional support and survival after myocardial infarction: A prospective, population-based study of the elderly. *Psychosomatic Medicine, 58,* 459–471.

Bourdieu, P. (1986). The forms of social capital. In J. Richardson (Ed.), *Handbook of theory and research for sociology of education* (pp. 241–258). New York: Greenwood.

Brownson, R. C., Jacobs, J. A., Tabak, R. G., Hoehner, C. M., & Stamatakis, K. A. (2013). Designing for dissemination among public health researchers: Findings from a national survey in the United States. *American Journal of Public Health, 103*(9), 1693–1699.

Brunson, E. K. (2013). The impact of social networks on parents' vaccination decisions. *Pediatrics, 131*(5) 1397–1404.

Centers for Disease Control and Prevention (CDC). (2011). State smoke-free laws for worksites, restaurants, and bars: United States, 2000–2010. *Morbidity and Mortality Weekly, 60*(15), 472–475.

Centers for Disease Control and Prevention (CDC). (2012). Comprehensive smoke-free laws: 50 largest U.S. cities, 2000–2012. *Morbidity and Mortality Weekly, 61*(45), 914–917.

Centers for Disease Control and Prevention (CDC). (January 2014). *State Tobacco Activities Tracking and Evaluation (STATE) system (data set).* Retrieved from http://apps.nccd.cdc.gov/statesystem/

Christakis, N. A., & Fowler, J. H. (2007). The spread of obesity in a large social network over 32 years. *New England Journal of Medicine, 357*(4), 370–379.

Christakis, N. A., & Fowler, J. H. (2008). The collective dynamics of smoking in a large social network. *New England Journal of Medicine, 358*(21), 2249–2258.

Christakis, N. A., & Fowler, J. H. (2009). Social network visualization in epidemiology. *Norwegian Journal of Epidemiology, 19*(1), 5–16.

Christakis, N. A., & Fowler, J. H. (2012). Social contagion theory: Examining dynamic social networks and human behavior. *Statistics in Medicine, 32,* 556–577.

Cunningham, S. A., Vaquera, E., Maturo, C. C., & Narayan Venkat, K. M. (2012). Is there evidence that friends influence body weight? A systematic review of empirical research. *Social Science & Medicine, 75*(7), 1175–1183.

Ferlander, S. (2007). The importance of different forms of social capital for health. *Acta Sociologica, 50,* 155–128.

Gillen, E. M., Lich, K. H., Yeatts, K. B., Hernandez, M. L., Smith, T. M., & Lewes, M. A. (2014). Social ecology of asthma: Engaging stakeholders in integrating health behavior theories and practice-based evidence through systems mapping. *Health Education & Behavior, 41*(1), 63–77.

Gladwell, M. (2002). *The tipping point: How little things can make a big difference.* New York: Back Bay Books.

Granovetter, M. S. (1973). The strength of weak ties. *American Journal of Sociology, 78*(6), 1360–1380.

Granovetter, M. S. (1983). The strength of weak ties: A network theory revisited. *Sociological Theory, 1,* 201–233.

Green, L. W. (2006). Public health asks of system science: To advance our evidence-based practice, can you help us get more practice-based evidence? *American Journal of Public Health, 96*(3), 406–409.

Green, L. W., Ottoson, J. M., Garcia, C., & Hiatt, R. A. (2009). Diffusion theory and knowledge dissemination, utilization, and integration in public health. *Annual Review of Public Health, 30,* 151–174.

Haider, M., & Kreps, G. L. (2004). Forty years of diffusion of innovations: Utility and value in public health. *Journal of Health Communications, 9,* 3–11.

Hanneman, R. A., & Riddle, M. (2005). Introduction to social network methods. Riverside: University of California, Riverside.

Hawe, P., Webster, C., & Shiell, A. (2004). A glossary of terms for navigating the field of social network analysis. *Journal of Epidemiology and Community Health, 58,* 971–975.

Institute of Medicine (IOM). (2013). *Evaluating obesity prevention efforts: A plan for measuring progress.* Washington, DC: National Academies Press.

Ivengar, R., Van de Bulte, C., Eichert, J., West, B., & Valente, T. W. (2011). How social networks and opinion leaders affect adoption of new products. *GfK Marketing Intelligence Review, 3*(1), 17–25.

Jumper-Thurman, P., Vernon, I. S., & Plested, B. A. (2007). Advancing HIV/AIDS prevention among American Indians through capacity building and the community readiness model. *Journal of Public Health Management & Practice, 13,* S49–S54.

Kadushin, C. (2012). *Understanding social networks: Theories, concepts and findings.* New York: Oxford University Press.

Kaiser Family Foundation (KFF), Kaiser Commission on Medicaid and the Uninsured. (2013). *Medicaid: A primer, 2013.* Retrieved from http://kff.org/medicaid/

Kawachi, I., & Berkman L. (2000). Social cohesion, social capital, and health. In L. F. Berkman & I. Kawachi (Eds.), *Social epidemiology* (pp. 174–190). Oxford: Oxford University Press.

Kelly, K. J., Edwards, R. W., Comello, M. L. G., Plested, B. A., Thurman, P. J., & Slater, M. D. (2003). The community readiness model: A complementary approach to social marketing. *Marketing Theory, 3*(4), 411–426.

Kincaid, D. L. (2004). From innovation to social norm: Bounded normative influence. *Journal of Health Communications 9*, 37–57.

Kobus, K. (2003). Peer and adolescent smoking. *Addiction, 98*(Suppl. 1), 37–55.

Lantz, P. M., & Pritchard, A. (2010). Socioeconomic indicators that matter for population health. *Preventing Chronic Disease, 7*(4). Retrieved from http://www.cdc.gov/pcd/issues/2010/jul/09_0246.htm

Luke, D. A., & Stamatakis, K. A. (2012). Systems science methods in public health: Dynamics, networks, and agents. *Annual Review of Public Health, 33*, 357–376.

Macinko J., & Starfield, B. (2001). The utility of social capital in research on health determinants. *Milbank Quarterly, 79*(3), 387–427.

Meadows, D. H., & Wright, D. (2008). *Thinking in systems: A primer.* White River Junction, VT: Chelsea Green Pub.

National Association of States United for Aging and Disability. (2013). *State Medicaid expansion tracker.* Retrieved from http://www.nasuad.org/documentation/State%20Medicaid%20Expansion%20Tracker%20February%202013.pdf

National Cancer Institute (NCI). (2000). *State and local legislative action to reduce tobacco use* (Smoking and Tobacco Control Monograph No. 11). Bethesda, MD: U.S. Department of Health and Human Services, National Institutes of Health, National Cancer Institute.

National Cancer Institute (NCI). (April 2007). Greater than the sum: Systems thinking in tobacco control (Tobacco Control Monograph No. 18; NIH Pub. No. 06–6085). Bethesda, MD: U.S. Department of Health and Human Services, National Institutes of Health, National Cancer Institute.

Papachristos, A. V. (December 3, 2013). Social networks can help predict gun violence. *Washington Post.* Retrieved from http://www.washingtonpost.com/opinions/social-networks-can-help-predict-gun-violence/2013/12/03/a15b8244-5c46-11e3-be07-006c776266ed_story.html

Papachristos, A. V., Braga, A. A., & Hureau, D. M. (2012). Social networks and the risk of gunshot injury. *Journal of Urban Health, 89*(6), 992–1001.

Papachristos A. V., & Wildeman, C. (2014). Network exposure and homicide victimization in an African American community. *American Journal of Public Health, 104*(1), 143–150.

Papachristos A. V., Wildeman, C., & Roberto, E. (2014). Tragic, but not random: The social contagion of nonfatal injuries. *Social Science & Medicine* (doi: 10.1016/j.socscimed.2014.01.056. [Epub ahead of print]

Plested, B. A., Edwards, R. W., & Jumper-Thurman, P. (April 2006). *Community readiness: A handbook for successful change.* Fort Collins, CO: Tri-Ethnic Center for Prevention Research.

Plested, B. A., Thurman, P. J., Edwards, R. W., & Oetting, E. R. (1998). Community readiness: A tool for effective community-based prevention. *Prevention Researcher, 5*(2), 5–7.

Robert Wood Johnson Foundation (RWJF). (2013). How can healthier school snacks and beverages improve student health and help school budgets? *Health Policy Snapshot: Childhood Obesity*. Retrieved from http://www.rwjf.org/content/dam/farm/reports/issue_briefs/2013/rwjf72649

Rogers, E. (2002). Diffusion of preventive innovation. *Addictive Behaviors, 27*(6), 989–993.

Rogers, E. M. (2003). *Diffusion of innovations* (5th ed.). New York: Free Press.

Sallis, J. F., Floyd, M., Cervero, R., & Kerr, J. (2008). *Welcome to ALR 101: Active living research.* Retrieved from http://www.activelivingresearch.org/files/ALR101_Sallis.pdf

Simons-Morton, B., & Farhat, T. (2010). Recent findings on peer influences on adolescent substance abuse. *Journal of Primary Prevention, 31*(4), 191–208.

Sliwa, S., Goldberg, J. P., Clark, V., Collins, J., Edwards, R., Hyatt, R. R., ... Economos, C. D. (2011). Using the community readiness model to select communities for a community-wide obesity prevention intervention. *Preventing Chronic Disease, 8*(6), 1–7.

Smith, K. P., & Christakis N. A. (2008). Social networks and health. *Annual Review of Sociology, 34,* 405–409.

U.S. Department of Health and Human Services (USDHHS). (2006) *The health consequences of involuntary exposure to tobacco smoke: A report of the surgeon general.* Atlanta: U.S. Department of Health and Human Services, Centers for Disease Control and Prevention.

Valente, T. W., Gallaher, P., & Mouttapa, M. (2004). Using social networks to understand and prevent substance use: A transdisciplinary perspective. *Substance Use & Misuse, 39*(10), 1685–1712.

Valente, T. W., & Pumpuang, P. (2007). Identifying opinion leaders to promote behavior change. *Health Education & Behavior, 34*(6), 881–896.

York, N. L., & Hahn, E. J. (2007). The community readiness model: Evaluating local smoke-free policy development. *Policy, Politics, & Nursing Practice, 8*(3), 184–200.

CHAPTER 8

Integrating Health Behavior Theories and Building a Theoretical Model

KEY TERMS

behavioral building blocks	milestone	reinforcing factors	theoretical logic model
enabling factors	PER worksheet	sequence	trial use
logic	predisposing factors		

LEARNING OBJECTIVES

1. Determine behavioral constructs common to multiple health behavior theories.
2. Classify health behavior constructs of seven theories by stage of change.
3. Express health behavior constructs in general lay terms.
4. Identify primary and secondary methods for determining behavioral antecedents in populations.
5. Diagram a theory-based logic model, synthesizing constructs from multiple health behavior theories.

IN THE NEWS ...

Cases of measles are on the rise in the United States. Even though it was eradicated from the United States in 2000, a record number of Americans are being diagnosed with this contagious disease. In 2013, there were 189 people who were reported to have developed measles. This represents the second largest number of cases in the United States since measles was eradicated. In 2014, the number of cases continued to grow at alarming rates. In the first quarter, 129 people in 13 states were infected. About a fourth of the Americans got measles while in other countries. The disease was brought into the United States and was spread to unprotected individuals. The Centers for Disease Control and Prevention (CDC) reported that most of the people infected (80–90%) were not vaccinated or had unknown vaccination status. In 1963, an extremely effective vaccine against measles was developed, and the measles vaccination program was started.

Stories of outbreaks in 11 communities filled the news in 2013. The largest outbreak was in New York City, where 58 people contracted measles. The virus spread through a close-knit Orthodox Jewish community. A second outbreak involved 25 Texans linked to the Eagle Mountain International Church. A visitor to a church who had recently traveled abroad started the outbreak.

Measles is still common throughout the world, including in some European, Asian, Pacific, and African countries. When people travel, they can be exposed to the virus and then return to the United States with the virus. High vaccination rates have impeded the spread of the virus once in the country.

Measles is a dangerous respiratory disease. It spreads quickly through coughing and sneezing. Approximately 40% of children who develop measles will be hospitalized. In rare cases, it can be deadly. Measles typically starts with a fever that is followed by a cough, runny nose, and red eyes. A rash of small red spots develops on the head and spreads to the rest of the body. Since measles had been eliminated from the United States, public health officials worry about delays in diagnosis. Newer health care professionals may not know what a case of measles looks like, which can delay treatment. The CDC recommends that children, teenagers, and adults be up-to-date on their measles vaccination, including before international travel.

Introduction

No single theory explains the broad scope of all health behaviors. Given a particular behavior, environmental conditions, and target audience, one theory may be more applicable than others. For example, the theory of planned behavior (TPB) explains or predicts intention to engage in a target behavior. In this decision-making theory, all the constructs reflect the cognitive and affective domains. The health belief model (HBM) explains the likelihood of single-act behaviors such as health screening and immunization, where the likelihood of the behavior is driven by perceived threat of the illness. Social cognitive theory (SCT) explains health behavior in a social context over time; it includes constructs from the cognitive domain but also includes the learning of target behavior–related skills and access to resources.

A combination of theories may be necessary to explain variations in behavior. For example, the literature shows a relationship between a construct of the HBM, perceived threat, and intention to use condoms consistently and correctly (Kirby, 2002); in addition, the behavioral capabilities construct of SCT has a relationship to actual condom use (Tortolero et al., 2005). Similarly, smoking cessation programs that demonstrate at least a 20% cessation rate are often stage-matched interventions (transtheoretical model). Stage-matched interventions target specific behavioral factors during select times in the process of quitting. Intentions to quit smoking (TPB), trigger management and refusal skills (SCT), and environmental support (social ecological model) are all targets through a stage-matched smoking cessation program (Ranney et al., 2006; Spencer et al., 2002).

Applying and combining theoretical constructs to specific behaviors and populations is challenging due to the abstract definitions of theoretical constructs and the duplication of similar constructs across multiple theories. Constructs are specific to theories, and theory creators may include some of the same concepts in the individual theories. The duplication of some concepts, and the exclusivity of other concepts, can confuse new theory users. For example, many theories propose that a person's confidence in performing a skill has a strong relationship with actual behavior performance. The HBM, the TPB, and SCT each include a confidence-type construct. To add to the confusion, similar terms may be given different names in a given theory. Self-efficacy in SCT is called perceived behavioral control in the TPB. The PER worksheet helps practitioners develop the best comprehensive understanding of a health behavior.

The PER Worksheet

The **PER worksheet** is a planning tool that provides lay term prompts for identifying health behavior antecedents (Langlois & Hallam, 2010). It encompasses eight common health behavior theories: health belief model, theory of planned behavior, social cognitive theory, social ecological model, social networks, social support, transtheoretical model, and diffusion of innovations. The PER worksheet is organized into three columns: **P**redisposing, **E**nabling, and

Reinforcing factors (which are terms of the PRECEDE/PROCEED model) (Green & Kreuter, 2005). After identifying a specific target behavior (e.g., parental decisions to immunize their children), program planners identify possible antecedents and record these on the PER worksheet. Planners can use the worksheet to cluster similar concepts and organize their understanding of the factors related to the behavior. After the antecedents are recorded, planners organize the antecedents into the theory logic model. Table 8-1 summarizes many of the constructs discussed in the previous chapters and shows the overlap and similarities across the health behavior theories.

Column 1: Predisposing Factors

Predisposing factors represent cognitive and affective antecedents related to motivation or rationale for the target behavior (Green & Kreuter, 2005). The category prompts include *know*, *believe*, *intention*, and *demographics*. In terms of the behavioral theories, predisposing factors encompass the HBM, TPB, SCT, and the social ecological model. Knowledge is part of most theories, including the HBM and SCT. Knowledge is captured as a modifying factor or individual differences in the HBM. In SCT, knowledge is necessary to perform a specific skill. Beliefs are fundamental parts of the HBM, TPB, and SCT. The core constructs of the HBM (perceived susceptibility, perceived severity, and perceived threat) are beliefs. Similarly, all the TPB constructs (subjective norms, perceived behavioral control, attitude toward the behavior, and intention) are beliefs. Outcome expectations, outcome expectancies, and self-efficacy are SCT belief constructs. Finally, the individual characteristics of the Predisposing column represent the intrapersonal level of the social ecological model.

Demographic variables can also act as predisposing factors. Age, gender, and race are variables that are commonly associated with changes in a range of behaviors or behavioral intentions. For example, older women are more likely to report an intention to breastfeed (Meedya, Fahy, & Kable, 2010). Yet, as women age, they are less likely to receive a mammogram (Schueler, Chu, & Smith-Bindman, 2008). Demographic factors can also be unique to populations. For example, for individuals with disabilities, the type of disability or extent of the disability can have a significant relationship with participation in preventative cancer screenings (CDC, 1998; Iezzoni et al., 2000; Martin, Orlowski, & Ellison, 2013). Innovativeness,

from the diffusion of innovation (DOI) theory, also predisposes individuals to action. The degree to which a person is willing to adopt new ideas and actions influences when he or she will take action in community adoption (Rogers, 2003). Few theories other than the HBM actually contain a specific demographic-type theoretical construct. The omission of demographic factors, though, makes them no less significant than any predisposing factor listed. Program planners will surely discover at least a handful of demographic factors that have relationships to behaviors of interest.

Column 1 of the worksheet represents the transtheoretical model's precontemplation and contemplation stages of change. In these first two stages of the TTM, an individual is in the cognitive and affective decision-making process. The individual must decide that the target behavior is "a good idea" (precontemplation) and then progress to "I can do this" (contemplation).

In the immunization example (Figure 8-1), knowledge of immunization schedules (what injection is needed and when follow-ups are due) and understanding threats of illness are documented antecedents for decisions to vaccinate (Brown et al., 2010). Luthy, Beckstrand, and Peterson (2009) report that 25.6% of parents said that they were confused about the vaccination schedule and were not sure when they should return to the primary care provider. Inconsistencies in providers' knowledge of vaccination schedules and inaccessible clinic locations lead to lower vaccination rates (Harris et al., 2007). Daley and colleagues (2006) report that 15% of parents they studied did not know whether influenza vaccination was recommended for their child.

Parents have numerous specific beliefs that influence their intention to vaccinate their children. Beliefs about the safety of vaccinations are consistent correlates of parent behavior. In a review of 31 published studies of parental decision making, lower vaccine uptake was typically linked with general side effects/safety concerns, lower perceived vaccine effectiveness and importance, belief that vaccine causes autism, own and others' experiences of vaccines and vaccine adverse events, belief in safety of single vaccines, belief in a danger of immune overload, and belief that children receive too many shots (Brown et al., 2010). Parents may have various types of intentions regarding childhood immunizations: to prevent disease, to comply with school regulations, and/or to benefit from herd immunity (Brown et al., 2010; Quadri-Sheriff et al.,

TABLE 8-1 Theoretical Constructs within the PER Worksheet

Predisposing	Enabling	Reinforcing
Know	**Be Able to Do (Skills)**	**Reminded**

Health Belief Model
  Knowledge
 	
Social Cognitive Theory
  Procedural knowledge
 	
Social Ecological Model
  Intrapersonal level
	Social Cognitive Theory
	  Behavioral capability
	  Self-regulation
		Health Belief Model
		  Cues to act
		
		Social Cognitive Theory
		  Observational learning
		
		Social Ecological Model
		  Interpersonal and community level

Believe/Value	**Access to**	**Positive Reinforcement**

Health Belief Model
  Perceived susceptibility
  Perceived severity
  Perceived threat
  Perceived benefits
  Perceived barriers
 	
Theory of Planned Behavior
  Attitude toward the behavior
  Subjective norm
  Perceived behavioral control
 	
Social Cognitive Theory
  Self-efficacy
  Outcome expectations
	Health Belief Model
	  Actual benefits
	
	Social Cognitive Theory
	  Environment
	  Observational learning
	  Facilitation
	
	Social Ecological Model
	  community and system
	  levels
	
	Social Networks
	  Social capital
	  Companionship
	
	Diffusion of Innovations
	  Innovation
		Social Cognitive Theory
		  Reinforcements
		  Incentive motivation
		
		Social Ecological Model
		  Interpersonal and community level

Intention	**Access Removed**	**Negative Reinforcement**

Theory of Planned Behavior
  Behavioral intention
	Health Belief Model
	  Actual barriers
	
	Social Cognitive Theory
	  Environment
	  Observational learning
	
	Social Ecological Model
	  community and system
	  levels
		Social Cognitive Theory
		  Reinforcements
		  Incentive motivation
		
		Social Ecological Model
		  Interpersonal and community level

continues

TABLE 8-1 *continued*

Predisposing	Enabling	Reinforcing
Demographic		**Social Support**

Health Belief Model
    Modifying factors: Age, sex,
    ethnicity, socioeconomic status
 	
Social Determinant Factors
		Social Cognitive Theory
		    Environment
		
		Social Ecological Model
		    Interpersonal and community level
		
		Social Support
		    Emotional support
		    Instrumental support
		    Informational support
		    Appraisal support

Other		

Diffusion of Innovations
    Innovativeness
 	
Health Belief Model
    Modifying factors		

Stage of: Precontemplation and contemplation	**Stage of:** Preparation and action	**Stage of:** Maintenance

Source: Adapted from Langlois & Hallam, 2010

2012). Finally, demographic factors associated with lower vaccination rates are education level, income level, and age and/or birth order of the child (Brown et al., 2010).

Column 2: Enabling Factors

Enabling factors represent environmental and skill antecedents that allow a person to accomplish the target behavior (Green & Kreuter, 2005). The category prompts include *be able to do (skills), access to,* and *access removed.* In terms of the behavioral theories, column 2 encompasses the health belief model (HBM), social cognitive theory (SCT), social networks (SN), the social ecological model (SEM), and diffusion of innovations (DOI). *Be able to do* reflects the skills one needs to successfully complete the target behavior. For example, keeping a food diary is a skill related to many nutrition-related behaviors. In SCT, this skill construct is called behavioral capability. Observational learning, also a construct in SCT, is a method of watching others and learning the skills. Access to resources and access removed from

resources is a construct of many theories. First, actual barriers and benefits are constructs of the HBM. Of note, *perceived* benefits and barriers are predisposing (cognitive) factors. For example, a perceived barrier may be lack of time; however, time may not be an actual barrier. This distinction is important from a programming perspective. Perceived barriers are often corrected through awareness strategies; actual barriers are addressed though environmental or skill strategies. Second, SCT constructs of the environment, observational learning, and facilitation are also resource-related constructs. Individuals are capable of watching others and learning the skills to engage in a specific behavior and gain access. Social networks, via capital and companionship, can also provide resources. People or groups can provide others with resources such as information, money, or services. Being exposed to an innovation is another resource-based construct from the DOI. Finally, environmental factors such as policy, regulations, and structures represent the community and system levels of the social ecological model.

TARGET BEHAVIOR Childhood vaccination: Decision making process of parents in accepting or refusing vaccines.

TARGET AUDIENCE Parents of children up to age 17.

OTHER KEY INDIVIDUALS Health care providers and network peers.

KNOW

Knowledge about *what*, *where*, and *when* to return for vaccination.

Parents' knowledge about threat of susceptibility especially in cases of eradicated diseases.

BELIEVE/VALUE

Safety and efficacy beliefs regarding single versus multiple injections.

Parental beliefs that vaccines are safe.

Perceived risk and severity of disease.

Preference for natural immunity.

Parental religious beliefs toward vaccination.

Perceived efficacy of other preventive actions: nutrition, hand washing and limited social contact.

Value of personal choice and social responsibility.

INTENTION

Intention to comply with immunization regulations and policy.

Expectations of herd immunity.

DEMOGRAPHIC

Parents' education level.

Age, income level, employment, ethnicity, family size, and residence.

OTHER

Prior experience with vaccinations.

Age of child.

Trust of healthcare and or government systems.

BE ABLE TO DO (SKILLS)

Communication skills to provide parents with appropriate information.

Language and cultural communication.

Health literacy particularly distinguishing anecdotal versus scientific information.

Record keeping of both provider and parents.

ACCESS TO/REMOVED

Health insurance.

Trusted, regular health care provider.

Opportunities (time) to discuss vaccinations with physician.

Attendance at school with their child: at school-located vaccination programs.

Well-child visits.

Beliefs and practices of others in the peer network.

Media, Internet, and other sources of information.

REMINDED

Reminders/prompts from physician's office.

Symptoms of disease.

POSITIVE REINFORCEMENT

Physician's recommendation/healthy relationship between parents and physician.

NEGATIVE REINFORCEMENT

Child's pain/anxiety/crying.

Social perceptions about sexually transmitted infections and related embarrassment.

Parental anticipated feelings of regret.

Side effects.

SOCIAL SUPPORT

Peer support for decisions.

Figure 8-1 PER Worksheet: Childhood Immunization Example

Source: Adapted from Narayan & Orlowski (2013)

Column 2 of the PER worksheet represents the preparation and action stages of change in the TTM. In these two stages, an individual is actively preparing to or actually performing the target behavior.

Immunization-related skills of both parents and providers influence childhood immunization rates. Health literacy, the ability to read and comprehend health-related information, and record-keeping skills of parents are associated with higher rates of immunization. Luthy and colleagues (2009) found that 23.3% of parents had difficulty in keeping their child's vaccination records up-to-date, and 9.3% had lost their child's vaccination record. Low health literacy is associated with lower immunizations rates for both children and adults (Berkman et al., 2011; Brown et al., 2010). Being able to understand and communicate in the primary language is especially challenging for minority groups and immigrants and often leads to a hesitation to vaccinate (Benin et al., 2006). Health care providers can facilitate immunizations by being able to communicate with parents about immunizations, provide opportunities for discussions, and establish a relationship of trust with the parents (Luthy et al., 2009; Smith et al., 2006). Benin and colleagues (2006) describe postpartum mothers' attitudes as existing along a continuum: vaccine accepters, vaccine hesitant, late vaccinators, or vaccine rejecters. Accepters stated that they had a trusting relationship with their pediatrician, were satisfied by the physician's dialogue about vaccination, and felt that their doctor was up-to-date on relevant information. By contrast, nonvaccinators stated that they sensed a feeling of alienation from their doctor, were unable to trust the physician, and felt as though the pediatrician did not have adequate knowledge about vaccines. Among the nonvaccinators, 75% specified that they wanted to trust their doctor and have proper communication with him or her (Benin et al., 2006). Media messages and peer networks also serve as antecedents for childhood immunizations (see Figure 8-1).

Column 3: Reinforcing Factors

Reinforcing factors come from others or the environment and promote the continuation or repetitiveness of the target behavior (Green & Kreuter, 2005). Some reinforcements and cues to act may be internal such as "a feeling of accomplishment" or "disease symptoms." The category prompts include *reminders, positive reinforcement, negative reinforcement,* and *social support.* In terms of the behavioral theories, column 3

encompasses the health belief model (HBM), social cognitive theory (SCT), social support (SS), and the social ecological model. Cues to act is a core construct of the HBM. Cues come before a behavior and nudge or remind us to complete an act. Behavioral reinforcements come after a behavior, as described in SCT. Social support is also a broad construct of SCT. Social support theory distinguishes the potential types of social support: emotional, instrumental, informational, and appraisal. These reinforcing factors come from two environmental levels of the social ecological model: interpersonal and the community.

Column 3 represents the maintenance stage of change in the TTM. This last stage involves the sustainability of the behavior and its integration into one's lifestyle.

In the childhood immunization example (see Figure 8-1), decision reminders include schedules as well as prompts by media and providers. Prompts by a provider, in particular, can facilitate action. Lin and colleagues (2006) compared immunization rates across years in the same parents. Rates dropped from 44 to 25% when the parents did not receive a recommendation for the annual influenza vaccine from their pediatrician. Negative outcomes after receiving injections can influence parental decision making for future childhood vaccinations. In one study, 20% of children reported clinically significant pain after receiving a vaccine (Cassidy et al., 2002). Pain can cause a high level of anxiety for the child, which transfers into anxiety for the parents, causing procrastination of additional vaccinations (Schechter et al., 2007). A child's pain, crying, and anxiety serve as negative reinforcements for future parental actions. In a study conducted by Luthy and colleagues (2009), 34.9% of parents whose child was late in receiving at least one vaccination and the parent reported concerns about the vaccination stated that the reason of their concern was because they were worried about the pain at the injection site and the child's anxiety. Finally, social support from a variety of sources is important for immunization continuation (Brown et al, 2010).

Introductory Strategies for Defining and Combining Theoretical Constructs

The PER worksheet and the method of grouping similar antecedents is an effective tool for organizing one's thought and promoting understanding of behavioral risk and protective factors. Over time, this process becomes a way of thinking about populations and behaviors, as well as a means of incorporating new knowledge into existing knowledge. Initially, the process of gathering information, grouping it, and then putting it into common categories can be a challenge. The following list provides rules of thumb that facilitate the early use of the PER worksheet.

Rules of Thumb

1. Knowledge consists of information related to the *target behavior*.

2. Beliefs are *specific*.

3. Other *important people* play roles in the target behavior.

4. Constructs exist on a continuum, and the behavioral direction does not need to be recorded.

5. Reinforcements can both positively and negatively influence behavior.

6. Interventions should *not* be listed.

Knowledge

Knowledge, as a behavioral antecedent, consists of information related to the target behavior. Typically, if one knows or learns certain information about a behavior, the likelihood of engaging in that behavior increases or decreases. Knowledge is a necessary prerequisite to health behavior change. Program planners, however, often overestimate the type and amount of knowledge necessary. As part of professional preparation, health clinicians and professionals acquire a great deal of knowledge on a variety of diseases and health behaviors. Furthermore, everyday print and electronic media contain significant amounts of factual health information. As a result, one can access a tremendous amount of information on most health behaviors. This access and volume can lead to an overemphasis on knowledge as a behavioral antecedent. For example, most individuals know that tobacco is responsible for many deaths in this country (USDHHS, 2010). Yet, knowledge of the number of deaths caused by smoking or the number of carcinogens is *not* a behavior antecedent. In a recent Gallup poll, 96% of American adults reported that they believe smoking is harmful to health, and 18% of American adults smoke. Thus, knowledge does not necessarily deter people from smoking. Similarly, in children and adolescents, knowing about the vitamin and mineral content of fruits and

vegetables is not associated with fruit and vegetable consumption (Taylor, Evers, & McKenna, 2005). As these examples demonstrate, statistical and similar types of information are rarely behavioral antecedents.

Knowledge antecedents tend to be related to risk, skills, or resources. First, knowledge of what puts an individual at risk for a potential health outcome is a behavioral antecedent. For example, in the tobacco research cited earlier in this discussion, smokers who reported incorrect knowledge about the health risks of newer tobacco products were less likely to attempt smoking cessation (USDHHS, 2010). Second, all skills have a knowledge component, identification of the elements of the skill, which precedes skill performance. For example, refusal skill development helps adolescents remain tobacco and alcohol free. To perform this skill, adolescents must be familiar with the different types of peer pressure and ways of using refusal skills. Finally, behavioral knowledge can involve knowing where or how to access resources. For instance, smokers who reported knowing that tobacco dependence treatment, such as counseling and pharmaceutical products, were covered by insurance were more likely to use the resources and more likely to attempt cessation (McMenamin, Halpin, & Bellows, 2006).

The number of items in the knowledge category may be limited for some health behaviors. Studies repeatedly document that knowledge has a small relationship with health behaviors. As previously mentioned, effective knowledge antecedents tend to be related to risk, skills, or resources and have a relationship with the target behavior. Given the narrowed focus of necessary knowledge to change a behavior, knowledge is the most difficult category to complete in the PER worksheet. In early use of the PER worksheet and behavioral mapping, the number of items in this category can make one uncomfortable. Many practitioners want to add factual knowledge or statistics as behavioral antecedents because this type of information is commonly targeted in education and clinical settings.

Beliefs

Beliefs are specific and most often focus on the expected outcomes of engaging in the behavior. For instance, an individual's beliefs related to physical activity are more likely to be "I believe that I'll make friends" and "I believe that I will lose weight," rather than "I have a positive attitude toward physical activity." Referencing the descriptions of the theoretical construct is helpful when defining specific types of beliefs. First, beliefs are outcome oriented: What does a person think will be an outcome from the behavior? This description comes from the construct of attitudes in the theory of reasoned action (TRA) and outcome expectations in SCT. A second powerful belief construct is self-efficacy, that is, one's confidence in performing a skill. Just as there are multiple outcome expectation beliefs, there are multiple forms of efficacy. Efficacy is skill and situation specific; an adolescent may be confident and anticipate success in refusing cigarette offers from a friend but less confident in refusing a cigarette offer from an older student at a party (Langlois, Petosa, & Hallam, 1999). Finally, beliefs involve others' expectations or perceived normative behavior, called social norms or subjective norms. There are multiple social norms as well. Family, friends, and employers can have different norms related to and acceptance of the same behavior. The perceived norms of friends, family, and employers will likely influence behavior differently. As a result of the different types of beliefs and the specificity of each belief, the number of items in the belief category can be large.

Important Others

Knowledge, beliefs, intentions, skills, and support offered by important others also should be considered in the development of the target behavior. Direct contact with individuals such as parents, coaches, or health care providers can have a significant indirect influence on an individual's health behaviors. For instance, a mother's intentions to breastfeed while in the hospital are strongly influenced by health care providers' cues, encouragement, and guidance (USDHHS, 2011). A new mother's health care providers' knowledge, beliefs, and skills can significantly influence the new mother's likelihood to breastfeed (Smith et al., 2006). As another example, parents' beliefs and skills influence childhood vaccination status. Likewise, the skills and resources of local health care providers influence parents' vaccination decisions (see Figure 8-1). Therefore, the knowledge, beliefs, intentions, skills, and support factors of important others should be captured in the PER worksheet.

Behavioral Direction

When completing the PER worksheet, individuals can get distracted by the "behavioral direction" or format of the antecedent. Behavioral direction refers to how an antecedent is

phrased. Terms can be phrased differently, often to reflect a particular relationship with the target behavior. In labeling antecedents, it helps to consider that all constructs exist on a continuum, and the variability in the construct explains a portion of the variability in the health behavior. On the PER worksheet, it is best to describe the antecedent in neutral terms. For example, one may wonder, "Is an antecedent (1) peers who smoke increase the likelihood of smoking or (2) peers who do not smoke decrease the likelihood of smoking?" The actual antecedent is peer smoking status.

In Figure 8-1, parents' education level is a predisposing factor in the decision to vaccinate children. In general, parents with higher education levels are more likely to vaccinate. Parents with less than a high school diploma are two times more likely to refuse childhood immunizations (Akis et al., 2011). As education levels increase, vaccination rates increase. However, the relationship between education level and vaccination is different for new vaccines such as the combination meningococcal-B and pneumococcal vaccine, and SARS. Parents with a higher level of education are 3.3 times more likely not to comply with new vaccination recommendations compared to parents of lower levels of education (Hak et al., 2005). The purpose of the PER worksheet is not to record all these variations, but to capture the antecedent. Parent education level is a predisposing factor for childhood immunizations. As it varies, so does the likelihood of vaccinations.

Reinforcements

By definition, positive reinforcements increase the likelihood of a future behavior, and negative reinforcements decrease the likelihood of a future behavior (see Chapter 6 for more information on this topic). A positive reinforcement might be praise from another, while a negative reinforcement might be embarrassment (see Figure 8-1). Both categories of reinforcements are important to the lifestyle integration of a behavior. Working definitions of reinforcements can be a bit more confusing. The confusion can arise from the behavioral direction as well as how the behavior is stated. A simple example can be seen in smoking and the "kick" that smokers feel from the first few puffs of a cigarette. The kick could be listed as a positive reinforcement for smoking. That immediate feeling increases the likelihood of future acts of smoking. Conceptually, this seems to be a negative reinforcement for the undesired behavior. Each behavior has a category of reinforcements that encourage the behavior and a second category of reinforcements that discourage the behavior. Similar to the strategy discussed in the behavioral direction section, individuals should not get distracted by the adjective. The positive and negative descriptors are used as reminders that reinforcements operate in opposition, but the descriptor terms can be changed to fit the working definitions. For example, reinforcement categories could be labeled "encouragement" and "discouragement" rather than "positive" and "negative." There can be similar confusion concerning the two categories of resources (access to and access removed). Resources can be made more accessible or restricted, and both categories should be captured on the PER worksheet.

No interventions

Finally, interventions are designed to change the antecedents listed in the PER worksheet. Thus, one should not list interventions in the worksheet. For example, researchers note that middle and high school students who participate in sex education are more likely to use contraception (Kirby, 2002). One may want to list "comprehensive sex education" as an access to resource for the behavior of consistent and correct condom use. The error in this thinking is that school-based health education is designed to change specific antecedents. It is changing the antecedents that is associated with change in health behavior. The mechanism or intervention by which the skills change is not an antecedent. In the comprehensive sex education example, the learning objectives of the Safer Choices curricula include building the following student skills: correct condom use, negotiation, refusal, and purchasing (Coyle at al., 1999; ETR Associates, 2004). Correct condom use, negotiation skills, refusal skills, and purchasing are the antecedents. When a student successfully participates in the Safer Choices program, he or she develops these skills. It is the student's acquisition of the skills that increases condoms use. These skills could be altered through another type of intervention, such as an online tutorial or parent education. The process of matching interventions to types of antecedents will be discussed in Chapter 9.

> **Check for Understanding**   Place the following factors in the correct categories of the PER worksheet: food label reading, fear of failure, price of fruit, and praise by parents.

Theoretical Logic Models

In addition to theory, the use of logic models is also recommended to increase and document program effectiveness (USDHHS, 1999; W. K. Kellogg, 2004). A logic model is a visual picture of how program planners expect a program to work; it illustrates the theory and the assumptions underlying the program. Programmatically, logic models display program resources, program activities, activity outputs, participant outcomes, and long-term impact. Models reflect the process of planning, implementation, and evaluation. It is the process of developing the model that creates stronger program plans and improved evaluations. "The clarity of thinking that occurs from building the model is critical to the overall success of the program" (W. K. Kellogg, 1998, p. 43).

One specific type of logic model, a **theoretical logic model**, is a detailed explanation of the target behavior or environmental condition (W. K. Kellogg Foundation, 2004). This type of model, also called a conceptual model, outlines the behavioral antecedents and the hypothesized relationship between the antecedents. This "visual explanation" helps planners map conceptual ideas or assumptions about the behavior. Assumptions include what the behavioral antecedents are, which are more important than others, and the relationship between the antecedents. It is from these assumptions about antecedents and relationships that all program activities are developed. Program activities are designed to change antecedents such as beliefs and skills. When these strategies are successful, changes in health behavior occur. These assumptions also map a sequence of the programming activities.

Activity logic models and outcome logic models are two other types of logic models. Activity logic models illustrate the specific activities that will be implemented in a program. They illustrate the work a team will actually *do* as part of a program (W. K. Kellogg, 2004). Outcome logic models illustrate the anticipated short-term and long-term outcomes from the program activities—what a team expects to *get* as a result of program activities. Therefore, activity and outcome logic models can be referred to as program logic models (Knowlton-Wyatt & Phillips, 2009). The theory model is the foundation of both the activities model and the outcome logic model. A theory model outlines the behavioral antecedents and the hypothesized relationship between the antecedents. An activity model adds activities a planner intends to do to change the antecedents and behavior; and finally, the outcome model projects the outcomes that will result if the activities work as intended. Because activities are designed around behavioral antecedents, many of the expected outcomes are changes in behavioral antecedents or processes related to changing antecedents. The ultimate goal of this process is the alignment of these three sections: theoretical assumptions, activities, and outcomes. Both activity and outcome logic models will be discussed in more detail in Chapter 9.

The final model should be linear and easy to follow. The logic model development process, however, is nonlinear and fluid. All models, logic and otherwise, represent a picture of one's understanding of a phenomenon. The understanding of complex phenomenon such as health behaviors evolves in stages. Models also likely evolve in stages. Clear, concise models are the result of multiple drafts and feedback from others.

The fundamental aspects of a model are sequence, grouped pieces, and relationships. To make the transition from the PER worksheet to building a conceptual model, program planners need to identify the big concepts that serve as model anchors. From the model anchors, sequence, grouped pieces, and relationships are formed. Behavioral anchors, sometimes called **behavioral building blocks**, represent antecedents or groupings of antecedents that are the foundation of the development of the logic model. Behavioral building blocks establish the initial framework from which other antecedents and relationships are displayed. Building blocks can be identified by answering one or more of the following questions:

1. What are the behavioral milestones?

2. What are the key antecedents?

3. Who are the important others?

Behavioral Milestones

Behavioral milestones represent stage transitions. In the process of behavior change, **milestones** are like gates that must be passed through in order for the later antecedents and processes to be meaningful. All behaviors have milestones. Two important and common milestones are intention and trial use. For example, if a young adult does not intend to use a condom consistently and correctly, then access to condoms and possession of the skills to use condoms are not important. Intention is also an important milestone in infant breastfeeding. A new mother must intend to breastfeed her infant

(USDHHS, 2011). Without intention, the skill and access to time and place is not important. The mother's intention can also change and thus may represent multiple milestones in the process of breastfeeding an infant for at least 12 months. A new mother's intentions may be specific in that she intends to breastfeed (1) while she is in the hospital, (2) once she and her infant go home, and (3) when she returns to work. These three intentions could represent three behavioral building blocks for breastfeeding an infant for 12 months.

Trial use of a target behavior is also an important behavioral milestone. Theoretically, if an individual tries a behavior and has a positive experience or does not have an expected negative experience, then efficacy and intention for repeating the behavior increase. **Trial use** is often the purpose of awareness interventions. For example, events such as National Walk to School Day encourage students to participate in the target behavior for one day. While one day of walking to school represents only a fraction of the desired behavior, getting a person to try a behavior and have a positive experience is a milestone to initiation and adoption of the behavior. Assuming the students enjoy themselves and find others to walk with, future walks to school are more likely (see Figure 8-2). Conversely, if a student walks to school and experiences undesired outcomes, that student is less likely to walk to school again. As demonstrated in Figures 8-2 and 8-3, one common sequence of behavioral milestones is intention, trial, and reinforcements.

After the behavioral building blocks are identified, antecedents remaining from the PER worksheet are placed logically around each behavioral building block. The **logic** of placing the remaining antecedents comes from the rich factual knowledge acquired from the individual theories. For example, if intention is a milestone, the next step is to reflect on the factors that drive intention. In the TPB, intention is influenced by attitudes toward the behavior, subjective norm, and perceived behavioral control (see Chapter 5 to review the TPB). These three constructs are all represented in the Beliefs category of column one in the PER worksheet. Therefore, many of the listed beliefs likely influence intention. Furthermore, beliefs can be grouped under headings such as beliefs about health outcomes or beliefs about social outcomes. For example, in new mothers, attitudes toward breastfeeding can be organized around (1) health outcomes for the infant as well as (2) comfort (see Figure 8-3).

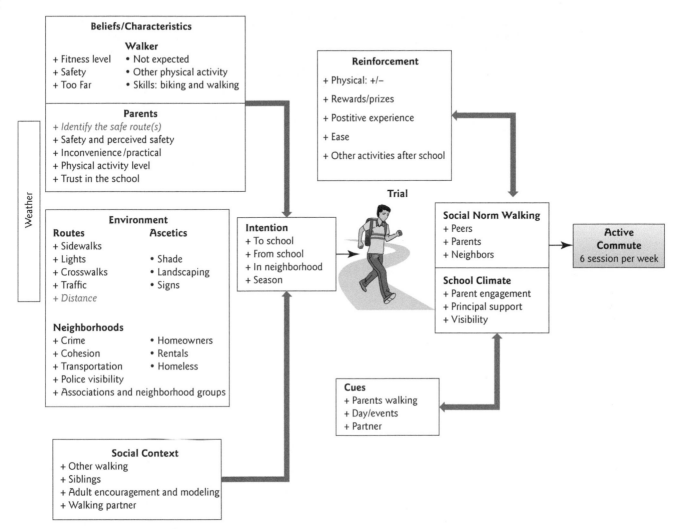

Figure 8-2 Finding a Route Theoretical Logic Model

Check for Understanding What antecedents might come after the trial use of a behavior?

Key Antecedents

Key antecedents are variables that have consistent and strong relationships with the target behavior or with another antecedent. Key antecedents are factors or variables that must change for the target behavior to change. The strength of relationships can be reported in a variety of ways. First, it is reported through statistical methods such as explained variance in the target behavior or the correlation between the behavior and the antecedent. Another way that strength of relationships can be reported is through descriptive information about the factor and the behavior. For example, antecedents or variables may be reported as the most common barriers to or facilitators of the target behavior. Another method by which to infer relationship strength and consistency is to read published meta-analyses

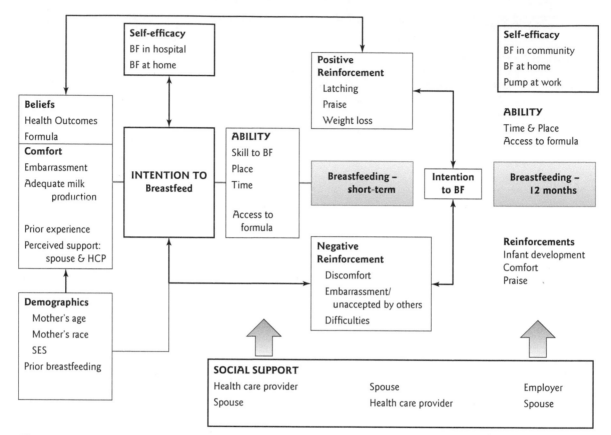

Figure 8-3 Breastfeeding for 12 Months Theoretical Logic Model

or comprehensive reviews of the literature. Studies and reports identify predictors of the target behavior across numerous studies and make conclusions as to the relationship between the antecedent and behavior. For example, McAuley and colleagues (2003) concluded that self-efficacy is the strongest predictor of physical activity and is consistently found to be the best facilitator of physical activity.

Key antecedents can fall into any category on the PER worksheet. After reviewing or assessing the behavioral antecedents in a population, key antecedents will stand out in the program planner's mind as *important*. In the case of adolescent fruit and vegetable consumption, the belief of unappetizing taste is arguably a must change antecedent (Glanz et al., 1998). In the case of breastfeeding, lack of social support and lactation difficulties are two must change antecedents (Meedya et al., 2010; USDHHS, 2011).

After the key antecedent behavioral building blocks are identified, the process is the same as that introduced with behavioral milestones. Remaining antecedents are placed logically around each behavioral building block. The logic of placing the remaining antecedents comes from the knowledge acquired from the individual theories.

Important Others

A third way to begin a conceptual model is to identify individuals who play a fundamental role in the behavior. Important others can be mapped as a pathway or story line through the model leading up to the target behavior. For example, in the walking and bicycling to school example, parents of young children play a fundamental role in the trial use and reinforcement of the behavior (Active Living Research, 2009; Kerr et al., 2006; National Center for Safe Routes to School, 2010).

A conceptual model may start with a parent block (or row of blocks) preceding the student trial use block (see Figure 8-2). The method of mapping important others is not as common as mapping by milestones or key antecedents; however, this method is valuable for select behaviors and populations. Behaviors that involve the beliefs, prompts, and resources of health care providers and parents of small children are two such examples.

Constructing a Conceptual Model

There are multiple ways to construct a theory or conceptual model. In some instances, a model will be based solely on milestones, key antecedents, and/or important others. However, in other instances, a model may use a combination of the three types of behavioral building blocks. For example, both milestones and important others are used as model anchors to illustrate the behavior of walking and bicycling to school (see Figure 8-2). Intention and trial use are illustrated as milestones, and parental beliefs and characteristics are factors of important others.

Models are organized around *big concepts* and groupings of antecedents, and they read in an *if–then* manner. Program planners group antecedents under the descriptive adjectives and present them sequentially. A team member, a funding agency, or a community stakeholder should be able to read the model from left to right, in a series of *if X, then Y* sentences. For example, in Figure 8-2, *if* parents believe the route is safe and that walking to school is not inconvenient, *then* they are more likely to encourage walking to school. Furthermore, *if* a child tries walking to school and experiences positive reinforcement, *then* he or she is likely to repeat the behavior.

Traditionally, sequencing is organized around time. As models move from left to right, time progresses. Persons are predisposed and over time, other factors enable and reinforce action. Sequencing can also be reflected be other big concepts. In a social ecological model, the big concepts are levels of the environment. These levels include the physical environment, social environment, political environment, and so on. In the examples of Chapter 4, the social ecological model for the behavior of bullying, antecedents were organized by levels of the environment: individual, peers, and then the school community.

Finally, because theory logic models are pictures of one's understandings and assumptions, no two models are the same. Figures 8-2 through 8-4 illustrate target behaviors as planners understood the behavioral antecedents and the hypothesized relationship between the antecedents. Other professionals may depict these behaviors differently.

The Model as a Communication Tool

The complete theory logic model serves as a communication tool. A one-page model communicates a tremendous amount of information. A well-designed model identifies a target behavior, influential factors, the assumed relationship of the factors, and future intervention targets. The model depicts two types of relationships. First, an effective model shows the relationship between the antecedents. For example, a model may illustrate a direct relationship between trial use and reinforcement. Second, and equally important, a theory model depicts how the pieces of the model fit together to form the whole model. Figure 8-3 outlines the assumed relationship between beliefs and intention (relationship of antecedents) and shows how intention is an essential milestone in breastfeeding (relationship to the whole). A theory model is a picture of the understanding of how the target behavior and the variables that influence that behavior are related. If one does not have a working understanding of the target behavior *and* the antecedents for that behavior, creating an effective model is unlikely to occur.

For models to be effective communication tools, they should be easy to follow and visually appealing. White space, color, and text boxes can make a model visually appealing. Graphics and design should be tools for communicating the content, though, and should not compete with the content. Use design and graphics as tools to help communicate **sequence**, grouped pieces, and relationships. Finally, when appropriate, one may consider using a graphic, color, or title that is innovative and memorable.

Table 8-2 outlines tips for creating a logical and visually appealing model. Keeping a model to one page and highlighting by color or design the fundamental aspects of the model are two important aspects of readability. A model cannot and should not be a complete representation of the behavior or one's understanding of the phenomenon. The model should be the big picture of the behavior, not the nuts and bolts (W.K. Kellogg, 2004). Teams will be able to supplement communication materials with text and with presentations.

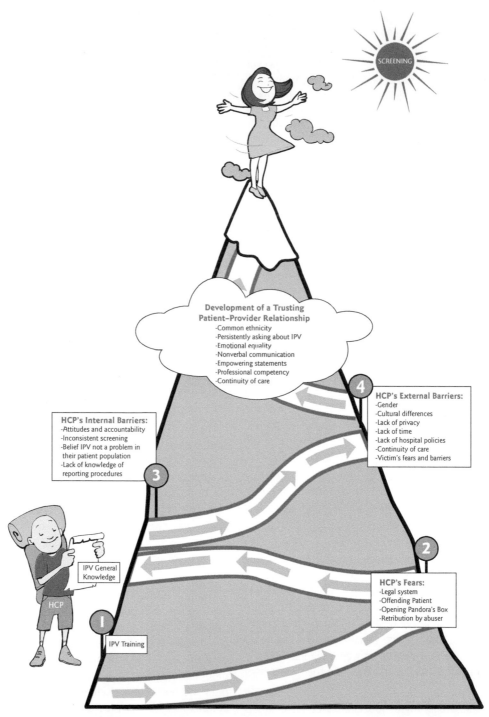

Figure 8-4 Screening for Intimate Partner Violence Theoretical Logic Model
Source: Ebron (2012)

TABLE 8-2 Tips for Constructing a Logic Model

Logical	Visually Appealing
Arrange antecedents in a time sequence.	Keep logic model to one page.
Group similar antecedents, such as beliefs or skills, around adjectives or themes.	Use white space on page.
Anchor model with two to three building blocks.	Color code regions of the model to communicate stages or building blocks.
Highlight milestone building blocks via color or bold text box lines.	Limit text to two to four words per antecedent box.
Place antecedents around building blocks.	Except for the title, frame text in a box or with a similar tool.
Link components with visual aids such as arrows or circles.	Include a graphic, design, color, or title to make readers enjoy and remember the message of the model.
Refine the model as understanding is refined.	Consider originality. Make it yours; there is not just one way to construct a model.

Identifying and Assessing Behavioral Antecedents

So how does one go about identifying the antecedents to list in the PER worksheet and developing the theoretical model? The methods are as similar, and as varied, as those employed in a community assessment. One can review the research of others, collect her own information, or incorporate a combination of these two methods. Literature reviews and published reports are useful methods for identifying factors reported by other researchers and professionals. Reviewing the work of others will help develop an initial understanding of behaviors and behavioral antecedents. Key assumptions or gaps in understanding are verified or filled via data collection. Focus groups, interviews, and questionnaires are traditional methods of primary data collection. Detailed content on assessment and evaluation is beyond the scope of this text; however, the following sections highlight content as it relates to studying behavioral antecedents.

Literature Review and Agency Reports

Reviewing the research of others is a helpful way to identify potential behavioral antecedents. Research findings about behaviors and behavioral antecedents are most frequently published in peer-reviewed journals, but one may also find helpful information in agency reports and on websites. Because researchers often focus on select categories of antecedents (e.g., beliefs and skills, and/or a particular population), it is strongly suggested that program planners use a variety of sources to conduct a comprehensive review of the literature. Locating published papers on behavioral antecedents requires searching by specific terms. Numerous combinations of search words will yield reports about behavioral factors; however, the following key words are a recommended starting point:

1. The target behavior *and*

2. One of the following: correlates, antecedents, factors, predictors

For example, in locating antecedents for breastfeeding, one would type into the key word search box *"breastfeeding"* and *"correlates."* "Breastfeeding" is the target behavior and "correlates" directs the search to behavioral antecedents. A PubMed search by these two terms yielded 234 articles. To search only by the behavior, "breastfeeding" yields over 36,000 hits, and the findings are primarily on the prevalence and benefits of breastfeeding. A similar keyword mistake is to search by health issue, which will produce articles related to the physiology of disease, prevalence, and risk factors—one ends up with a tremendous number of citations. One may also use theoretical construct names, such as attitudes or cues to action, to narrow a search. For example, a search in PubMed using the terms "breastfeeding" and "intentions" yielded 470 articles, 21 of which are reviews of literature. Finally, adding a specific population will narrow the search further.

Some behaviors are well researched, and antecedents can be identified by population and/or a specific form of the behavior. Physical activity is a well-researched behavior. The initial surgeon general's report on physical activity was published in 1999, and since then, thousands of physical activity studies have been published. A PubMed search using the words "physical activity" and "correlates" produced close to 4500 articles. However, adding the audience of "children" reduced the number to 568; "preschoolers" narrowed the relevant articles to 118. Searching by a specific form of physical activity also reduced the number of article citations. A search using the terms "walking to school" and "correlates" yielded 185 citations.

Table 8-3 includes a list of health behaviors, key words, and examples of relevant articles. When conducting a review of literature, articles published more recently tend to have more up-to-date information. Research and understanding in particular areas of focus evolve and trend by topic. Some "landmark" studies and/or reviews of behavioral factors may not be the most recent articles. To develop a scope of understanding of a behavior, the body of research should be read and processed. Rarely can a professional develop a rich understanding of a phenomenon through reading one or two articles. The articles listed in Table 8-3 serve as examples of the types of articles one should locate and the key words that can help locate them.

A comprehensive review of the behavioral literature may also include reports from credible agencies. Agencies can include federal organizations such as the Centers for Disease Control and Prevention and the National Highway Traffic Safety Administration. Agencies with health behavior and behavioral antecedent research briefs may also include foundations like the Robert Wood Johnson Foundation (www.rwj.org), research centers like Active Living Research (www.activeliving.org), federally funded centers like National Center for Safe Routes to School (www.saferoutesinfo.org), or advocacy groups like Susan G. Komen for the Cure (www.komen.org).

Primary Data Collection

Focus groups, key informant interviews, and questionnaires are common methods for assessing information about behaviors and behavioral antecedents.

Focus Groups and Key Informant Interviews

Focus groups are small groups of individuals that come together for a brief period to discuss behavior, attitudes, beliefs, and other antecedents in a group setting (Krueger & Casey, 2009). The individuals included in the focus group typically have a trait or behavior in common, such as being registered voters, cigarette smokers, or parents of children who attend the same school. The purpose of the focus group is to assess individual perceptions about particular behaviors. Knowledge, beliefs, and demographic and other predisposing factors can be assessed via focus groups. Focus groups are facilitated by a trained moderator and follow a semistructured facilitator's guide. Information from multiple groups can then be analyzed for topical themes (Krueger & Casey, 2009).

Key informant interviews are similar in style to focus groups but are conducted in a one-on-one format. An interviewer facilitates a discussion with an individual who is considered to have direct information about the behavior, the antecedents, and/or the settings in which the behavior takes place. Like focus groups, key informant interviews are intended to assess the interviewee's individual perceptions about particular behaviors; however, the key informant may or may not be a member of the target audience. For example, in the walking and bicycling to school example, a target audience member to be interviewed may be a parent. However, a school principal or police officer, neither of whom is a member of the target audience, may have equally valuable insight into the predisposing and reinforcing factors related to walking and biking to school. The interviews are facilitated by a trained interviewer and follow a semistructured facilitator's guide with set themes and planned probing questions (Patton, 2002). To develop a multidimensional understanding of perceived factors, multiple key informant interviews should be completed. Interviews should be conducted with individuals who engage in the behavior, program planners, policy makers, and others who have important information about the behavior. The qualitative methods of focus groups and key informant interviews have the potential to elicit information that is rich in context, meaning, and detail. The open-ended format of these

TABLE 8-3 Health Behaviors, Search Words, and Sample Published Articles

Content Area	Health Behavior	Possible Search Terms	Articles[a]
Nutrition	Fruit and vegetable intake	• Correlates • Vegetable intake • Children	**Characteristics of family mealtimes affecting children's vegetable consumption and liking.** Sweetman, C., McGowan, L., Croker, H., & Cooke, L. (2011) in *Journal of American Dietetic Association, 111*(2), 269-73. **Correlates of fruit and vegetable intake in US children.** Lorson, B. A., Melgar-Quinonez, H. R., & Taylor, C. A. (2009) in *Journal of the American Dietetic Association, 109*(3), 474-8.
Nutrition	Breastfeeding	• Breastfeeding • Intention	**Factors that positively influence breastfeeding duration to 6 months: A literature review.** Meedya, S., Fahy, K., & Kable, A. (2010) in *Women and Birth, 23*(4), 135-45. **Influence of partner support on an employed mother's intention to breastfeed after returning to work.** Tsai, S.Y. (2014) in *Breastfeeding Medicine, 9*(4), 222-230.
Physical Activity	Walking to and from school	• Walk to school • Parental beliefs	**Active transportation and acculturation among Latino children in San Diego County.** Martinez, S. M., Ayala, G. X., Arredondo, E. M., Finch, B., & Elder, J. (2008) in *Preventive Medicine, 47*(3). 313-8. **Parental safety concerns and active school commute: Correlates across multiple domains in the home-to-school journey.** Oluyomi, A. O., Lee, C., Nehme, E., Dowdy, D., Ory, M. G., & Hoelscher, D. M. (2014) in *International Journal of Behavioral Nutrition and Physical Activity, 11*(1), 11-32.
Alcohol and other drugs	Binge drinking	• Binge drinking • Predictors	**Underage drinking: A developmental framework.** Masten, A. S., Faden, V. B., Zucker, R. A., & Spear, L. P. (2008) in *Pediatrics, 121*, S235-S251. **Determinants of sustained binge drinking in young adults.** Wellman, R. J., Contreras, G. A., Dugas, E. N., O'Loughlin, E. K., & O'Loughlin, J. L. (2014) in *Alcoholism: Clinical and Experimental Research, 38*(5), 1409-1415.
Physical activity (PA)	Organized PA in individuals with a disability	• Individuals with a disability • Physical activity • Barriers	**A review of social and environmental barriers to physical activity for adults with intellectual disabilities.** Bodde, A. E., & Seo, D. C. (2009) in *Disability & Health, 2*(2). 57-66. **Barriers associated with exercise and community access for individuals with stroke.** Rimmer, J. H., Wang, E., & Smith, D. (2008) in *Journal of Rehabilitation Research & Development, 45*(2), 315-22.

continues

TABLE 8-3 *continued*

Content Area	Health Behavior	Possible Search Terms	Articles[a]
Injury prevention	Emergency preparedness	• Emergency preparedness • Predictors	**Predictors of emergency preparedness and compliance.** Murphy, S. T., Cody, M., Frank, L. B., Glik, D., & Ang, A. (2009) in *Disaster Medicine and Public Health Preparedness, 3*(Supplement 2). S1–S9. **Family emergency preparedness plans in severe tornadoes.** Cong, Z., Liang, D., & Luo, J. (2014) in *American Journal of Preventive Medicine, 46*(1), 89-93.
Injury prevention	Health care provider screening for intimate partner violence	• Domestic violence screening • Physician attitudes	**Barriers to domestic violence screening in the pediatric setting.** Erickson, M., Hill, T., & Siegel, R. (2001) in *Pediatrics, 108*(1), 98-102. **"They told me to leave": How health care providers address intimate partner violence.** Rse, D. S., Lafleur, R., Fogarty, C. T., Mittal, M., & Cerulli, C. (2012) in *Journal of the American Board of Family Medicine, 25*(3), 333-42.
Tobacco	Smoking cessation in pregnant women	• Smoking cessation • Pregnancy • Correlates	**Smoking cessation during pregnancy: A systematic literature review.** Schneider, S., Huy, C., Schütz, J., & Diehl. K. (2010) in *Drug and Alcohol Review, 29*(1), 81-90. **Pregnancy smoking in context: The influence of multiple levels of stress.** Weaver, K., Campbell, R., Mermelstein, R., & Wakschlag. L. (2008) in *Nicotine & Tobacco Research, 10*(6), 1065-73.
Sexual behaviors	Adherence to HIV treatment	• Determinants • Treatment adherence HIV	**Impact of HIV-related stigma on treatment adherence: A systematic review and meta-synthesis.** Katz, I. T., Ryu, A. E., Onuegbu, A. G., Psaros, C., Weiser, S. D., Bangsberg, D. R. & Tsai, A.C. (2013) in *Journal of the International AIDS Society, 16*(Suppl. 2). 1-25. **A systematic review of barriers to medication adherence in the elderly: Looking beyond cost and regimen complexity.** Gellad, W. F., Grenard, J. L. & Marcum, Z. A. (2011) in *American Journal of Geriatric Pharmacotherapy, 9*(1), 11-23.

Source: a) Located in PubMed, April 2014.

methods produces findings that are harder to score and summarize and thus may be supplemented with survey methods of understanding, such as questionnaires.

Questionnaires

Questionnaires can be administered via written surveys, telephone, face-to-face questioning, or the Internet. One can use questionnaires to examine knowledge, beliefs, demographics, and behavior patterns, as well the relationship among these factors. With a computer and a few hours, questionnaires are easy to construct (Gillham, 2007); however, the ease with which one can now create and distribute questionnaires has contributed to their misuse and even abuse (Gillham, 2007). Valid and reliable questionnaires need to be developed following specific procedures. Typically, a pool of questions, or items, is generated from the literature and/or other questionnaires. Not only should there be consideration as to the purpose of the questions, the format of the items should receive careful consideration and testing. Questionnaire items can be open ended or close ended. Close-ended items require an individual to pick a response from a list of options. Common close-ended formats include multiple choice, true/false and Likert scales. These forced responses allow the items to be scored and tallied. Early drafts of questionnaires need to be reviewed by a panel of experts, and they also need to be field tested with a population similar to the target population. Prior to final administration, a questionnaire should also be pilot tested for a measure of reliability, that is, is the questionnaire formatted such that it consistently gathers responses? Once the instrument is documented as valid and reliable, it can be used to collect data from the target population. Given this process, a practitioner may consider using an existing questionnaire. For example, the National Center for Safe Routes to School has posted on its website a questionnaire for assessing both parents' and students' perceptions regarding walking to and from school (National Center for Safe Routes to School, 2012).

Observation

Observation is another category of primary data collection used to assess need, evaluate program outcomes, and understand behavioral antecedents. Observation is the direct recording of behaviors, events, or traits. Observation eliminates the need to ask participants to answer questions through interviews, focus groups, or questionnaires. Observations and counts can assess health behavior frequency, and they can assess numerous behavioral antecedents. For example, in the walking and bicycling to school example (see Figure 8-2), the number of students walking to and from school can be observed and counted (Pedestrian and Bicycle Information Center, 2007). A volunteer can stand at the school entrance on select days and record the number of students who arrive via walking or bicycling. The observer can also record many other variables, such as gender, age, walking partners, and disposition. Observations, like the walking tally, can be the sole form of data collection or can supplement other methods, such as self-reported walking (Gillham, 2008). Observation, via a walkability audit, may also be a tool to assess features of routes that facilitate or create barriers to walking. Audits and similar counts most often reveal antecedents in the Enabling and Reinforcement columns of the PER worksheet.

Mixed-Method Approach

For practitioners, a mixed-method approach to behavioral understanding is ideal and realistic. Reviewing the work of others will help planners develop an initial understanding of behaviors and behavioral antecedents. Primary data collection can then verify key assumptions or fill in gaps in understanding. This approach captures the best of both worlds. One can learn a great deal about a behavior from the work of others; however, to rely solely on secondary information may lead to a false or incomplete understanding of behavioral factors in a particular population or context. Similarly, a practitioner is unlikely to have the time and resources to complete a significant amount of primary data collection. Safe Routes to School, a national program of the U.S. Department of Transportation's Federal Highway Administration, endorses such a mixed-methods approach to planning. There are Safe Routes programs in 15,000 schools across all 50 states and the District of Columbia (National Center for Safe Routes to School, 2012). Funded Safe Routes programs are designed around five areas, called the 5 Es. The 5 Es model includes engineering, enforcement, education, encouragement, and evaluation (Pedestrian and Bicycle Information Center, 2007). These very specific intervention areas are based on research from the national center and others. This research has identified perceptions of safety and convenience, route infrastructure and design, route safety, and social networks as common behavioral correlates of walking and/or bicycling to school (Active Living Research, 2009). Local programs are more likely to be successful and use resources efficiently if there is an assessment of the particular correlates that are influencing the local behavior. For example, one community may have safe and aesthetically pleasing routes, but most of the students live outside a 1-mile radius. A second community may have a true neighborhood school, with most children living within close proximity to the school; however, parents may have concerns about traffic, sidewalks, and safety. Completing some primary data collection will help a planner distinguish the differences in context.

The process of behavioral understanding begins with determining the scope and purpose of the assessment (Price, Dake, & Ward, 2010). The categories on the PER worksheet serve as a guide to developing the scope, purpose, and objectives. Through the research of others and primary data collection, program planners develop an understanding of the knowledge, beliefs, intentions, demographics, resources, skills, cues, reinforcements, and/or support networks that influence the desired behavior.

SUMMARY

Health promotion programs are best designed around more than one health behavior theory. Multilevel interventions blend concepts from intrapersonal, interpersonal, and community-level theories. The PER worksheet is a planning tool that provides lay term prompts from eight health behavior theories and one planning model. The PER worksheet is organized into three columns: **P**redisposing, **E**nabling, and **R**einforcing factors (which are terms of the PRECEDE/PROCEED model). Predisposing factors represent cognitive and affective antecedents related to motivation for the target behavior. The category prompts include know, believe, intent, and demographic factors. Enabling factors represent environmental and skill antecedents that enable a person to accomplish the target behavior. The category prompts include be able to do (skills), access to, and access removed. Reinforcing factors come from others or the environment and promote the continuation or repetitiveness of the target behavior. The category prompts include reminders, positive reinforcement, negative reinforcement, and social support. A theory logic model provides a visual picture of these antecedents and their hypothesized relationship to the target behavior. To make the transition from the PER worksheet to building a theory model, program planners need to identify the big concepts that serve as model anchors.

IN THE CLASSROOM ACTIVITIES

1) Take the list of factors that influence one of your health behaviors (from Chapter 2, activity #5). Classify the factors into the categories of the PER worksheet. Knowing the general prompts and the rich information from the behavioral theories, add additional factors to each column.

2) Select and read one article from Table 8-3. Classify health behavior factors into the categories of the PER worksheet. Compare with another student.

3) Identify "key antecedents" or the behavioral milestones in the practice of childhood immunizations. Reference Figure 8-1 as needed.

4) Work with another student, and using Figure 8-1, create a theory-based logic model, synthesizing constructs from multiple health behavior theories.

5) Refer to Table 8-2, refine the theoretical model, and share the model with the class.

WEB LINKS

Centers for Disease Control and Prevention, Vaccines & Immunizations: http://www.cdc.gov/vaccines/

Office of Behavioral and Social Sciences Research: http://obssr.od.nih.gov/index.aspx

Safe Routes to School: http://www.saferoutesinfo.org/

W. K. Kellogg Foundation: http://www.wkkf.org/resource-directory

REFERENCES

Active Living Research. (2009). *Walking and biking to school: Physical activity and health outcomes.* Robert Wood Johnson Foundation. Retrieved from http://www.activelivingresearch.org/files/ALR_Brief_ActiveTransport.pdf

Akis, S., Velipasaoglu, S., Camurdan, A. D., Beyazova, U., & Sahin, F. (2011). Factors associated with parental acceptance and refusal of pandemic influenza A/H1N1 vaccine in Turkey. *European Journal of Pediatrics, 170*(9), 1165–1172.

Benin, A. L., Wisler-Scher, D. J., Colson, E., Shapiro, E. D., & Holmboe, E. S. (2006). Qualitative analysis of mothers' decision-making about vaccines for infants: The importance of trust. *Pediatrics, 117*(5), 1532–1541.

Berkman, N. D., Sheridan, S. L., Donahue, K. E., Halpern, D. J., & Crotty, K. (2011). Low health literacy and health outcomes: An updated systematic review. *Annals of Internal Medicine, 155*(2), 97–107.

Brown, K. F., Kroll, J. S., Hudson, M. J., Ramsay, M., Green, J., Long, S. J., et al. (2010). Factors underlying parental decisions about combination childhood vaccinations including MMR: A systematic review. *Vaccine, 28*(26), 4235–4248.

Cassidy, K., Graham, J. R., McGrath, P.J., Finley, G. A., Smith, D.J., Morley, C., et al. (2002). Watch needle, watch TV: Audiovisual distraction in preschool immunization. *Pain Medicine, 3*(2), 108–118.

Centers for Disease Control and Prevention (CDC). (1998). Use of cervical and breast cancer screening among women with and without functional limitation: United States, 1994–1995. *Morbidity and Mortality Weekly, 47*(40), 853–856.

Centers for Disease Control and Prevention (CDC). (1999). Framework for program evaluation in public health. *Morbidity and Mortality Weekly, 48*(No. RR-11), 1–40.

Coyle, K., Basen-Engquist, K., Kirby, D., Parcel, G., Banspach, S., Harrist, R.,...Weil, M. (1999). Short-term impact of safer choices: A multicomponent, school-based HIV, other STD, and pregnancy prevention program. *Journal of School Health, 69*(5), 181–188.

Daley, M. F., Crane, L. A., Chandramouli, V., Beaty, B. L., Barrow, J., Allred, N., Berman, S., & Kempe, A. (2006). Influenza among healthy young children: Changes in parental attitudes and predictors of immunization during the 2003 to 2004 influenza season. *Pediatrics, 117*(2), e268–e277.

Ebron, D. (2012). *Conquering health care provider barriers to intimate partner violence screening: Theoretical logic model* (Unpublished graduate project). Dayton, OH: Wright State University.

ETR Associates. (2004). *Safer choices preventing HIV, other STDs and pregnancy*. Scotts Valley, CA: ETR Associates.

Gillham, B. (2007). *Developing a questionnaire* (2nd ed.). New York: Continuum International.

Gillham, B. (2008). *Observation techniques: Structured to unstructured*. New York: Continuum International.

Glanz, K., Basil, M., Maibach, E., Goldberg, J., & Snyder, D. (1998). Why Americans eat what they do: Taste, nutrition, cost, convenience, and weight control concerns as influences on food consumption. *Journal of the American Dietetic Association, 98,* 1118–1126.

Green, L. W., & Kreuter, M.W. (2005). *Health promotion planning: An educational and ecological approach* (4th ed.). Boston: McGraw Hill.

Hak, E., Schönbeck, Y., Melker, H. D., Van Essen, G. A., & Sanders, E. A. M. (2005). Negative attitudes of highly educated parents and health care workers towards future vaccinations in the Dutch childhood vaccination program. *Vaccine, 23*(24), 3103–3107.

Harris, K. M., Hughbanks-Wheaton, D. K., Johnston, R., & Kubin, L. (2007). Parental refusal or delay of childhood immunization: Implications for nursing and health education. *Teaching and Learning in Nursing, 2*(4), 126–132.

Iezzoni, L. I., McCarthy, E. P., Davis, R. B., & Siebens, H. (2000). Mobility impairments and use of screening and preventive services. *American Journal of Public Health, 90*(6), 955–961.

Kerr, J., Rosenberg, D., Sallis, J. F., Saelens, B. E., Frank, L. D., & Conway, T. L. (2006). Active commuting to school: Associations with environment and parental concerns. *Medicine and Science in Sports and Exercise, 38*(4), 787–794.

Kirby, D. (2002). Antecedents of adolescent initiation of sex, contraceptive use, and pregnancy. *American Journal of Health Behavior, 26*(6), 473–485.

Knowlton-Wyatt, L., & Phillips C. C. (2009). *The logic model guidebook: Better strategies for great results*. Los Angeles: Sage.

Krueger, R. A., & Casey, M. A. (2009). *Focus groups: A practical guide for applied research* (4th ed.). Thousand Oaks, CA: Sage.

Langlois, M., & Hallam, J. (2010). Integrating multiple health behavior theories into program planning: The PER worksheet. *Health Promotion Practice, 11*(2), 282–288.

Langlois, M., Petosa, R., & Hallam, J. (1999). Why do effective smoking prevention programs work? Student changes in social cognitive theory constructs. *Journal of School Health, 69*(8), 326–331.

Lin, C. J., Nowalk, M. P., Zimmerman, R. K., Ko, F., Zoffel, L., Hoberman, A., & Kearney, D. H. (2006). Beliefs and attitudes about influenza immunization among parents of children with chronic medical conditions over a two-year period. *Journal of Urban Health, 83*(5), 874–883.

Luthy, K. E., Beckstrand, R. L., & Peterson, N. E. (2009). Parental hesitation as a factor in delayed childhood immunization. *Journal of Pediatric Health Care, 23*(6), 388–393.

Martin, S., Orlowski, M., & Ellison, S. (2013). Sociodemographic factors that predict cervical cancer screenings in Ohio women with a disability. *Social Work in Public Health, 28*(6), 583–590.

McAuley, E., Jerome, G. J., Marquez, D. X., Elavsky, S., & Blissmer, B. (2003). Exercise self-efficacy in older adults: Social, affective, and behavioral influences. *Annals of Behavioral Medicine, 25*(1), 1–7.

McMenamin, S. B, Halpin, H. A., & Bellows, N. M. (2006). Knowledge of Medicaid coverage and effectiveness of smoking treatments. *American Journal of Preventive Medicine, 31*(5), 369–374.

Meedya, S., Fahy, K., & Kable, A. (2010). Factors that positively influence breastfeeding duration to 6 months: A literature review. *Women and Birth, 23,* 135–145.

Narayan, R., & Orlowski, M. (2013). *Parental decision-making process in accepting or refusing childhood vaccination: PER worksheet* (Unpublished graduate project). Dayton, OH: Wright State University.

National Center for Safe Routes to School. (2010). *Safe Routes to School travel data: A look at baseline results from parent surveys and student travel tallies.* Retrieved from http://saferoutesinfo.org/resources

National Center for Safe Routes to School. (2012). *Safe Routes to School 2011–2012 annual report.* Retrieved from http://saferoutesinfo.org/

Patton, M. Q. (2002). *Qualitative research & evaluation methods* (3rd ed.). Thousand Oaks, CA: Sage.

Pedestrian and Bicycle Information Center. (2007). *Safe Routes to School guide.* Retrieved from http://www.saferoutesinfo.org/resources

Price, J. H., Dake, J. A., & Ward, B. (2010). Assessing the needs of program participants. In C. I. Fertman & D. D. Allensworth (Eds.), *Health promotion programs: From theory to practice* (pp. 91–108). San Francisco: Jossey-Bass.

Quadri-Sheriff, M., Hendrix, K. S., Downs, S. M., Sturm, L. A., Zimet, G. D., & Finnell, S. M. (2012). The role of herd immunity in parents' decision to vaccinate children: A systematic review. *Pediatrics, 130*(3), 522–530.

Ranney, L., Melvin, C., Lux, L., McClain, E., & Lohr, K. N. (2006). Systematic review: Smoking cessation intervention strategies for adults and adults in special populations. *Annals of Internal Medicine, 145*(11), 845–856.

Rogers, E. M. (2003). *Diffusion of innovations* (5th ed.). New York: Free Press.

Schechter, N. L., Zempsky, W. T., Cohen, L. L., McGrath, P. J., McMurtry, C. M., & Bright, N. S. (2007). Pain reduction during pediatric immunizations: Evidence-based review and recommendations. *Pediatrics, 119*(5), e1184–e1198.

Schueler, K. M., Chu, P. W., & Smith-Bindman, R. (2008). Factors associated with mammography utilization: A systematic quantitative review of literature. *Journal of Women's Health, 17*(9), 1477–1498.

Smith, O. J., Kennedy, A. M., Wooten, K., Gust, D. S., & Pickering, L. K. (2006). Association between health care providers' influence on parents who have concerns about vaccine safety and vaccination coverage. *Pediatrics, 118*(5), e1287–e1292.

Spencer, L., Pagell, F., Hallion, M. E., & Adams, T. B. (2002). Applying the transtheoretical model to tobacco cessation and prevention: A review of literature. *American Journal of Health Promotion, 17*(1), 7–71.

Taylor, J., Evers, S., & McKenna, M. L. (2005). Determinants of healthy eating in children and youth. *Canadian Journal of Public Health, 96*(Supple 3), S20–S26.

Tortolero, S. R., Markham, C. M., Parcel, G. S., Peters, R. J., Jr., Escobar-Chaves, S. L., Basen-Engquist, K., & Lewis, H. L. (2005). Using intervention mapping to adapt an effective HIV, sexually transmitted disease, and pregnancy prevention program for high-risk minority youth. *Health Promotion Practice, 6*(3), 286–298.

U.S. Department of Health and Human Services (USDHHS). (2010). *How tobacco smoke causes disease: The biology and behavioral basis for smoking-attributable disease; A report of the surgeon general.* Atlanta: U.S. Department of Health and Human Services, Centers for Disease Control and Prevention (CDC), National Center for Chronic Disease Prevention and Health Promotion, Office of the Surgeon General.

U.S. Department of Health and Human Services (USDHHS). (2011). *The surgeon general's call to action to support breastfeeding.* Washington, DC: U.S. Department of Health and Human Services, Office of the Surgeon General.

W. K. Kellogg Foundation (1998). *W. K. Kellogg Foundation evaluation handbook.* Battle Creek MI: Author.

W. K. Kellogg Foundation (2004). *Logic model development guide.* Retrieved from http://www.wkkf.org/resource-directory

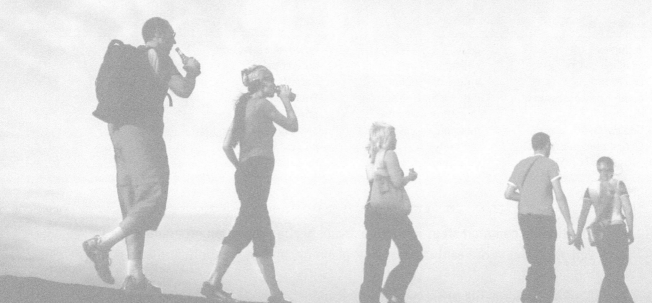

Applying Theory to Improve Practice

CHAPTER 9

Outcome Logic Models: The Picture of Program Planning and Evaluation

KEY TERMS

activities	goal	outcome evaluation	short-term objectives
baseline	indicator	outcomes	target
coalition	influential factors	outputs	triangulation
community assessment	intermediate objectives	Photovoice	
disability	long-term objectives	prioritization	
fidelity	morbidity	process evaluation	
Geographic Information System (GIS)	mortality	process measures	
	objective	resources	

LEARNING OBJECTIVES

1. Identify the common steps in the process of health promotion programming.
2. Link the process of health assessment, planning, implementation, and evaluation to logic modeling.
3. Identify components of an outcome logic model.
4. Explain a program's assumptions and anticipated outcomes illustrated in an outcome logic model.
5. Construct an outcome logic model, aligning behavioral targets to activities and outcomes.

IN THE NEWS ...

The Human Genome Project was completed in 2003. Researchers from the National Human Genome Research Institute explain that a genome is all of a person's genetic material, including the genes and the smaller genomic elements. Genes are made up of DNA, the chemical compound that directs the activities of every organism. DNA molecules are made of two twisting paired strands referred to as a double helix. The DNA code is written with four letters, each representing a different base. The four bases are adenine (A), which pairs with thymine (T), and cytosine (C), which pairs with guanine (G). "The human genome was found to contain approximately 3 billion of base pairs, which reside in the

23 pairs of chromosomes within the nucleus of all our cells. Each chromosome contains hundreds to thousands of genes, which carry the instructions for making proteins. Each of the estimated 20,000–25,000 genes in the human genome makes an average of three proteins" (National Human Genome Research Institute, n.d.).

The Human Genome Project has given rise to new understandings about health and opportunities for diagnosis, treatment, and prevention. The first human sequence took 6 to 8 years with an estimated cost of $1 billion. As a result of the mapping, there are now over 2000 genetic tests for human conditions. A human genome can now be sequenced in a few days, costing around $4000. Understanding a person's genome sequence allows for individualized genetic counseling and encouragement of preventive behaviors. In 2013, the Smithsonian Institute in Washington, DC, opened an exhibit to celebrate the tenth anniversary of the first complete human genome sequence.

The HeLa cells were instrumental to the Human Genome Project and similar cell-based discoveries. The HeLa cells were from a 31-year-old African American woman named Henrietta Lacks and were the first human cells ever to be grown in culture. A book about the life and cells of Henrietta Lacks, *The Immortal Life of Henrietta Lacks*, debuted on the New York Times Bestseller list in 2010 and remains on the list at the time of this writing, in 2014. The cells were extracted and cultivated from Lacks in 1951 without her permission. In 2013, the National Institutes of Health, the federal agency responsible for biomedical research, announced an agreement with members of the Lacks family. The agreement outlines new policies on cell use consent and privacy as well as family involvement in further use of the HeLa cells.

Introduction

Logic models are pictures of how planners think a program will work to improve the health of a community. Logic models communicate a program's assumptions, designed activities, and expected outcomes. An outcome logic model is a graphic depiction of the health promotion planning process. These one-page models represent a significant amount of work and clarity in thought. Advocates of outcome logic models state that they improve program evaluation by identifying evaluation targets during the planning process. Outcome logic models also promote the alignment of clearly identified activities to clearly defined outcomes as well as serve as communication tools. The models themselves are tools for understanding and planning. They map planned work and the process for achieving expected outcomes. The framework of the model is useful during the process of planning a health improvement project. Teams start with what is known or assumed and then create plans for the unknown and/or missing pieces.

This chapter will introduce the outcome logic model as both a planning and a communication tool, and discuss the individual components represented in the model. Outcome logic modeling graphically maps the process of program planning and evaluation.

Program Planning and Evaluation

The *process* represented in outcome logic models is health promotion program planning and evaluation. Health promotion is achieved through the process of planning, implementing, and evaluating multilevel interventions. Numerous planning models are developed by various organizers. Actual steps in the process might be tailored to the needs of an audience or the language of a discipline. Each model, however, reflects the four basic steps in a generic planning process: assessing and prioritizing community need, planning strategies of change, implementing targeted strategies, and measuring change (see Figure 9-1). Community

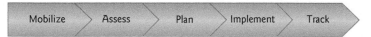

Figure 9-1 MAP-IT Generic Program Planning and Evaluation Model

Source: Adapted from Healthy People 2020, U.S. Department of Health and Human Services

health improvement is a large undertaking, so coalition and/or partnership building is typically imbedded in one of the early stages of the process. The work involved in these basic steps is completed and then represented in a visual organizer: the outcome logic model.

Assessing and Prioritizing

Health promotion programs are designed to maintain and/or improve the health of individuals and communities. As described previously, the health of populations is managed by altering risk and protective factors. This improvement process begins with an assessment of the health of individuals and their communities. Assessment work answers the question "What is needed?" and is sometimes called a needs assessment. Priorities are selected from information collected in the assessment, and programs of change are implemented and evaluated.

Collectively, a community health assessment paints a picture of the health, the factors influencing health, and the resources of a community. On an individual level, as in health care, this process might be more uniformly defined. A person makes an appointment with a health care provider, and a health history and physical are completed. Through that process, priorities are selected, and strategies for health improvement or maintenance are prescribed. The individual may take some medication, watch his diet, or quit smoking. Months later, the individual returns for follow-up, and the indicators of concern identified in the initial office visit are reassessed. The process is the same in population-level health, but due to the size of a particular population, availability of data, resources, and time constraints, the assessment means and indicators vary.

Describing the Community

All **community assessments** describe the community, the health status of the community, health-related factors, and community resources. Descriptions of the community, health-related factors, and resources are based on data from a broad range of sources. While the categories of information are similar across assessments, the **indicators** used to describe the population can vary by setting. Indicators are measures that have been selected to represent a targeted variable. Worksites, schools, health care organizations, and public health departments collect different information. In a community wide

assessment, information would be used from across all those settings. However, assessments of more defined populations may use more setting-specific indicators. For example, information on weight status and fitness levels varies significantly by setting. In a neighborhood setting, Behavioral Risk Factor Surveillance System (BRFSS) data collected by state health departments may be one of the main data sources. In a school setting, Fitnessgram™ or similar types of data collected in physical education might be a more accurate source. At worksites, health screenings may be the best source of data about weight status and fitness.

Data sources may be available, but they also need to be accessible for community use. Student fitness data may be available to teachers and staff in the school system, but it may not be readily accessible for use by those who are not on the school staff or wellness team. Similarly, worksite wellness programs, safety programs, and health insurance claims contain information that is useful when describing the health of the worker population. A team approach to the assessment can help identify and access a variety of health indicators. Generally, the more types of agencies or groups represented in the process, the wider the scope of available information. Regardless of agency representation, though, some information may not be available.

See Table 9-1 for examples by community assessment category descriptor. As a reminder, Chapters 1 and 2 also include information on existing secondary health and health behavior data sources.

Describing the community involves describing *who* is in the community as well as *how* the community is defined. *How* a community is defined is often the starting point in a community assessment. What are the unifying traits in the community of interest? Communities can be simply defined by a geographical location, for example, a school district, a worksite, a congregation, or a county. Community boundaries can also be defined by a common need or interest, for example, caregivers of children with disabilities, individuals living with chronic diseases, or pregnant women. A community's unifying trait does not have to be health related, for example, incoming freshman on a college campus are a community in which health status and health behaviors may be of interest, yet the property that defines the community is not defined by health. After the unifying trait or community boundary is established, it is important to describe the number of

TABLE 9-1 Community Health Assessment Indicators

Community Description	
Number of community members	Average household income
Participants by subgroups: gender, age, marital status, neighborhood, job classification	Children receiving free or reduced lunch
Geographical or other boundaries of the community	Unemployment rates
Community leaders: formal and informal	Neighborhood occupancies: rental, ownership, vacancy, other
Education attainment: third grade reading scores, high school graduation rates, college degrees	Crime or policy violations
Number of Medicaid/Medicare beneficiaries	

Physical, Mental, and Social Health	
Leading causes of death	Calls to counseling and support centers
Average life expectancy	Reported acts of intentional violence: fighting, domestic violence, and murder
Infant mortality rates	Acts of unintentional violence: automobile, falls, and drowning
Low birth weight babies	Sexually transmitted infections
Rates of chronic disease: heart disease, cancers, stroke, obesity, diabetes, and hypertension	Influenza
Planned and unplanned pregnancies	Dental caries among children
Health care expenditures by diagnosis	Enrollment in support services for children with disabilities (Help Me Grow, March of Dimes, and others)
Worker compensation claims	Enrollment in nonprofit caregiver support programs (e.g., for caregivers of people with Alzheimer's disease)
Sick days used by employees	Number of weekly Meals on Wheels

Health Behaviors	
Physical activity	Adult vaccinations
Rates of fitness facility use	Childhood vaccinations
Bikeway, walking trail, or track use	Prenatal visits
Fruit, vegetable, and other food purchase: cafeterias, area stores, and/or markets	Percentage of mothers breastfeeding for 6 months

continues

TABLE 9-1 *continued*

Food consumption or waste	Injury-related emergency department visits: bicycles, sports, fires, automobile, and fighting
Contraceptive use	Self-reported youth sexual activity
Adult tobacco use	Underage alcohol use
Calls to tobacco quit line or services	Alcohol sales
Smoking ban violations	Property damage

Health Care Utilization

Number of Medicaid and Medicare providers	Immunization rates
WIC program enrollment	Emergency and urgent care visits
Medication use	Participation in preventive screenings: mammography and other cancer screenings, hypertension, and glucose
Number of members with a primary care physician	School health center visits

Environment and System Supports

Air pollution/ozone days	Neighborhood Watch or similar associations (worksites, teachers)
Population density	Access to recreation facilities and shared spaces
Water quality	Fast-food restaurants
Emergency services response times	

Community Resources

Key places of community congregation: places of worship, senior centers, art studios, military veteran clubs, and child care centers	Community organizations: services clubs, parent organizations, alumni groups, and nonprofit health organizations
Fitness and recreation facilities	Community health centers
Intergenerational programs	Smoking cessation programs
City and county agencies: public health, city planning, volunteer programs, senior outreach	Grocery stores, restaurants, and food pantries

Sources: Adapted from the following:

Community Health Status Indicators Working Group (2009)

USDHHS (n.d.)

County Health Rankings and Roadmaps (2014)

members, their traits, and their connections. A good description will create a picture of the members, highlighting both their similarities and differences. Standard information includes demographics such as of sex, age, race, educational attainment, and income.

A description of a community's health should reflect the continuum of health (wellness as well as acute and chronic conditions) as well as the various categories of health (physical, mental, and social). **Mortality** indicators reflect the leading causes of death and infant mortality (County Health Rankings & Roadmaps, 2014; USDHHS, n.d.). Disease indicators, called **morbidity**, include categories of infectious diseases, chronic disease, birth outcomes, and environmental health indicators (Community Health Status Indicators Working Group, 2009; County Health Rankings & Roadmaps, 2014; Metzler et al., 2008). Examples of infectious diseases include influenza, sexually transmitted infections, and West Nile virus. Other specific morbidity indicators include rates of low birth weight babies, diabetes, Autism spectrum disorder, unplanned pregnancies, self-rated health status, and air quality. Local **disability** indicators often include measures of agency enrollment and participation. Some of those agencies include Councils on Aging, Medicaid services, school programs, developmental disability services, and counseling and medical assistance services. Further, the American Community Survey, part of the U.S. Census, collects information about disability. Table 9-1 lists common health status indicators.

Ideally, descriptions of population health report indicators of "the five Ds"—death, disease, disability, discomfort, and distress. Describing population-level discomfort and distress is a challenge, though. These community attributes are important, and the challenge is more often the availability of information. Death and disease data are routinely quantitatively recorded, but measures of discomfort and distress are not uniformly defined or collected. Actual measures of emotional health, distress, and discomfort can be measured through use of services and/or survey information collected by a coalition.

Health-related factors include behavioral, environmental, social, and demographic risk factors. Behavioral factors of interest include tobacco and alcohol use, physical activity, diet, sexual activity, and drug and/or medication use (County Health Rankings & Roadmaps, 2014; Kottke & Isham, 2010). Health care utilization, a specific behavioral category, can include treatment compliance, preventive screenings, and

prenatal care. Social factors are harder to quantify and much less likely to exist in a current data set, but they are nonetheless important. Categories of social-related factors include social cohesion, social structure, and social capital (Lantz & Pritchard, 2010). Actual indicators may include measures of poverty, educational attainment, housing market characteristics, household makeup, perceived social connectedness, and civic involvement (Lantz & Pritchard, 2010). The importance of selecting measures of meaning in a community assessment cannot be overstated. Communities select and tailor measures to the purpose and community of the assessment. For example, the protective factor of social connectedness could be measured in a school environment via the percentage of the student body active in at least one extracurricular group, club, or team.

Community assessments are based on the objective data. **Objective** data can be observed and measured, and it is unbiased. Good descriptions use information from a variety of sources and from sources of information as close to the community of interest as possible. Rarely can one or two indicators accurately describe most members of a community. In the process of understanding community strengths and needs, it is important to drill down into subgroups and subgroup differences. Multilayer information can create a more detailed picture of a community's needs and opportunities.

An example of analyzing data by smaller community segments is the U.S. Census data. Census data is reported on the national level, followed by state- and county-level information. Users can drill down to a zip code (an area within a county that may have part of a city or parts of multiple towns) and even a census block (an area that may be as small as a city block). Community assessors may not be able to report information equivalent to that of a census block but are encouraged to describe subgroup differences. Disease or age-specific mortality rates are broad examples of drilling down to subgroups. In a school district, drilling down may involve reporting information by buildings or grade levels. Again, analyzing information by geographic location, age, and other demographic information allows communities to target very defined subgroups.

In addition to using existing data, coalitions may choose or need to collect additional information during the community assessment. Information may not exist on certain aspects of a community, and/or data in its current form may not accurately capture a feature of the community. Additional information can be collected through surveys, observations, audits, and key informant interviews. Photographs and mapping are two particularly interesting tools that can be used to describe properties of a community. A method called **Photovoice** enables community members to use photographs and narratives to communicate a setting or experience (Community Tool Box, n.d.; Wang & Burris, 1997). Photovoice can give a voice to members of a population but has especially powerful potential with vulnerable populations such as those who face poverty, language barriers, social isolation, cultural barriers, or other challenging circumstances. The goals are to record and reflect on current conditions, encourage community consensus on issues, and bring about change in conditions by reaching decision and policy makers (Community Tool Box, n.d.). Photographers can produce powerful, moving images that foster awareness and communication. Figure 9-2 shows a photo used to describe healthy options in a school cafeteria.

Photographers need to be directed by a question, prompt, or issue. Prompts and questions reflect the issue that is being assessed and described. For example, in a somewhat famous use of Photovoice, children of sex workers living in Calcutta were asked to use cameras to document a day in their life. The powerful photos became the inspiration for the Academy Award–winning documentary *Born into Brothels*. Other prompts can be more specific, such as "document occupational work hazards" (Flum et al., 2010), "capture barriers to healthy eating and active living" (Kaiser Permanente, 2013), or "identity barriers to and facilitators of community participation after a spinal cord injury" (Newman, 2010). After individuals take photographs, an important step in the process is to share the photos *and* reflections with others. First, photos are shared with the other photographers and community members. Four prompts, or versions of these prompts, can guide meaningful dialogue. Photographers describe the contents of the photos (describe the photo). Next, photographers give a personal meaning to the photo or tell why they took the photo (what is really happening). Third, photographers state how the images of the photo relate to their lives (impact on lives). And finally, photographers and future advocates describe what they can do about the conditions depicted in the photo (suggested actions). A second step in photo sharing is to share the collective messages and themes with others *outside* the community. The purpose of this sharing is to raise awareness and seek collective action. There are a variety of ways collective action can be facilitated: a community developed work plan, letter writing campaigns, an exhibit, or a meeting with policy makers (Community Tool Box, n.d.). Community members can use the images to document the current issue and ask for change.

Mapping, through **Geographic Information Systems (GIS)** or old-school paper and pencil methods, also creates visual pictures of communities as indicators are plotted on a

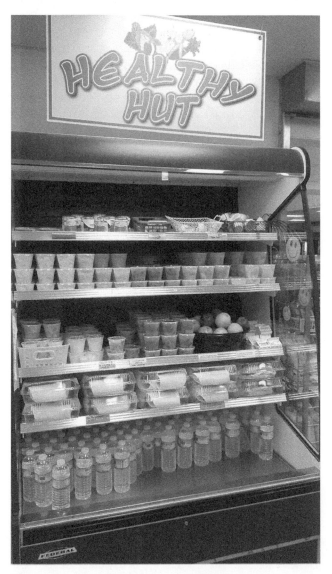

Figure 9-2 Healthy Options in the School Cafeteria

map of a defined community. GIS is widely used in public health to map various disease incidences and, more recently, to map neighborhood properties such as connected streets, public transportation, and retail establishments. With mapping, patterns of place can be become visually identifiable (Kirschenbaum & Russ, 2002). The Behavioral Science in Action feature at the end of the chapter includes additional information on GIS.

The last section within a community assessment is a description of resources within a community. Resources (and the lack thereof) are important as coalitions determine priorities and action steps. Resources are multilevel, starting with individuals and extending to private and nonprofit organizations, businesses, public institutions, and physical resources. A possible sixth category—that of community identity—is important to consider in an assessment. Factors such as reputation, pride, and history can serve or hinder community improvement initiatives. After the prioritizing phase of the assessment concludes, it is useful for coalitions to revisit the resources phase of the assessment and extend the level of understanding of existing, developing, and lacking resources.

Prioritizing

Prioritizing is typically the last step in a community health assessment. Prioritizing is putting the work of the community assessment into practice. **Prioritization** involves interpreting the information within the community health assessment and selecting priorities of action. Choosing priorities of action involves selecting a focus area or areas, as well as identifying targeted members of the community. There are many considerations in selecting these priorities, such as:

- Importance: What is the impact on the health of the community?

- Timing: What is the current public interest in the issue?

- Resources: Are there appropriate resources for addressing the issue?

Coalition members will likely identify multiple issues to be addressed. Rarely is there *the* one issue that stands clearly above the rest. As teams process and deliberate health and health-related issues, importance, timing, and resources may be ways to organize thoughts and discussions. The importance of an issue relates to its level of impact on a community's health. Are people dying prematurely or suffering? What

are the quality of life or economic impacts of the issue? Who is and how many people are affected by the issue, and what will be the consequences of not acting? The issues of timing and resources together address the concept of *winnablility*. If a community takes action, is it likely to produce the desired change? As discussed in Chapter 7, timing is hard to quantify, but it involves determining whether it is the "right time" for a community to take action on an issue. What is the public will or interest in an issue? The process of enacting state-level smoking bans provides a good example of the importance of timing. States have pursued statewide public indoor smoking bans at different times over the past decade. To date, 27 states and the District of Columbia have legislated comprehensive statewide bans (Americans for Nonsmokers' Rights Foundation, 2014). States' decisions to enact the bans have been based on overwhelming data on the ill effects of secondhand smoke, for example, lung cancer, heart disease, and other adverse health effects (Americans for Nonsmokers' Rights Foundation, 2014). Resources that can be devoted to an issue should also be considered. First, communities may choose to take action because resources, such as a grant or a business partner, have become available. The availability of evidence-based interventions for an issue is also a consideration. See the discussion of community readiness in Chapter 7 for additional information.

Mobilizing Coalitions

Community health assessments are best completed in a collaborative process (IOM, 1997; NACCHO, n.d.; USDDHHS, n.d.). Community engagement improves the accuracy of the assessment as well as the implementation of forthcoming interventions. Accuracy of the assessment is improved by bringing multiple viewpoints, sources of information, resources, and skills to the assessment, as well as increasing the number of persons available to complete the work. Furthermore, when coalition members work together to set priorities, it can lead to successful collaborations for addressing the community's health needs. Productive and meaningful community engagement throughout the process can also lead others in the community to take ownership of needs that cannot be addressed by the one agency or funder (Catholic Health Association of the United States, 2013).

The health of a community is everyone's business. Time and consideration should be put into identifying and recruiting partners from across multiple sectors of the community. Community residents, community groups and leaders, public and other organizations, educational institutions, nonprofits, businesses, health care providers, and public health agencies are sectors that should be considered for membership in a coalition. When recruiting and operating coalitions, members can serve in various capacities and at various levels of commitment. **Coalitions**, groups of people or agencies who have formed around a common purpose, are often guided by large representative steering or advisory committees. Steering committees meet less frequently than other work groups and serve to provide vision, community buy-in, and agency cooperation. The process and product of the community assessment and interventions is completed by work groups of smaller more specialized teams.

Facilitating large meetings with diverse perspectives can be challenging, and the use of trained facilitators may be helpful. The *MAPP User Handbook* and related tools, developed by the National Association of County & City Health Officials (NACCHO) and the Centers for Disease Control and Prevention (CDC), have material that is useful to help with developing coalitions and facilitating the process.

> **Check for Understanding** Define a community, then list three possible indicators for the following sections of a community health assessment: (1) community characteristics, (2) health status, (3) health-related factors, and (4) resources.

Planning Strategies of Change

After priorities are selected, a plan for change is developed. A good plan includes clear objectives and specific strategies for reaching those objectives. Objectives are statements that communicate the targets of intended change. All programs should be guided by objectives. Objectives say to the team and others, "This is what we are working on; these are our priorities." The terminology related to these objectives can vary slightly across population health disciplines and planning models. This text uses the language of the Centers for Disease Control and Prevention Healthy People 2020 Framework and Framework for Program Evaluation in Public Health: *goals, objectives, strategy, baseline,* and *target.* In other settings, terms may vary slightly.

Goals

A **goal** is a statement that explains what a program wishes to accomplish (USDHHS, CDC, 2011). Goals tend to be future oriented, with a time frame longer than the actual program. A goal may also be called the vision. The goal is the reason coalitions or communities have come together.

Objectives

Objectives break a goal down into the smaller pieces of the work (USDHHS, CDC, 2011). Objectives define the intended work on each level of the program and align to the hierarchy of relationships depicted in the disease prevention model. Objectives take the target from the model and state the target in measurable forms (see Figure 9-3). The evaluation framework of the Centers for Disease Control and Prevention delineates the different objectives by the time frame of the work and outcome:

- **Short-term objectives** are typically the direct work of intervention. Specific strategies are designed to change these short-term objectives. Objective targets include knowledge, beliefs, skills, resources, support, and/or reinforcements.

- **Intermediate objectives** result from changes in the short-term objectives. Intermediate targets are the risk or protective factor of interest, such as the behavior of medication compliance. Because of the target, these objectives may also be called a behavioral objective or outcome objective (Green & Kreuter, 2005).

- **Long-term objectives** are the expected outcome of the program. Long-term objectives clearly identify the health issue to be altered.

The terms "baseline" and "target" are also used with reference to the various levels of objectives. **Baseline** refers to the starting point or value of the indicator. **Target** refers to the desired amount. If the work of the group is successful, the target level will be achieved. For example, a school wellness committee may seek to take action because 60% of the vegetables from school lunches are thrown away uneaten. The committee sets a target of less than 30% of vegetables being served will be thrown away uneaten.

Objectives are also broadly described as either process measures or outcome objectives. **Process measures** are indicators of program implementation, reach, and quality.

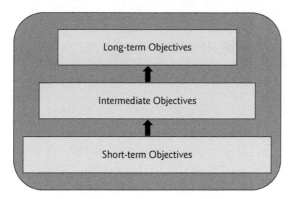

Figure 9-3 Objectives by Level of the Disease Prevention Model

Process measures are the immediate outputs of implementation. Process measures can reflect actions that a program planner assumes will happen: classes are held, instructors follow the lessons, reminder calls get made, or consumers like the materials. Evaluators are interested in process measures because they speak to degrees of program implementation and **fidelity**. Two broad categories include participation and reaction (USDHHS, CDC, 2011). Short-term, intermediate, and long-term evaluations depend on the assumptions represented in process measures. Process objectives are used to improve programs through the feedback loop they provide. Collecting information along the way allows coalitions to adjust resources and/or strategies of change as indicated.

SMART Objectives

Objectives state the desired target and anticipated degree of change. A well-stated objective is one sentence of 15 to 20 words that includes the following information: *who is going to do what*, *when* and to *what extent*.

SMART is a helpful acronym to keep in mind when writing measurable objectives. "Specific," "measurable," "action," "relevant," and "time" are the key words to remember with SMART objectives (see Figure 9-4). Specific objectives use concrete words to describe who and what are the targets. Measurable objectives are quantifiable, meaning the target can be counted. Establishing measurable forms of a behavior was discussed in Chapter 2. Action describes the act that will be completed. Something happens to create change—people attend, prompt others, comply, quit, or report. Action describes the planned something. "A" is occasionally described as "achievable." However, "action" is the preferred term, with the reasoning that all objectives require some type of action. Realistic objectives are reachable. They should represent the next step in the process of change. Time refers to the time frame during which the objective will be accomplished. Time frames can be any block of time: a day, a week, a month, or a year. Table 9-2 includes examples of the three types of objectives written in the SMART format.

Strategies of Change

Strategies of change are specific actions designed to accomplish an objective. Programs consist of a collection of strategies. They can include a media campaign, a class, product distribution, a smoking ban policy, a tax, a support group, and much more. Types of strategies fall into one of the five general categories of health promotion interventions. The categories consist of health education, health communications, health engineering, health policy, and community mobilization. Each of these intervention types tends to be most successful in altering particular types of antecedents.

Health education is any combination of planned learning experiences designed to facilitate voluntary changes in behavior that are conducive to health (Green & Kreuter, 2005). The

Specific	State *what* is trying to be accomplished.
Measurable	State the desired *level* of the behavior.
Action	State in terms of actions that are *behaviors*, not to be confused with outcomes.
Realistic	Realistic goals are *individualized* and represent the next step for that behavior.
Time	State the time *frame* for the action and measurement. The time frame can be by occurrence, daily, or weekly. Shorter time frames are ideal.

Figure 9-4 Components of SMART Objectives

TABLE 9-2 Examples of SMART Objectives

Type of Objective	Incorrect Format	SMART Format
Short-term	Pregnant mothers will be taught how to breastfeed a newborn.	By the end of the prenatal class, all pregnant women will be able to demonstrate the correct positioning for breastfeeding an infant.
Intermediate	Increase the number of women who breastfeed their newborn.	100% of the women leaving the hospital after delivery will be breastfeeding their newborn.
Long-term	Improve the well-being of children living in Apple County.	At least 85% of newborns will be within ideal weight range at the 4-week well child visit.

targets of health education are knowledge, belief, and skill antecedents (Joint Committee on National Health Education Standards, 2007; Joint Committee on Terminology, 2001). The strategies within health education are endless, ranging from self-help materials to intensive one-on-one coaching. *Health communication* interventions use communications strategies to inform and influence decisions that affect health (USDHHS, NIH, & NCI, 2008). Health communication strategies include media, advertising, and/or public relations. Like health education, the interventions seek to alter knowledge and beliefs and also provide reminders (USDHHS, NIH, & NCI, 2008).

Health engineering involves altering a product or the environment to meet a behavioral objective. Engineering strategies target access type antecedents and enable persons to take action. Products or physical environments are built or redesigned to increase access to behavior facilitators as well as to limit access to counter-facilitators. Engineering strategies can also target behavior-related skills, making it easier for a skill to be performed. Examples of engineering-based strategies include single-size food packages, fluoridated water, and speed bumps.

Health policy is the fourth category of health promotion interventions. Policies are laws, regulations, or formal and informational rules established by government or organizations (Association of State and Territorial Directors & CDC, 2001; Story et al., 2008). Policies can be implemented on all levels of the environment: interpersonal, organizational, and within the larger systems such as state and federal laws. Policies influence access and reinforcements.

Involving the target audience in the implementation of a program is an additional intervention category called *community mobilization*. Trusted members of the community are recruited and trained to provide health education, advocate for policy, or facilitate media campaigns. The roles of the enlisted community members can include providing correct information, motivating others to take action, providing resources, and reinforcing behavior changes (Merzel & D'Afflitti, 2003; USDHHS, CDC, n.d.). Community mobilization is rarely an independent intervention; rather, it is a method to enhance the impact of other strategies targeting knowledge, beliefs, skills, reminders, and **resources** (Community Preventive Services Task Force, 2005; Merzel & D'Afflitti, 2003).

Successful risk reduction programs employ strategies from more than one type of intervention. It is the complement of the interventions that allows program planners to address the multiple and varied types of antecedents that drive health behavior. No one type of intervention can change and/or sustain health behavior change.

Implementing Strategies of Change

Implementation involves taking plans that were developed in the assessment and planning phases and putting them into practice. Implementation is moving from planning to doing. Examples of implementation include teaching the health education classes that were selected, altering the environmental attributes in a manner that promotes the desired behaviors, and passing and enforcing policies. Programs consist of numerous strategies that are designed to work synergistically to produce changes, and the best-practice methods of implementation vary by intervention category. The methods and resources required for implementing a health communication campaign differ from the methods and resources for changing the physical and social environment. Implementing evidence-based programs is a large subject area and is the topic of Chapter 10.

Evaluating Change

The purpose of evaluation is to assess a program's effectiveness and to improve the program for future use. In linear models, evaluation is shown as the last step in the process; however, it is more accurately described as a thread that is woven throughout. Evaluation begins in the planning phase of the program and is an ongoing part of health promotion. Program evaluation requires clearly defined targets. The targets of change are identified in the planning process and then collected during and after program implementation. Good program planning not only improves evaluation but also makes for easier program evaluation. When evaluation measures are identified from the start, processes for collection can be built into the implementation plan.

Objective-Driven Evaluation

Evaluation is the comparison of an object of interest against a standard of acceptability (Green & Lewis, 1986). In an objective-driven evaluation, objects of interest are the *what* in the stated objective. Objects of interest can include health incidence such as new infections, behavior rates such as condom use, predisposing factors such as knowledge, and process measures such as program participation rates. Standards of acceptability reflect the *who* and *how much* of a stated objective. Standards of acceptability are set by an outside body, such as accreditation bodies, through professional guidelines, and/or by teams in setting objectives. Thus, in an objective-driven program, evaluation is the process of answering the question "Did we accomplish what we said we would accomplish?"

Measures collected during the process of implementation are collectively called process evaluation. **Process evaluations** are also called formative and implementation evaluations. All these terms ("process," "formative," and "implementation") imply that the measures are collected during the process of the intervention (phase of implementation). Measures collected after the intervention, as outcomes of the intervention, are collectively called outcome evaluations. **Outcome**

evaluations are also called summative evaluations (Green & Kreuter, 2005).

Measures of Change

With clear program objectives, the focus of evaluation becomes the selection of indicators for those objectives. Objectives identify the target of change, and indicators will be the actual measures of change. In population health, indicators are often proxy measures of the actual target and/or phenomenon. For example, Healthy People Access to Health Care Objective 3 (AHC-3) is to increase by 10% the proportion of persons with a usual primary care provider. The selected indicator is the number of persons who report in the Medical Expenditures Panel Survey that they have a usual primary care provider (USDHHS, n.d.). The Medical Expenditures Panel Survey is a national survey commissioned by the Agency for Healthcare Research and Quality (AHRQ). Due to sampling and data availability, a local community project would choose different indicators for a similar objective.

> **Check for Understanding**   What might be three possible indicators for a countywide initiative to increase persons with a usual primary care provider?

Local coalitions and planners often choose the measures of change. There is no one right indicator, but some indicators are better than others. Indicators should be accurate sources of information about the target, and they need to be able to be collected in a reliable, timely manner. Choosing authentic and manageable indicators is important because indicators are how we make conclusions about a program. If there are poorly defined, unreliable, and/or missing sources of information, coalitions may make inaccurate conclusions about their programs.

The standards for evaluation outlined in the CDC Evaluation Framework can guide the indicator selection process. The standards do not prescribe a method of evaluation; rather, they serve as a guide for people who are considering actual indicators (USDHHS, CDC, 2011). Properties of measures of change to be considered include:

- Utility: Who will use these results, and will the indicator(s) provide *relevant* information in a timely manner?

- Feasibility: Are the indicators *realistic* given the available time, resources, and expertise?

- Propriety: Do the indicators engage those most directly affected by the program and changes in the program, such as participants or the surrounding community? Are the rights of individuals and the community protected?

- Accuracy: Will the indicators produce information/findings that are *valid and reliable*?

Gathering credible evidence about program objectives can involve triangulation. **Triangulation** is the use of multiple sources of data for the same indicator. Triangulation is useful when outcomes are difficult to measure and/or the data sources have limitations. Difficulty in measurement can be due to the nature or complexity of the target, the availability of instruments, and/or the scope of the population. Further, using multiple methods helps increase the accuracy of the measurement and the certainty of conclusions when the various methods yield similar results (USDHHS, CDC, 2011). If communities select and track three measures of a behavior, and all three measures move in a positive direction, other people have increased confidence in the conclusion of positive outcomes.

Triangulation should also be considered as a strategy for drawing conclusions about the important program indicators. There are certainly outcomes that program stakeholders and staff are more interested in than others. Changes in the influential factors and the actual behavioral target are typically deemed as important evaluation measures; however, stakeholders may also be equally interested in consumer satisfaction and/or degree of community implementation. Information from a variety of sources will increase the accuracy of conclusions about the target factor. Using multiple sources of information will also enable information to be captured from different subgroups or audiences.

Returning to the ACH-3 objective to increase by 10% the proportion of persons with a usual primary care provider, what three local indicators did you identify? Would the use of three indicators, as opposed to just one, allow for a more accurate conclusion? The following list provides a few ideas of local indicators of access to primary care providers (Berk & Schur, 1998; County Health Ranking & Roadmap, 2014; IOM, 1993):

- Percentage under the age of 65 without health insurance

- Population per primary care provider

- Hospitalization rates for select preventable conditions

- Emergency department visits for unusual source of care

- Prenatal care usage

- Free clinic usage

- Use of school health services

- New patient visits at select health care facilities

- Employee surveys of primary care

- Waiting lists for select types of care

An outside agency or funder can also prescribe the indicators to be collected. If a program is part of a larger project, the measures of change need to be the same so that information can be aggregated and compared across programs. Hospital systems, school districts, and public health departments have numerous outcome indicators required by outside agencies. For example, hospitals report readmission rates, condition-related mortality, and catheter-associated urinary tract infections to accreditation bodies. School districts report attendance, participation in free and reduced cost lunch programs, and academic testing results to state departments of education. Public health districts are required to report children's lead poisoning test results and various measures of public water use and quality. The indicators are set by outside agencies so that information can be summarized and compared across organizations and sites. Health promotion initiatives may have indicators set by funders or outside agencies that also allow for summarizing results and comparisons. Even when indicators are prescribed by funders or decision makers, coalitions may choose to collect information on additional indicators that are also meaningful to the community, stakeholders, or program staff.

Using Questions to Focus the Evaluation Process

In addition to clearly defined program objectives and corresponding indicators, evaluators recommend the use of evaluation questions. Key evaluation questions are related to program impact and are to be answered through the process of evaluation (USDHHS, CDC, 2011; W. K. Kellogg, 2004). Questions include, but also extend beyond, measures of process implementation and outcome indicators. Questions posed by others may include financial considerations, ease of use of program services and materials, community response to the program, and links to other services. The use of questions can also help focus the evaluation and ensure that teams speak to conclusions about the program that are meaningful to communities, participants, funders, staff, and self.

Teams or coalitions of diverse backgrounds, skills, and roles assemble early in the health promotion planning process to assess, plan, and implement an initiative. It is likely that members of a diverse group would be interested in different aspects of program outcomes and experiences. Members' and outside stakeholders' expected *use* of the program evaluation information also vary and will likely be reflected in the scope of evaluation questions posed. Participants, the end users of a program, tend to be interested in the quality and accessibility of the activities. Staff and team members typically want to answer questions about changes in risk factors and health outcomes. Program partners may ask questions about reach and links to their services and/or business. Administrators are interested in the sustainability of a project and other business considerations, such as market share and return on investment. Evaluation questions exist on every segment of the of the health promotion process (see Figure 9-1), yet they can be grouped into the following categories: implementation, effectiveness, efficiency, cost-effectiveness, and attribution (USDHHS, CDC, 2011).

The development of evaluation questions is not a separate procedure in evaluation. It is a step to help focus the team's efforts as well as ensure buy-in and use of the evaluation (Martin & Heath, 2006). As teams consider indicators and methods of collection, they should check in with stakeholders, community members, future participants, funders, and staff. Ask each potential reader of the evaluation, "In the end, what do you want or need to know about the program?" The evaluation plan will, most likely, not answer every posed question. However, an evaluation should address questions deemed important by stakeholders and decision makers.

Outcome Logic Models

Activity logic models and outcome logic models are the two types of logic models. Activity logic models illustrate the specific activities that will be implemented in a program. They illustrate the work a team will actually *do* as part of a program (W. K. Kellogg, 2004). Outcome logic models illustrate the anticipated short-term and long-term outcomes from the program activities, that is, what a team expects to *get* as a result of the program activities. Thus, activity and outcome logic models can be referred to as program logic models

(Knowlton-Wyatt & Phillips, 2009). The theory model is the foundation of both the activities and the outcome logic models. A theory model (discussed in Chapter 8) outlines the behavioral antecedents and the hypothesized relationship between the antecedents. An activity model adds activities a planner intends to do in order to change the antecedents and behavior. Finally, the outcome model projects the outcomes that will result if the activities work as intended. Because activities are designed around behavioral antecedents, many of the expected outcomes are changes in behavioral antecedents, or processes related to changing antecedents. The ultimate goal of the model process is the alignment of these three sections: theoretical assumptions, activities, outcomes.

Benefits of Outcome Logic Models

Outcome logic modeling improves program evaluation. Good program evaluation requires clearly defined targets or measures. These measures of change are identified in the planning process and are stated as program objectives. In an outcome logic model, the indicators of those measures are also clearly defined and bulleted. Both objectives and indicators are defined before the program is implemented, thereby increasing the likelihood of a meaningful evaluation.

Logic models also encourage alignment of the program components. By placing resources, activities, and outcomes side by side and reading them in an "if–then" order, alignment of those components emerges. The same alignment can occur in a paragraph- or text-style plan, but it can easily get lost or be seen as separate pieces of the plan.

Placing resources, activities, and outcomes side by side can also highlight gaps in the program plan and/or evaluation. The big picture approach of creating an outcome logic model forces teams to focus on the big picture items and whether those components are aligned to one another. Early drafts of a program model function as a gap analysis, where empty boxes in the model identify missing links in the program plan and evaluation. Again, the *process* of creating and modifying the model is actually the process of clarifying program assumptions, activities, and intended outcomes.

Once completed, the logic model becomes a communication tool. The one-page document tells the program's story, much like a photograph. It communicates the behavior to be changed, mediators' assumptions, the designed activities of change, as well as the outcomes one may expect—and the resources required to achieve the model. The model also communicates the assumed relationship of the components. To a first-time reader, such as an administrator, a community member, or a funder, a model can easily communicate the big picture of a program. It forms the program's conceptual framework, with details of the plan and assumptions communicated elsewhere in text. This big picture model is also helpful for communicating the relationship and sequence of events, as this type of framework can become lost or hard to track in longer forms of text.

A program outcome logic model also fosters team consensus and accountability. It clearly communicates the activities and intended outcomes of the team's collective work, and it puts members on the same page. It can demonstrate to team members their role in a larger picture and how their work is linked to the work of others and important outcomes. The simplicity of the communication tool also allows members to clarify misconceptions about team priorities and roles while keeping teams focused on the big picture of community health improvement. Finally, the clarity of the single-page written model, with aligned pieces and clear outcomes, aids in accountability.

Components of Logic Models

The fundamental aspects of a logic model are grouped pieces, sequence, and relationships. The grouped pieces of outcome logic models include theoretical assumptions, inputs, and outputs (see Figure 9-5). Broadly, inputs are the resources and activities that we do, and outputs are the results from our work. The W. K. Kellogg Foundation (2004) and the Centers for Disease Control and Prevention (USDHHS, CDC, 2011) have further delineated the components into the specific pieces shown in Table 9-3.

Influential Factors and Assumptions

Influential factors and assumptions are the primary factors or forces influencing a behavioral target and the assumed relationship between factors. Influential factors are based on research, best practices, past experience, and common sense, and they are described in the theoretical model of the target behavior or factor. *It is from these assumptions about antecedents and relationships that all program activities are developed.* Program activities are designed to change these predisposing, enabling, and reinforcing factors. When strategies are successful, changes in health behavior occur. These assumptions also map a sequence of programming activities. The outcome logic model does not include all the details depicted in the theoretical model; rather, it contains the behavioral building blocks (see Chapter 8) and other key factors or assumptions.

Resources

Resources are the financial, human, material and other inputs from outside the program that are used to deliver the program activities. Common resources include staff with specialized skills and responsibilities, money, space, time, equipment, and communication materials.

Activities

Activities are the planned actions initiated to achieve the desired outcomes in the target groups. Strategies of change will vary by type of program. As previously described in this chapter, activities fall into five broad categories: health education, health communication, health policy and enforcement, health engineering, and community mobilization/outreach. Within each category, specific types of activities are listed, such as screenings and case management.

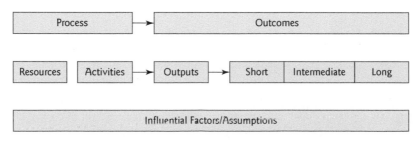

Figure 9-5 General Logic Model

TABLE 9-3 Components of Outcome Logic Models

Model Component	Definition	Link to Program Planning and Evaluation Process
Influential Factors or Assumptions	Primary factors influencing a behavioral target.	Community assessment and theoretical logic model
Resources or inputs	The financial, human, material, and other inputs going into the program.	Community assessment
Activities	The strategies, events, and actions of the planned program. Can include products, services, and infrastructure.	Program planning and implementation
Outputs	The direct results (effects) of program activities. They are typically described in terms of the size and/or scope of the activities. Examples include number of participants at an event (size), actual distribution of materials (size and scope), and degree of classroom lessons implemented (scope).	Process evaluation Implementation evaluation
Short-term outcomes	Changes in the behavioral antecedents or targets of the intervention activities. Should be tied to the influential factors and include knowledge/awareness, beliefs, skills, resources, social support, and/or reinforcements.	Outcome evaluation
Intermediate outcomes	Changes in the risk or protective factor targeted collectively by the program.	Outcome evaluation
Long-term outcomes	Organizational-, community-, and/or system level changes, including community-level measures of change in health or the conditions of health.	Outcome evaluation Community assessment

Sources: Adapted from the following:

W.K. Kellogg (2004)

USDHHS, CDC (2011)

In Figure 9-6, planned activities include a health communications campaign directed at health care providers, a baby-friendly hospital policy initiative, new mother health education, and the creation of breastfeeding-friendly physical and social environments. Within each category, numerous strategies are planned. For example, the media campaign will include social media, a mass media campaign, community outreach, and health care provider outreach. Within each of the strategies are detailed action plans.

Outputs

Outputs are the immediate measurable outcomes of activities. Outputs are process measures of program implementation, fidelity, and reach. Common measures can include number of sessions or events held, requests for information, attendance, attrition, actual media coverage, number of community partners, participant demographics, and customer satisfaction. It is from outputs that statements about program implementation are made.

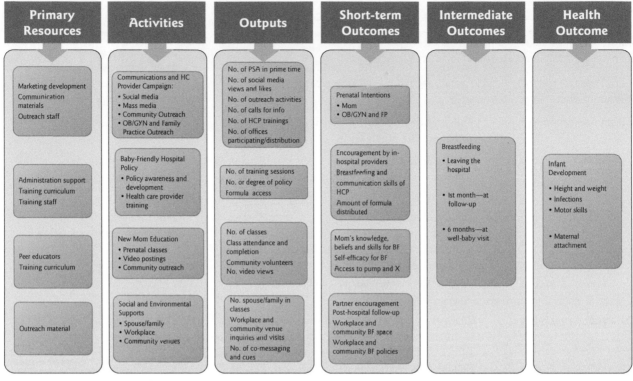

Box Influential factors (For example, see Figure 9-5 in this chapter).

Figure 9-6 Breastfeeding Outcome Logic Model

Short-Term Outcomes

"**Outcomes** are the changes in someone or something (other than the program and its staff) that you hope will result from your program's activities" (USDHHS, CDC, 2011). Short-term outcomes are typically the direct results of an intervention. Measures include knowledge, beliefs, skills, resources, support, and/or reinforcements. Short-term outcomes are closely aligned to the influential factors identified earlier. Short-term outcomes precede changes in a risk or protective factor.

Intermediate Outcomes

Intermediate outcomes are the risk or protective factors of interest stated in an operational, measurable form. Intermediate outcomes are commonly the behaviors of individuals that will be altered or an environmental risk condition, such as exposure to environmental toxins.

Long-Term Outcomes

All health promotion programs align to health outcomes. Long-term outcomes are organizational-, community-, or system-level changes in health or the conditions of health.

The sequence or order of the grouped pieces is an important feature of outcome logic models. A team member, funding agency, or a community stakeholder should be able to read the outcome model from left to right, in a series of "*if* X, *then* Y" sentences. The assumption about the relationship of X to Y is that item X precedes Y. For example, before physicians prompt pregnant patients about breastfeeding (short-term outcome), physicians need to receive training and literature about talking to women regarding breastfeeding (activity with outputs). Sequencing often represents a time line of action and expected outcomes.

Constructing a Logic Model

Logic models are pictures of how planners think a program will work to improve the health of a community. Logic models are only as good as the logic that the program is built upon. If the program is built on a hodgepodge of activities, the "logic" in the model may be lacking. In constructing a logic model, the focus is to capture the big picture of the intervention and is often completed in a process of backward design.

What: The Big Picture

For models to be effective communication tools, they should be easy to follow and visually appealing. The model should be the big picture of the program, not the nuts and bolts (W. K. Kellogg, 2004). A model cannot be a complete representation of the program or one's understanding of the phenomenon. Teams will be able to supplement the model with other communication materials such as text and presentations. Keeping a model to one page and highlighting the fundamental aspects of the model with color or design are two important aspects of model readability.

How: Backward Design

One common method for developing an outcome logic model is through backward design. Backward design requires starting with the end in mind (Wiggins & McTighe, 2005). In backward design, teams start with the purpose of the project, select indicators that would indicate progress, *and then* plan the activities and outputs that precede. As mentioned earlier, logic models read from left to right (if X, then Y); however, in a backward design planning process, work starts at the far right of the model and moves to the left. The practice of starting with desired outcomes is not uncommon. Total quality improvement, curriculum design, and product design are other processes that start with identifying the desired outcomes (Wiggins & McTighe, 2005).

Developing an outcome logic model is a skill that develops with practice and experience. Like program planning and evaluation, professionals develop their own techniques and personalization. For those new to outcome logic modeling, the following section includes a suggested step-by-step process. The W. K. Kellogg Foundation (2004) also has numerous planning forms and model templates to guide the backward design process. The following sections provide general steps for completing an outcome logic model in a backward design

process. These general steps reflect a starting point. In practice, the steps are not as linear as presented here. Teams and coalitions will circle back and forth to various components of the model, refining their plan as thoughts about assumptions, relationships, and outcomes become more refined and clarified.

Step 1: Identify the Goal   State the purpose of the project or coalition. The purpose can be based on the community assessment and prioritization process, or it can be partially predefined based on the community-based organization, division, department, or special project that one works within.

Step 2: Identify the Long-Term Outcome   State the health issue that the program intends to change. Health issues should be stated in an operational form, distinguishing between the various types of change desired—primary, secondary, or tertiary. The final version of the model includes the agreed upon indicator(s).

Step 3: Select the Intermediate Outcome   State the risk or protective factor(s) that will be shaped. Risk and protective factors are behavioral and/or environmental targets that have strong relationships to the long-term outcome. Again, in the final version of the model, the outcome should be stated in an operational, measurable form.

Step 4: Influential Factors and Assumptions   Identify the primary factors in your target community that influence the behavior. The assumption is that if these factors are changed, the behavior or environmental risk factor will change. This step is crucial for designing appropriate strategies of change.

Step 5: Select the Short-Term Outcomes   Short-term outcomes precede changes in a risk or protective factor and are extended from the influential factors stated in step 4. There will be multiple short-term outcomes that include knowledge, beliefs, skills, resources, support, and/or reinforcements. There is fluidity with steps 5 and 6. Some planners may begin with identifying types of activities that will alter the influential factors (step 6) and then identify the short-term outcomes of these activities.

Step 6: Identify Types of Activities   List types of interventions and possible strategies that will be planned to alter the short-term outcomes. Remember to consider existing resources and established interventions. It works best to group similar types of strategies with a unifying title (such as new mom education) and then align the nested boxes with their respective short-term outcome(s).

Step 7: Review Resources List the "big picture" resources needed to accomplish the planned activities. Without being redundant, group resources with a unifying title and align the nested boxes to their respective activity or activities.

Step 8: Outputs Select and bullet outputs for each nested box of interventions. Using evaluation questions will be helpful to identifying meaningful process indicators. Output measures should speak to the degree and reach of the activities listed in step 6.

Step 9: Revisit the Entire Model The last step is to revisit the full model and make adjustments as needed. As a whole, is the model coherent and the components aligned? Read the model from left to right in the *if–then* format. Does the model flow? Are the assumptions and intended outcomes clear? In the development of steps 1 through 8, relationships and assumptions are binary between two pieces or elements. The last step is to evaluate the whole model: Does it accurately tell the story of your intended work? If not, make adjustments as needed.

Make it Interesting

Design and graphics are tools to help communicate the program's story. Color and nested boxes can be used to group pieces, highlight assumed relationships, and show sequence. White space, color, and art make a model visually appealing and easy to read. Graphics and design should be tools for communicating the content; they should not compete with the content. Finally, one may consider using a graphic or title that is innovative and memorable when appropriate. Table 8-2 outlines tips for creating a logical and visually appealing model.

SUMMARY

Logic models are visual representations of how program planners think their program will work in a community to address a particular health behavior. A logic model allows planners to map and organize their thoughts in a way that will ensure program objectives and goals are properly aligned. A logic model can include short-term, intermediate, and long-term objectives for a project, and models are an excellent way to communicate these objectives to all involved in program planning. Logic models are also incredibly flexible, allowing planners to tailor them to the needs of the program and target audience, as well as adjust and edit the model as program planning occurs and changes.

BEHAVIORAL SCIENCE IN ACTION

Using GIS to Map Disease and Health Determinants

Geographic information system, commonly referred to as GIS, is a system that combines maps, databases, and statistical analysis in a way that lets users select and view data in a number of ways. In most fields, the data that have been collected also have a location connected to it. GIS technology takes the data and combines them with the science of cartography, allowing users to see the data in relation to a location they choose. Traditional roadmaps are combined with aerial photos, satellite images, and other digital information to create a fuller picture of the location. GIS software is usually tailored to users and their preferences, so there is not just one single GIS software or interface.

Grouping individuals by where they reside allows researcher to examine trends in income, age, health status, and any number of other characteristics. By combining multiple maps, GIS users are able to select locations in a number of ways depending on what works best for their research. Common locations include zip codes, census tracts, school districts, and city limits.

GIS lets users view many types of data. Experts and students use the technology in the fields of seismology, meteorology, economics, transportation, and health. Users can search for many types of data to fulfill their research objectives, but some of the most common types of data are listed in the following sections (ESRI, n.d.).

Where things are: Users can search for locations that have specific features or qualities, which will allow patterns to emerge. For example, a search could be done for zip codes with a diabetes prevalence greater than 20%.

Quantities: Knowing how many of something are in a specific area can be useful information. When trying to plan a healthy eating intervention, knowing how many supermarkets, farmers' markets, convenience stores, and restaurants are in a specific area will be useful to aid in understanding how easy it is to access food in the community.

Densities: GIS can show the user the distribution of a feature across a geographic area. For example, searching for Supplemental Nutrition Assistance Program (SNAP) beneficiaries by census tract would allow a user to see where those receiving food stamps are clustered in an urban area.

What's nearby: A user can search for specific features that are located within a certain region. This is a useful function for researchers interested in the walkability of a neighborhood because it is possible to see the location of supermarkets, schools, and other pertinent features in a given location.

What's happening nearby: GIS technology allows users to search for various types of activities of interest that occur in a specific area. A user may want to know about driving under the influence (DUI) or drug offenses that occur within a school zone.

The Centers for Disease Control and Prevention's Division for Heart Disease and Stroke Prevention recently used national data to explore heart health by state. Using data from the Behavioral Risk Factor Surveillance System (BRFSS) and GIS software, researchers were able to create the most complete picture of heart health in the United States to date (CDC, 2014). The Interactive Atlas of Heart Disease and Stroke (http://nccd.cdc.gov/DHDSPAtlas/) allows users to create their own maps and has heart disease-related data, demographic information, and social determinants of health that are able to be viewed by county and state. The following nationwide map (Figure 9-7) showing diabetes prevalence by county is one of many maps generated by the CDC.

The uses of GIS are expanding, and more fields are using this informative and flexible program to help in research and project planning. As the amount of data and uses increase, GIS will become an integral part of health promotion and program planning.

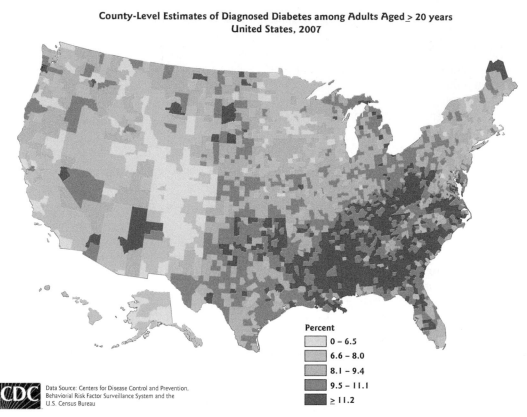

Figure 9-7 GIS Map of County-Level Estimates of Diagnosed Diabetes

Courtesy of Centers for Disease Control and Prevention

IN THE CLASSROOM ACTIVITIES

1) Identify the common steps in the process of health promotion programming.

2) Visit the website of the County Health Rankings & Roadmaps Project at the University of Wisconsin Population Health Institute. Locate and summarize a state's health rankings. Explain county-level trends within the state.

3) As a class, use the Photovoice method to assess and describe one campus issue. Pick one of the following prompts (or create your own): identify and categorize campus safety concerns, document opportunities to enhance student connectedness, or discuss factors that influence food and beverage choices. Each person should take three photos related to the selected prompt and pick the one photo that most accurately captures the issue. Share that photo with the class, addressing the following:

(a) what is seen in the photo, (b) what is really happening, (c) how this relates to the campus experience, and (d) what can be done about the issue.

4) Using a theoretical model from Chapter 8, construct an outcome logic model, aligning behavioral targets to activities and outcomes.

5) Take a campus or other community project and diagram the work and outcomes in an outcome logic model. Are there gaps in the logic? Are the outcome indicators clearly identified?

6) Using the model from class activity number 4 or another outcome logic model, explain three assumptions depicted in the model. What might be three influential factors of the intermediate outcome? Share your conclusions with another student.

WEB LINKS

County Health Rankings & Roadmaps Project at the University of Wisconsin Population

Geographic Information Systems (GIS) at the Centers for Disease Control and Prevention: http://www.cdc.gov/gis/

Health Institute: www.countyhealthrankings.org

Healthy People Leading Health Indicators: www.healthypeople.gov

Human Genome Project at the Smithsonian National Museum of Natural History: http://unlockinglifescode.org

National Institute of Justice: http://www.nij.gov

U.S. Census Bureau: http://www.census.gov

REFERENCES

Americans for Nonsmokers' Rights Foundation. (2014). *U.S. tobacco control laws database*. Retrieved from http://www.no-smoke.org/goingsmokefree.php

American Lung Association (ALA). (2014). *State of tobacco control, 2014*. Retrieved from http://www.stateoftobaccocontrol.org

Association of State and Territorial Directors of Health Promotion and Public Health Education & Centers for Disease Control and Prevention (CDC). (2001). *Policy and environmental change: New directions for public health*. Atlanta: Centers for Disease Control and Prevention.

Berk, M. L., & Schur, C. L. (1998). Measuring access to care: Improving information for policymakers. *Health Affairs, 17*, 180–186.

Catholic Health Association of the United States. (2013). *Assessing and addressing community health needs*. Retrieved from http://www.chausa.org/communitybenefit/

Centers for Disease Control and Prevention (CDC), Division for Heart Disease and Stroke Prevention. (2014). *Chronic disease GIS exchange*. Retrieved from http://www.cdc.gov/dhdsp/maps/index.htm

Community Health Status Indicators Project Working Group. (2009). *Data sources, definitions, and notes*. Department of Health and Human Services. Retrieved from http://wwwn.cdc.gov/CommunityHealth/HomePage.aspx

Community Preventive Services Task Force. (2005). Tobacco. In S. Zaza, P. A. Briss, & K. W. Harris (Eds.), *The guide to community preventive services: What works to promote health?* (pp. 3–79) New York: Oxford University Press.

Community Tool Box. (n.d.). *Assessing community needs and resources: Implementing Photovoice in your community* (Chapter 3, Section 20). Retrieved from http://ctb.ku.edu/en/tablecontents/chapter3_section20_main.aspx

County Health Ranking & Roadmaps. (2014). *2014 measures and data sources*. University of Wisconsin, Population Health Institute & Robert Wood Johnson Foundation. Retrieved from http://www.countyhealthrankings.org/

ESRI. (n.d.) *What is GIS?* Retrieved from http://www.esri.com/what-is-gis

Flum, M. R., Siqueira, C. E., DeCaro, A., & Redway, S. (2010). Photovoice in the workplace: A participatory method to give voice to workers to identify health and safety hazards and promote workplace change – a study of custodians. *American Journal of Industrial Medicine, 53*(11), 1150–1158.

Green, L. W., & Kreuter, M. W. (2005). *Health promotion planning: An educational and ecological approach* (4th ed). Boston: McGraw Hill.

Green, L. W., & Lewis, F. M. (1986). *Measurement and evaluation in health education and health promotion*. Palo Alto, CA: Mayfield.

Institute of Medicine (IOM). (1993). *Access to health care in America*, edited by M. Milliman. Washington, DC: National Academies of Science.

Institute of Medicine (IOM). (1997). A community health improvement process (CHIPS). In Institute of Medicine, *Improving health in the community: a role for performance monitoring*. Washington, DC: National Academy of Science.

Joint Committee on National Health Education Standards. (2007). *National health education standards: Achieving excellence* (2nd ed.). Atlanta: American Cancer Society.

Joint Committee on Terminology. (2001). Report of the 2000 Joint Committee on Health Education and Promotion Terminology. *American Journal of Health Education, 32*(2), 89–103.

Kaiser Permanente. (May 2013). *Our stories: Photovoice*. Retrieved from http://share.kaiserpermanente.org/article/our-stories-photovoice/

Kirschenbaum, J., & Russ, L. (2002). *Community mapping: Using geographic data for neighborhood revitalization: A tool from the equitable development handbook*. Oakland, CA: Policylink.

Knowlton-Wyatt, L., & Phillips, C. C. (2009). *The logic model guidebook: Better strategies for great results*. Los Angeles: Sage.

Kottke, T. E., & Isham, G. J. (2010). Measuring health care access and quality to improve health in populations. *Preventing Chronic Disease, 7*(4), A73. Retrieved from http://www.cdc.gov/pcd/issues/2010/jul/09_0243.htm

Lantz, P. M., & Pritchard, A. (2010). Socioeconomic indicators that matter for population health. *Preventing Chronic Disease, 7*(4), A74. Retrieved from http://www.cdc.gov/pcd/issues/2010/jul/09_0246.htm

Martin, S. L., & Heath, G. W. (2006). A six-step model for evaluation of community-based physical activity programs. *Preventing Chronic Disease.* Retrieved from http://www.cdc.gov/pcd/issues/2006/jan/05_0111.htm

Merzel, C., & D'Afflitti, J. (2003). Reconsidering community-based health promotion: Promise, performance and potential. *American Journal of Public Health, 93*(4), 557–574.

Metzler, M., Kanarek, N., Highsmith, K., Bialek, R., Straw, R., Auston, I.,... Klein, R. (2008). Community Health Status Indicators Project: The development of a national approach to community health. *Preventing Chronic Disease, 5*(3). Retrieved from http://www.cdc.gov/pcd/issues/2008/jul/07_0225.htm

National Association of County & City Health Officials (NACCHO). (n.d.). *Mobilizing for Action through Planning and Partnerships: Achieving healthier communities through MAPP.* National Association of County & City Health Officials. Retrieved from http://www.naccho.org

National Human Genome Research Institute. (n.d.). *A brief guide to genomics.* Retrieved from www.genome.gov

Newman, S. D. (2010). Evidence-based advocacy: Using Photovoice to identify barriers and facilitators to community participation after spinal cord injury. *Rehabilitation Nursing, 35*(2), 47–59.

Story, M., Kaphingst, K. M., Robinson-O'Brien, R., & Glanz, K. (2008). Creating healthy food and eating environments: Policy and environmental approaches. *Annual Review of Public Health, 29*, 253–272.

U.S. Department of Health and Human Services (USDHHS). (n.d.). *Healthy people 2020.* Retrieved from http://www.healthypeople.gov

U.S. Department of Health and Human Services (USDHHS), Centers for Disease Control and Prevention (CDC). (n.d.). *Community health worker training materials for cholera prevention and control.* Retrieved from http://www.cdc.gov/cholera/materials.html

U.S. Department of Health and Human Services (USDHHS), Centers for Disease Control and Prevention (CDC). (2011). *Introduction to program evaluation for public health programs: A self-study guide.* Atlanta: Centers for Disease Control and Prevention.

U.S. Department of Health and Human Services (USDHHS), National Institutes of Health (NIH), National Cancer Institute (NCI). (2008). *Pink book: Making health communication work* (2nd ed.). Bethesda, MD: National Cancer Institute. Retrieved from http://www.cancer.gov/pinkbook/

Wang, C., & Burris, M. A. (1997). Photovoice: Concept, methodology, and use for participatory needs assessment. *Health Education & Behavior, 24*(3), 369–387.

Wiggins, G., & McTighe, J. (2005). *Understanding by design.* Upper Saddle River, NJ: Pearson.

W. K. Kellogg Foundation. (2004). *Logic model development guide.* Retrieved from http://www.wkkf.org/resource-directory/resource/2006/02/wk-kellogg-foundation-logic-model-development-guide

CHAPTER 10

Evidence-Based Interventions

KEY TERMS

community health worker	evidence	health engineering	small media
community mobilization	experiential evidence	health policy	social marketing
contextual evidence	health communication	mass media	strategy
default	health education	program	

LEARNING OBJECTIVES

1. Discuss strategies within the five categories of health promotion interventions.
2. Match intervention strategies to type of antecedent and anticipated population health impact.
3. Locate evidence-based health promotion programs.
4. Complete the process for creating evidence-based programs.

IN THE NEWS ...

The National School Lunch Program (NSLP) feeds about 32 million children a school day. It is the second largest federal assisted feeding program in the country, second only to the Supplemental Nutrition Assistance Program (SNAP). In 2010, Congress passed the Healthy, Hunger-Free Kids Act of 2010 that includes significant policy changes to school lunch programs. The policy altered access to healthy choices in the school environment. The new meal guidelines and competitive food guidelines were the most significant changes in the program in over 15 years and have filled the news of the past years. The NSLP is administered by the U.S. Department of Agriculture.

In January 2012, new school meal requirements were released. The new meal guidelines required schools to offer *both* a fruit and a vegetable, provide only low-fat (1%) or nonfat milk, set calorie limits for meals, and increase the use of whole grains and red and dark green vegetables. The meal pattern guidelines went into effect in the fall of 2012, and newspapers across the country carried student and parent reactions to the new foods, servings, and calorie limits. According to the new guidelines, a reimbursable meal had to include a fruit or a vegetable. Schools worked to include fruits and vegetables in each meal; but with this work came reports of high amounts of waste. Some reports estimated that more than half of the served vegetables were being thrown away. Opposition to the meal calorie limits was also a news item, particularly the limits of 700 calories for sixth through eighth graders and 850 calories for high school students. One concern was that there were too few calories for growing adolescents.

The following year also began with school food, this time snacks, making headlines. On February 1, 2013, the federal government released for public comment additional guidelines to address snacks and a la carte food items, including items sold in vending machines. Under the new rules, snack items (i.e., foods that are not part of reimbursable meals) are low in fat, salt, sugar, and calories. More specifically, snacks need to be a fruit, a vegetable, a dairy product, a protein food, a product rich in whole grains, or a combination food with at least a quarter cup of fruit or vegetable. Alternatively, a snack food can be no more than 200 calories per serving and low in fat and sodium. Beverages with calories are limited to 8 ounces (elementary) to 12 ounces (middle and high schools). The list of allowable beverages has changed dramatically, too. Sugary sodas and similar sugary beverages are out. Food from bake sales, fund-raisers, and other school traditions is not included in the new restrictions. The Smart Snacks in School standards took effect in the fall of 2014.

Introduction

Successful risk reduction programs employ strategies from more than one type of intervention. It is the complement of the interventions that allows program planners to address the multiple and varied types of antecedents that drive health behavior. No one type of intervention can change or sustain population-level health behavior change. Specific types of interventions are better suited for altering specific types of antecedents. In the opening example, school meal policy was used to address children's access to food. The policy mandated that certain foods (fruits, vegetables, whole grains, and low-fat milk) be made available to students as part of the meal selection. As will be discussed later in the chapter, access alone cannot alter actual eating behaviors. Strategies to address the appeal and convenience of foods can work synergistically with improved access to then improve student eating behaviors.

This chapter discusses the various categories of health promotion interventions and a hierarchy of anticipated impacts from the various types of interventions. The five broad categories of interventions, illustrated in level 4 of the disease prevention model, align to specific antecedents (see Figure 10-1). Within each of the broad categories of intervention, there are numerous specific types of strategies. Strategies are the implemented actions to produce change in the facilitating factor. In addition to targeting different types of antecedents, strategies should also be selected based on anticipated impact. The health impact pyramid suggests that interventions that target population-wide factors produce larger and longer-lasting change in behavior and health status.

Categories of Health Promotion Interventions

Programs are defined as a set of planned activities implemented over time to achieve specific objectives (Green & Kreuter, 2005). In the outcome logic models discussed in the

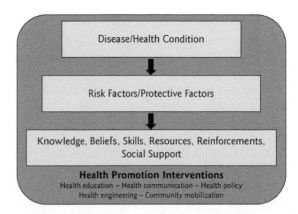

Figure 10-1 Interventions within the Disease Prevention Model

previous chapter, programs were represented by resources, activities, and anticipated outcomes. Examples of national programs include the Breast and Cervical Cancer Program (administered by the Centers for Disease Control and Prevention); Safe Routes to School (Federal Highway Administration, U.S. Department of Transportation); Freedom from Smoking (American Lung Association); Play 60 (National Football League), and the Healthy Homes Program (U.S. Department of Housing and Urban Development). Programs consist of numerous **strategies** that are designed to work synergistically to produce changes in the many influential factors driving behavior. Strategies are the general tactics programs use to achieve their stated objectives and goals, and they should be "based on knowledge about effective communication, the intended audience's needs and characteristics, and the program's capabilities, timelines, and resources" (NCI, 2008). Within programs, strategies can be grouped by type, such as media campaigns and policy advocacy.

Successful risk reduction programs employ strategies from more than one type of intervention. The strategies employed to change awareness of an issue or available resources are different from strategies employed to alter environmental context. In general, there are five categories of health promotion interventions: health education, health communications, health engineering, health policy, and community mobilization. Each of these intervention types is successful in altering select types of antecedents.

Health Education

Health education is any combination of planned learning experiences designed to facilitate voluntary changes in behavior that are conducive to health (Green & Kreuter, 2005). The specific targets of health education are knowledge, belief, and skill antecedents (Joint Committee on Health Education and Promotion Terminology, 2001; Joint Committee on National Health Education Standards, 2007). Voluntary changes in behavior are facilitated by changes in behavior-specific knowledge, beliefs, and skills. Learning activities implemented to change particular knowledge, belief, and skill antecedents are important to changing behavior. In the breastfeeding outcome logic model (Figure 9-6), prenatal classes and videos were shown as health education activities.

The strategies that can be used within health education are endless. Health education strategies can be organized around classroom-based instruction such as lectures, case studies, demonstrations, and role-plays. Strategies may be incorporated into events such as health fairs, community forums, and health care services. Strategies may be offered in a consumer on-demand format, such as telephone counseling and informational kiosks. Finally, print health education materials can include brochures, newsletters, displays, and web pages (Gilbert, Sawyer, & McNeill, 2011). Strategy decisions consider the antecedent, the target audience, and the program resources.

Current technologies provide opportunities to offer traditional health education programs in nontraditional venues. For example, general skills for smoking cessation are well researched and evaluated. Smokers need to develop trigger management and refusal skills, be able to correctly use pharmacological aids, manage stress, and be supported to remain smoke free (Ranney et al., 2006; USDHHS, 2000; Villanti et al., 2010). The Become an EX smoking cessation program (www.becomeanEX.org) is an example of a contemporary smoking cessation program that targets traditional cessation skills via the Internet. The target audience is long-term smokers who have previously tried to quit smoking. Intervention strategies are organized around three main blocks: relearning habit (trigger management), relearning addiction (pharmacological management), and relearning social support (stress and social support). This online format addresses traditional learning objectives, but the online format lends itself to accessibility and convenience (American Legacy Foundation, 2012). For example, in traditional programs, a recent ex-smoker may have a designated person to call in times of cravings; in the online format, a participant activates an "emergency button" for immediate social support.

School-Based Health Education

School-based health education targets the same antecedents as general health education (knowledge, beliefs, and skills), but the instruction is associated with the classroom setting and school-affiliated events. The National Health Education Standards further define the targets of school instruction as informational concepts related to health promotion and disease prevention (Standard 1) as well as seven behavior-related skills (Joint Committee on National Health Education Standards, 2007). Within content areas, the standards define outcome behaviors along with the content-specific functional content and related skills (see Table 10-1). For example, in an injury prevention content area, one K-2 target behavior is evacuation during fires and fire drills. Key concepts (Standard 1) include listing indicators of a fire and identifying fire escape routes. The primary skills (Standard 4) are the ability to map one or more routes from each bedroom and to locate the family meeting place (Joint Committee on National Health Education Standards, 2007). Theory guides the development of content-specific instruction, with special attention called to theoretical constructs of risk perception, social pressures, and group norms. Other characteristics of effective health instruction include skill and behavior reinforcement, personalized messaging, and links to other school and community resources (CDC, DASH, 2011)

Motivational Interviewing

Motivational interviewing is a specific health education–type program associated with health care–affiliated patient education. Motivational interviewing (MI) uses patient-centered techniques to assess ambivalence and support a person in the process of voluntary behavior change (Rollnick, Miller, & Butler, 2007). This approach to voluntary change is different from traditional health education approaches in that the participant shares information, and the health professional listens in one-on-one exchanges. The strategies of MI are not lecture, information dissemination, or role-play; rather, they are open-ended questions, expressing empathy, and reflective listening (Rollnick et al., 2007). The targets of MI are beliefs, particularly self-efficacy and motivation. Self-efficacy, defined as one's confidence in performing a specific task, is seen as a potential motivator of change. Motivation is defined as a discrepancy between one's perception of how things are and the expectation of how things should be (Rollnick et al., 2007). The average participant–professional interaction is brief, approximately 15 minutes, and occurs over several meetings; thus, MI interventions are also called brief interventions (Rubak et al., 2005).

The brief and individualized approach of MI lends itself to health care provider settings. Brief screenings and

TABLE 10-1 National Health Education Standards

Standard Number	Standard Objective
Standard 1	Students will comprehend concepts related to health promotion and disease prevention to enhance health.
Standard 2	Students will analyze the influence of family, peers, culture, media, technology, and other factors on health behaviors.
Standard 3	Students will demonstrate the ability to access valid information and products and services to enhance health.
Standard 4	Students will demonstrate the ability to use interpersonal communication skills to enhance health and avoid or reduce health risks.
Standard 5	Students will demonstrate the ability to use decision-making skills to enhance health.
Standard 6	Students will demonstrate the ability to use goal-setting skills to enhance health.
Standard 7	Students will demonstrate the ability to practice health-enhancing behaviors and avoid or reduce health risks.
Standard 8	Students will demonstrate the ability to advocate for personal, family, and community health.

Source: Joint Committee on National Health Education Standards (2007)

interventions are integrated into the care settings of emergency departments, primary care and specialty clinics, and prenatal centers (Emmons & Rollnick, 2001; NIAAA, 2005; Rubak et al., 2005). In these settings, brief interventions have successfully facilitated change of alcohol use disorders in adolescents and adults as well as smoking cessation in adolescents, pregnant women, and other adults (Heckman, Egleston, & Hofmann, 2010; Lai et al., 2010; NIAAA, 2005).

Health Communications

Health communication interventions use communication strategies to inform and influence decisions that affect health (NCI, 2008). Health communication strategies include media, advertising, and/or public relations. Like health education, the interventions seek to alter knowledge and beliefs and also provide reminders (NCI, 2008). Because of these targets, health communication campaigns are commonly referred to as awareness and information campaigns and are information based. For example, breast, cervical, and colorectal screening campaigns may describe screening procedures, remind individuals of the benefits of early detection, or suggest means to overcoming specific barriers to action (Community Preventive Services Task Force, 2012).

Well-designed messages are a critical element of health communication campaigns. Well-designed messages originate from a clearly defined communication goal, that is, what will be achieved through the campaign (NCI, 2008). A message is then developed around a main idea or point that a planner wants to convey to the intended audience. Effective messages *target particular antecedents* and are communicated in a culturally appropriate and audience-appealing manner (NCI, 2007). For example, the 5 a Day message was part of a communications campaign to increase fruit and vegetable consumption (NCI, 2001).

The 5 a Day campaign targeted *knowledge of the number of recommended servings*. In 1991, when this campaign was initiated, a popular phrase was "An apple a day keeps the doctor away." An apple represents one fruit serving, a number well below the recommended five. In 1991, only 8% of the population reported knowing that five was the recommended number of fruit and vegetable servings per day (NCI, 2001). Knowledge of servings per day was a barrier and needed to be changed before other antecedents could be altered. In the awareness campaign, the number five was front and center in

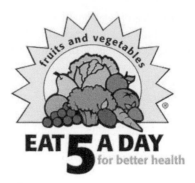

Figure 10-2 5 a Day Logo

Source: Courtesy of U.S. Department of Agriculture

the logo and all other messaging (see Figure 10-2). The 5 a Day message was distributed via numerous media, including posters, public service announcements, and grocery store trial events. This health communication campaign evolved over time to include classroom health education curricula, cookbooks, and industry promotions (NCI, 2001).

There are numerous specific strategies within health communication. One way to organize communication strategies is by the following categories: mass media, small media, and interpersonal communication (Community Preventive Services Task Force, 2012). Interpersonal communication is the transfer of information between small groups of people; phone calls, e-mails, letters, and personal visits are examples of activities in which individuals share information. **Mass media** campaigns are characterized by the use of radio, television and/or print media with broad distribution channels. In public health, space or time in mass media channels can be bought or donated to a campaign by television networks, radio stations, and newspapers for public service advertisements (Randolph & Viswanath, 2004). Mass media messages can create general awareness and are often supplemented with other approaches, such as the distribution of health education materials, patient reminders, or campaign events (Community Preventive Services Task Force, 2012).

Small media campaigns are smaller in scope and distribution and include patient education materials, fact sheets, newsletters, posters, displays, presentations, and promotional items such as pencils, magnets, and T-shirts (Community

Preventive Services Task Force, 2012). Messages still target a particular antecedent in a culturally appropriate and audience-appealing manner, but small media campaigns are also an ideal opportunity for tailored messaging. Mass media can draw statewide or national attention, with local media providing messaging tailored to address audience-specific local barriers or cues. For example, mass and small media campaigns have been used in combination to increase participation in breast, cervical, and colorectal cancer screenings (Community Preventive Services Task Force, 2012; Sabatino et al., 2012). National campaigns such as the Susan G. Komen Foundation's Race for the Cure®, the American Cancer Society's Movement for More Birthdays, and pink ribbon campaigns are well-known mass media awareness campaigns that have been successfully supplemented by patient reminders, patient education materials, and local campaign events.

Effective health communication campaigns also involve multiple communication objectives and evolve as audience characteristics change. First, audiences should be segmented, meaning grouped by similar properties. Segmenting may occur by demographics, cultural beliefs, and/or behavioral stage. Messages are designed for particular segmented audiences. For instance, the age of a woman, along with her ethnicity, level of education, and income, can play a role in how likely she is to receive an annual mammogram (Meissner et al., 2006). Similarly, women can be at different stages of breast screening behavior: never having had a mammogram, nonresponders to reminders, and/or relapsers (NCI, 2007). Small media messages should communicate to these women differently because the attitudinal and/or resource barriers are unique. Audiences also need multiple exposures to the same messages, but as knowledge or attitudes change, so should messaging. With the 5 a Day campaign discussed earlier, as knowledge about the recommended number of servings improved, the messages within that campaigned also changed. Past and current nutrition messages related to fruit and vegetables include Fruits & Veggies: More Matters, Eat Your Colors, and Make Half Your Plate Fruits and Vegetables (USDA, 2011; USDHHA, 2010).

Social Marketing

Social marketing is a particular form of health communication that applies commercial marketing techniques to campaigns designed to promote voluntary behavior change conducive to health (Andreasen, 1995). Social marketing applies the marketing elements called the four Ps: product, price, place, and promotion (CDC, n.d.c.; Cheng, Kotler, & Lee, 2011). In social marketing campaigns, the product is not typically the actual health behavior; rather, it is an attitude, outcome, expectation, or desired consumer outcome related to the behavior. Tobacco advertisements are a great example of selling a desired outcome, not the actual tobacco use. The images and written messages communicate perceived social outcomes such as attractiveness, independence, and/or masculinity. The product gets a lot of attention in the campaign planning process, but price, place, and promotion are equally important to a successful campaign. Price reflects the monetary and nonmonetary costs to the intended audience. Place and promotion are closely linked: place reflects the locations and means through which a person can be reached, while promotions are the actual mediums used to carry the campaign messages.

Act against AIDS is a national communication program that employs social marketing to raise awareness among all Americans and increase HIV testing in high-risk groups. The initiative implements multiple campaigns targeted to specific audiences: health care professionals, the general public, and various high-risk groups. The primary behavioral goal is the same—to increase the number of persons who are tested for HIV—yet the campaigns use different messages to address the barriers unique to each target audience. Overall, messages tend to address the stigma related to and complacency about testing, and support physician efforts to counsel and test patients. For example, Testing Makes Us Stronger encourages black gay and bisexual men to get tested. The product of the campaign is strength and control (USDHHS, CDC, 2012). The bold image and large words both highlight personal strength (see Figure 10-3). Testing is not an act of weakness or fear; testing gives a person strength. Campaign ads are featured in national magazines, as television public service announcements, and on websites. Billboards, radio spots, and media coverage are also distributed in targeted cities. There are Facebook pages, YouTube videos, and a dedicated website. At the local level, materials are available for individuals and organizations to download and distribute. Partnerships are also an important strategy when building community-specific promotions and placements. *Act against AIDS* has developed partnerships with 19 leading national civic and social organizations that represent the populations hardest hit by HIV and AIDS. Partners are selected for their ability to reach specific

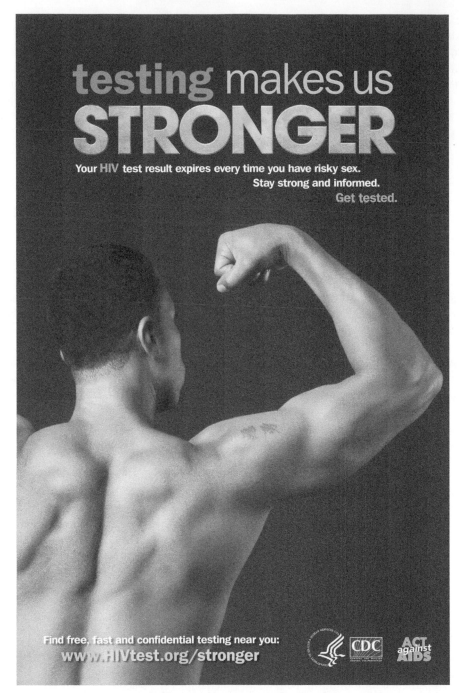

Figure 10-3 Act against AIDS Social Marketing Campaign Poster

Source: Courtesy of Department of Health and Human Services and Centers for Disease Control and Prevention

populations at increased risk at the national and/or local level (USDHHS, CDC, 2012). Current partners include the Magic Johnson Foundation, Black Entertainment Television (BET) Networks, Kaiser Family Foundation, National Hispanic Council on Aging, and Black Atlanta AIDS Institute (USDDHHS, CDC, 2012).

The Centers for Disease Control and Prevention has developed online toolkits for social marketing in the areas of violence prevention, cardiovascular health, tobacco prevention, diabetes, and emergency risk (CDC, n.d.c.).

Health Engineering

Health engineering involves altering a product or the environment to meet a behavioral objective. Engineering strategies target access-type antecedents and enable persons to take and maintain action. Products or physical environments are built or redesigned to increase access to behavior facilitators as well as to limit access to counterfacilitators. For example, adding fluoride to the product of city water is one way to provide near universal access to fluoride. Engineering strategies can also target behavior-related skills, making it easier for a skill to be performed. Self-monitoring, (goal setting and record keeping) is a behavioral skill associated with nutrition, physical activity, tobacco use, sleep, and numerous other health behaviors. Behavioral rates of record keeping are less than ideal, though, due to the complexity and inconvenience of the skill. Mobile applications have been introduced to make record keeping easier. With Meal Snap one merely takes a picture of a meal, and the kilocalories are calculated and loaded into a food diary. Finally, engineering can be a mechanism for providing reminders. The dinging sound of a seat belt reminder and prompts in an electronic medical record are two examples of health engineering reminder strategies.

Engineering a health-promoting environment is about manufacturing function and appeal. Environmental function focuses on the utility of the space and structures within the space. Usefulness of a space is both the presence of necessary structures within the space as well as the minimization of barriers or counterfacilitators. Environmental appeal focuses on the aesthetic value of the space. Appealing environments have properties that may be perceived as attractive, exciting, and/or calming. Behavior-promoting environments contain amenities that support the behavior and are both functional and appealing. For instance, a physical activity–friendly environment would include functional amenities such as sidewalks, lighting, and connectedness, and appealing amenities might include well-landscaped neighborhoods, outdoor art, and colorful business districts (see Figure 10-4). A breastfeeding-friendly environment would include functional amenities such as a dedicated area in which to breastfeed and privacy. Aesthetic amenities would include cleanliness, comfortable seating, and music.

Functional and appealing environments can occur in all settings and through simple design strategies. In the workplace, modest environmental changes to stairwells have led to documented increases in the use of stairways (Kerr et al., 2004). The StairWELL to Better Health program makes stairwells more appealing with paint, carpet, natural light, framed artwork, and music. Motivational signage placed at stairwell entry points also serve as cues to enter (see Figure 10-5). In one study, by making worksite stairwells attractive and visible, stair use increased by about 9% (Kerr et al., 2004). In an extension of these engineering principles, individuals can modify their own environments to promote behavior change. For example, when a smoker is preparing to quit smoking, he or she is encouraged to remove all cigarettes, ashtrays, and lighters from his or her environment and add items such as mints and air fresher. Such strategies create a behavior-supporting environment by decreasing access to smoking-related products and adding substitutions.

Like environments, products can also be altered to provide health-promoting action. Product engineering can increase access to behavior facilitators and/or limit exposure to counterfacilitators. Product engineering strategies can be both highly technical and everyday simple. Mobile applications (apps), such as the Meal Snap are an example of a product manufactured to promote a behavior-related skill of self-monitoring intake. Program planners may not have the skills or resources to develop applications or technical retail products. However, products can be redesigned more simply. Stocking vending machines with only low-fat snacks and offering smaller servings of food are examples of simple product changes to influence behavior-related access, skills, and reminders.

Health engineering along with health policy is a powerful strategy of change because of the type and magnitude of change that is facilitated. When environments, or contexts, are changed so that the healthy choice is the easier or default

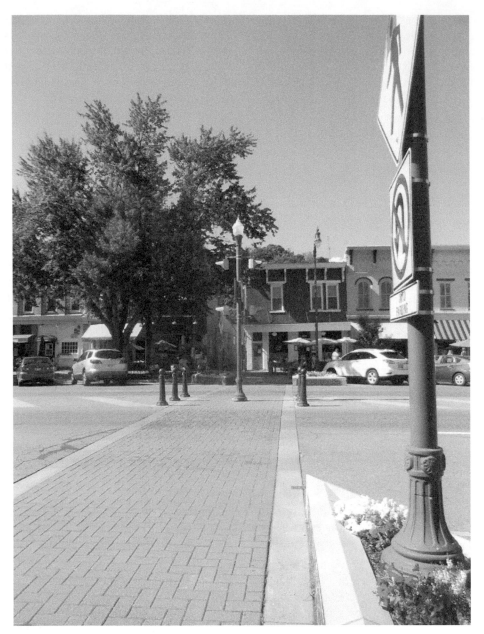

Figure 10-4 Physical Activity–Friendly Environment

choice, completing the desired healthy action becomes relatively certain (Frieden, 2010). For example, the addition of speed bumps and traffic circles to roadways decreases automobile speed. Structurally, the environment makes speeding in those particular areas very challenging, if not impossible. Strategies that change physical and social environments also reach greater numbers of individual than other strategies. A class or media campaign about speeding may reach between

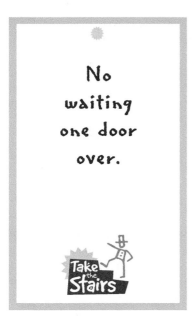

Figure 10-5 StairWELL to Better Health Campaign Poster

Source: Courtesy of Centers for Disease Control and Prevention

20 and 100 people a day. By contrast, a speed bump reaches every person who drives that path. Finally, the powerful impact of policies and engineering also comes from creating environments that support individual behaviors. When an individual changes a behavior, he or she is more likely to continue that behavior change in a physical and social environment that supports the behavior. Without supportive environments, individual behavior changes are unlikely to be sustained.

The topic of the Behavioral Science in Action feature at the end of this chapter is engineering choice in the school cafeteria. Read there how schools implement environmental strategies that work strategically with the new school meal guidelines to improve students' fruit, vegetable, whole-grain, and caloric intakes.

Check for Understanding   Look at column two of the PER worksheet (refer to Table 8-1 and Figure 8-1 as needed). What antecedents could be changed via product or environmental engineering?

Health Policy and Enforcement

Health policy is the fourth category of health promotion interventions. Policies are laws, regulations, or formal and informational rules established by government or organizations (Association of State and Territorial Directors of Health Promotion and Public Health Education & CDC, 2001; Story et al., 2008). Policies can be implemented on all levels of the environment: interpersonal, organizational, and within the larger societal systems via state and federal laws. Policies influence access and reinforcements. Like engineering, policies work to create physical and social environments that promote and sustain health behavior. Reinforcements may include consequences for a behavior, such as penalties for impaired driving or paying higher insurance premiums for select behaviors. Because policies are often used to create physical environments, alter products, or create access to services, policy interventions are closely tied to health engineering interventions.

Policies, like health engineering, also reach a greater number of individuals than do other types of interventions and thus have the potential to impact or create societal behavioral norms. Tobacco control policy dictates the places people can smoke, the price of tobacco products, the age of purchaser, and incentives or costs related to health insurance. State smoking bans and federal regulatory rules are policies commonly associated with smoking control; however, smaller environments' policies and rules be equally important. Rules within a family and among friends influence daily access and reinforcements and are strongly associated with remaining smoke free. Household bans or space restrictions are also associated with lower smoking prevalence rates (Biener et al., 2010). Household rules provide behavioral reinforcements and restrict access. The antismoking norm created by these policies can also encourage others to quit. For example, workplaces with smoking bans report a higher number of employees who quit smoking.

Implementation and enforcement are essential pieces of policy interventions. A policy must be implemented and enforced before it can alter access and/or produce reinforcements. Implementation is the degree to which a policy is implemented. Degrees of implementation can vary greatly in organizations and systems. Enforcement is the monitoring of the policy implementation and the assignment of the expected consequences. Implementation and enforcement are often erroneously assumed in interventions. Monitoring implementations and enforcing that implementation are necessary for all levels of implementation: interpersonal, organizational, and systemic. Household rules, workplace and community policies, and state and federal regulations are less effective in altering access and reinforcements without implementation and enforcement.

Numerous allied health behaviors have been facilitated by policy and system interventions. Childhood immunization rates are a set of behaviors that have clearly been affected by state and federal policies. All states have school immunization laws that define the immunizations children must have before they can enter school (USDHHS, CDC, 2011). Students must receive the required vaccinations before school entry, unless they have a health condition or religious objection that prevents immunization. Furthermore, the Vaccines for Children Program (VFC) and Section 317 of the Public Health Services Act improved access to immunizations by funding 95% of publicly provided immunizations (National Conference of State Legislatures, 2011). Prior to school laws and federal funding, childhood immunization rates ranged from 60% to 70%. Rates have since increased to well over 90% (Hinman, Orenstein, & Schuchat, 2011). Other medical-type health behaviors influenced by state and federal access policies include mammography, cervical cancer screenings, colorectal cancer screenings, HIV screenings, and medication compliance. Table 10-2 provides samples of policies employed across health promotion settings.

Community Mobilization

Involving the target audience in the implementation of a program is an additional intervention category called **community mobilization**. Trusted members of the community are recruited and trained to provide health education, advocate for a particular policy, or facilitate media campaigns. The roles of the enlisted community members can include providing correct information, motivating others to take action, providing resources, and reinforcing behavior changes (Merzel & D'Afflitti, 2003; USDHHS, n.d.a.). Community mobilization is rarely an independent intervention; rather, it is a method to enhance the impact of other strategies targeting knowledge, beliefs, skills, reminders, and resources (Community Preventive Services Task Force, 2005; Merzel & D'Afflitti, 2003). By involving trusted community members as messengers, social norm, reinforcement, and social support antecedents that are harder to shape may also be altered.

A significant benefit of community mobilization is gaining access to a harder-to-reach community. Harder-to-reach populations are often members of minority groups, and typical mainstream public health initiatives do not reach or do not appeal to them. *Reach* can be a matter of geography, isolation, health status, or socio-demographic characteristic. The audience is physically or organizationally not easily accessible. Health characteristics that might create vulnerability and isolation include disability, addiction, chronic illness, and mental illness (RWJF, 2011). *Appeal* can be a matter of trust, language, or cultural practices. In appeal, barriers are not space and distance, but socio-cultural factors. Community members who are ethnically or culturally similar to the target audience can serve as a bridge for overcoming appeal barriers. Reach and appeal can act independently or synergistically. A community may be receptive to public health initiatives, but reach is the obstacle for program implementation. In addition, reach and appeal can act synergistically when a community is physically difficult to reach and distrusting of health care providers. Immigrants, individuals who speak English as a second language, adolescents, men who have sex with men, rural residents, and older black men are just a few populations for whom community mobilization is a recommended intervention component (Community Preventive Services Task Force, 2005; Merzel & D'Afflitti, 2003; Shults et al., 2009; USDHHS, n.d.a.; Victor et al., 2010).

Community mobilization also creates a capacity for sustainability. First, the recruited community members receive training in preparation for and continuation of their project role. They develop health and disease prevention knowledge, skills in navigating community organizations, advocacy skills, and others. Training occurs on the job as well as through structured training sessions (Global Health Workforce Alliance & WHO, 2010; Kash, May, & Tai-Seale, 2007). In approximately half the community mobilization programs, trainees complete a structured education program (USDHHS, 2007a). In some instances, education programs are extended into certificate training programs that involve community college classes and a state-level certification (Kash et al., 2007). Because members are recruited from the community, the members and their new skills remain in the community after a program's funding is over. Those community workers continue as a source of health-related knowledge and advocacy within the community. Second, the relationships between agencies and community members continue as well. That means those relationships do not leave the community.

TABLE 10-2 Sample Health Promotion Policies By Setting

	Sample Policies
Public	Excise taxing and minimum pricing of tobacco and alcohol
	Nutrition labeling of restaurant and fast food
	Smoking bans and enforcement
	Primary versus secondary safety belt laws
	Minimum age driving laws
	Alcohol impaired driving laws
Worksite	Guidelines on fat and calorie content of vending machine foods
	Health insurance premiums paid by health risk
	Reimbursement for fitness club membership
	Smoke-free campuses
	Designation of clean and comfortable lactation areas for nursing mothers
	Influenza vaccine requirements for health care workers
School	Limits on fat and calorie content of a la carte foods
	Provision of space and equipment for indoor recess
	Definition of bullying to include verbal bullying, physical violence, and cyber bullying
	Distance and school busing eligibility
	Restrictions on alcohol retail outlet density around campus
	School day start time
	Annual body mass index (BMI) screenings of a school district's students
Allied Health	Adoption of National Heart, Lung, and Blood Institute (NHLBI) Guidelines for the Assessment of Overweight & Obesity in Adults by a provider system
	Formula provision to new mothers
	Chart review policy for provider guideline adherence
	Designation of funds for breast and cervical cancer screenings for underinsured women
	Helmet and mouth guard use during athletic practice and games

The use of community health workers is a specific form of community mobilization. Trusted members of the community are recruited and trained for a particular role within a public health initiative. Community health workers (CHW) are involved in programs seen by the target audience as medical in nature, with CHWs serving in an allied health care capacity. The World Health Organization (2007) discusses **community health workers** in the following way: CHWs should be members of the communities where they work, should be selected by the communities, should be answerable to the communities for their activities, should be supported by the health systems but not necessarily a part of its organization, and have shorter training than professional workers. Specific roles can include serving as a navigator of complex health systems, health and self-care educator, outreach and member recruitment, or event organizer (USDHHS, 2007a). In the United States, CHWs play an active role in achieving behavioral outcomes such as increasing participation in cancer screenings and improving diabetes and hypertension management (Fernandez et al., 2009; Norris et al., 2006; USD-HHS, 2007a; Victor et al., 2010; Viswanathan et al., 2009).

Community health workers play a vital role in the attainment of global health improvement goals. CHWs fill gaps between understaffed medical professionals and population access. In a recent review of 266 global programs, CHWs were found to play key roles in nutrition, maternal health, birth and newborn care, breastfeeding, immunizations and well-child care, malaria control, tuberculosis control, HIV/AIDS prevention and control, and mental health interventions (Global Health Workforce Alliance & WHO, 2010). More successful CHW programs recruit well, have good selection and recognition programs, provide initial training and continuing education, are based on community need, and are integrated into the health care system. Factors that limit the success of CHWs are shortages of basic drugs, immunizations, and commodities (like condoms); lack of or nonfunctional equipment, adequate supervision, continuing education, and links to the health system; and low status of CHWs (Global Health Workforce Alliance & WHO, 2010).

The Community Health Agents program in Brazil is a featured program in the World Health Organization report. Family health teams are assigned to a specific geographic region and complete home visits to families in that area. Each team consists of a physician, nurse, nurse's aid, and four to six community health workers. A unique aspect of this program is that the CHWs are paid health professionals who are supervised by a salaried nurse. CHWs receive a salary funded by the state government. CHWs receive 8 weeks of initial training followed by monthly and quarterly continuing education. Currently, there are more than 30,000 family health teams and more than 240,000 CHWs across the country covering about half of Brazil's population. Program outcomes include expanded vaccination coverage, breastfeeding promotion, increased use of oral rehydration salts, management of pneumonia, and growth monitoring. The program has also been associated with declines in infant mortality (Global Health Workforce Alliance & WHO, 2010).

Frisbee or Flying Disc?

Is it a Frisbee or a flying disc? An iPod or a digital music player? A tissue or Kleenex? Products and processes may have the same function but be called by different names. In the preceding pairs, both names in the set are correct, but one is a brand name and the other is a generic term. Frisbee is the trademarked name of a flying disc. An iPod is the trademarked name of Apple's digital music player, and Kleenex is the trademarked name for tissue. The categories of health promotion interventions are no different—organizations may apply a specialized name for one or more health promotion intervention categories, but the functions or meaning are the same. Personalizing intervention terms to specific programs can help communities remember as well as apply the scientific concepts into practice.

An example of this personalization of intervention terms to a specific context is the 5 Es model of the Safe Routes to School program. In the Safe Routes to School Program, local planners are required to organize program and funding requests in a 5 Es model: education, encouragement, engineering, enforcement, and evaluation (Pedestrian and Bicycle Information Center, 2007). Education activities teach students pedestrian and bicycling safety skills, as well as the benefits of active commuting. Education strategies also communicate the location of the routes and resources, and remind parents and school neighbors of safety precautions. Similarly, encouragement activities generate excitement for and reinforce walking and bicycling to school. In the 5 Es model, education and encouragement categories are similar to the generic categories of health education and health communications. Enforcement activities monitor policy compliance and encourage drivers, walkers, and neighbors to follow rules that make active commuting safe. Enforcement in the 5 Es model has the same function as health policy and enforcement. Finally, engineering activities build safe and aesthetically appealing routes.

A second example of this personalization of intervention terms is the categorical terms within the Community Guide. The Community Guide is an informational resource for public health practitioners and researchers (www.thecommunityguide.org). Teams of independent researchers, called Community Preventive Services Task Force, review intervention evaluations and published studies. The task force is an independent panel of public health and prevention experts from universities, health departments, health care settings, and foundations. The work of the task force is then summarized by content and behaviors to help communities select public health interventions. For instance, intervention categories in physical activity are (1) awareness/information, (2) behavioral/social, and (3) environmental/policy. Within awareness and information campaigns, the interventions of community-wide campaigns, mass media, and classroom-based health education are summarized. Within behavioral and social approaches, health education by different audience and settings are reviewed. Finally, environmental design, land use, and travel policies are reviewed. The Centers for Disease Control and Prevention provides administrative, research, and technical support to the Community Preventative Services Task Force.

The Health Impact Pyramid

The health impact pyramid is another way to organize thoughts and decisions about health promotion interventions. This framework consists of five tiers of possible public health interventions and the anticipated population-level impacts of the associated interventions. The pyramid shape is used to reflect a hierarchy of the potential impact on population-level health (see Figure 10-6). More effective interventions are those that reach broader segments of a population (more people) in a community and require less individual effort (Frieden, 2010).

Interventions at the base of the pyramid have the potential to impact some of the most powerful and long-lasting correlates on community health, the social factors discussed in Chapter 3. Moving up from the base, environmental, clinical, and education-based interventions are described as interventions with smaller impacts on community-level health. As the pyramid narrows, the public health impact decreases; however, the ease of intervention implementation and the likelihood of individual change often improve. A community

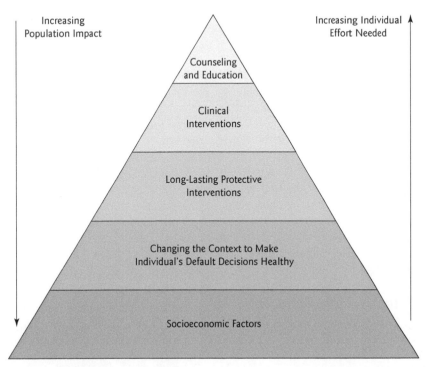

Figure 10-6 Health Impact Pyramid
Source: Adapted from Frieden (2010)

immunization program is easier to implement than a program to improve housing conditions. Arguably, though, providing safe housing with acceptable air quality and access to transportation can have greater impacts on the long-term health status of a greater number of individuals.

Socioeconomic Factors

Socioeconomic factors are the foundations from which people connect to work, others, recreation, and health care. Socioeconomic factors are "the basic foundations of a society," including factors like poverty, employment, education, and housing (Frieden, 2010). Although the actual mechanisms by which they influence health vary, and at times are very complex, the correlations between socioeconomic factors and health status are strong. Interventions of change at this level of the pyramid involve significant paradigm shifts in government, resource allocation, and the willingness of communities. Addressing disparities in socioeconomic factors would theoretically close gaps in numerous disparities in health outcomes, though this alone will not cure communities of health status issues.

Changing the Context and Environment

Tier 2 of the health impact pyramid includes interventions that alter the context beyond the person. As discussed throughout this book, the physical and social environment from which the health behavior operates and/or originates has a powerful influence over behavior. Changing the context so that the healthy or desired behavior becomes the "default" or easier choice can significantly influence the health actions, and thus the health status, of many. Contextual changes that have made healthier choices "easier" and more sustainable include indoor smoking bans, transfat regulations, seat belt laws, fluoridating water, walkable communities, and clean water and air initiatives. Tier 1 and tier 2 interventions are often achieved through policy and engineering strategies of change.

Long-Lasting Protective Interventions

Tier 3 of the pyramid consists of long-lasting protective interventions. Long-lasting protective interventions promote action by an individual, with the necessary action occurring one time or infrequently. The actions of the individual do not require ongoing clinical care or attention but protect or improve health long after the desired behavior has occurred.

Immunizations, colonoscopies, and male circumcision are examples of clinical actions that occur infrequently but protect health for years (Frieden, 2010).

Clinical Interventions

Tier 4 of the pyramid consists of clinical interventions, such as blood pressure and cholesterol control. With technological and pharmaceutical advances, as well as the documentation of evidence-based medicine, there is a greater understanding of clinical interventions that can improve health. Clinical interventions are higher up on the impact pyramid. This is not due to treatment efficacy; rather, it is more attributable to the access and adherence to these types of interventions. Nonadherence to treatment and limited access to regular care diminish the impact of clinical interventions on the health of populations.

Counseling and Education

Health education and counseling represent the tip, or fifth tier, of the pyramid. Health education facilitates voluntary change in behavior via changes in knowledge, beliefs, and skills. Again, evidence-based public health initiatives have documented several education and counseling programs that facilitate change in behavior (see the next section about evidence-based programs). Impact, or change, often occurs on an individual level, and it takes considerable time and resources to achieve widespread population change, that is, to reach comparable numbers of individuals exposed to a contextual change such as fluoridated water. Nonetheless, health education interventions represent an important tool in improving community health; certain health issues require individual behavior change that cannot be facilitated by a policy or contextual change. Use of condoms and meal preparation are two such examples. Furthermore, it is often the behavior change of an individual that becomes a catalyst for change in a community, for example, mothers change the health practices (and contexts) of their families, principals change those of their schools, chief executive officers (CEOs) those of their companies, and so forth.

Successful risk reduction programs employ strategies from more than one type of intervention. The health impact pyramid reinforces the concept that community-level changes in health status require multilevel interventions. No matter how interventions are categorized or organized, it is the complement of the interventions that addresses the multiple and varied types of factors that drive and sustain health behavior.

With the exception of socioeconomic factors, no one type of intervention can change and/or sustain health behavior change. Likewise, certain behaviors, or stages of behavior, lend themselves better to certain interventions.

Existing Evidence-Based Programs

Previous sections of this chapter have explained the various categories of health promotion interventions and described the anticipated population-level impact of categories of interventions. Knowledge of intervention categories, their ideal targets, and expected impacts has evolved through the collection and evaluation of data. The understanding and knowledge gathered are then applied to the program planning process. The remainder of this chapter will discuss the selection and implementation of actual health promotion programs.

In Chapter 1, evidence-based public health (EBPH) practice was described as the use of the best available scientific evidence, using data and information systems systematically, applying program planning frameworks, engaging the community in decision making, conducting sound evaluation, and disseminating what is learned (Brownson, Fielding, & Maylahn, 2009). There are numerous resources to aid one in identifying evidence-based programs, allowing professionals to plan the most effective programs possible for the community or other intended audience.

What Is Evidence?

All health promotion programs should be evidence based. **Evidence** is some form of data for use in making judgments and decisions (Brownson et al., 2009). Practitioners want to use the *best available* data in their decision making but recognize that the best type of data may not be available due to the nuances of working with people in their communities or in emerging fields or populations. Therefore, good public health practice is using "the best available data," and these data fall into various categories.

Puddy and Wilkins (2011) introduced a continuum from which evidence can be evaluated. Evidence can be well supported, supported, promising, emerging, and undetermined (see Figure 10-7). The continuum of evidence is based on the effectiveness of the program or strategy (outcomes) and the strength of the evidence (quality of the information). Well-supported and supported programs are those programs with effective desired outcomes and with studies completed with a rigorous design and method. Promising and emerging evidence has some evidence of effectiveness, but additional studies are needed. Programs of undetermined evidence may have anecdotal community information about outcomes, but additional information is needed. Finally, evidence can also indicate that use of the practice is unsupported or harmful. In these cases, the practice should not be used.

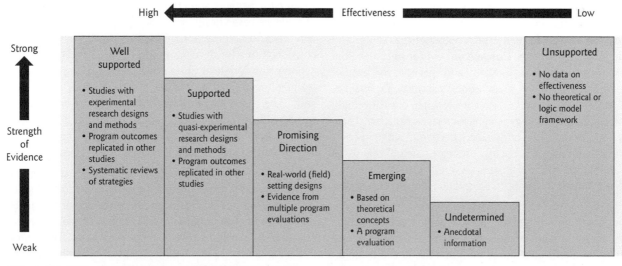

Figure 10-7 Continuum of Program Evidence

Source: Adapted from Puddy and Wilkins (2011)

Professional organizations use the continuum of evidence to make recommendations. The labels and terms differ, but the method typically involves reviewing the body of available evidence on effectiveness, benefit, and sometimes cost and then making practice recommendations. To communicate the effectiveness of data and strength of evidence about clinical preventive care to health care practitioners, the U.S. Preventive Services Task Force (USPSTF) (2008) adopted a letter grade system. After reviews of published research, clinical behaviors are assigned one of five letter grades. Grade A recommendations are highly recommended. Grade B actions are also recommended with high certainty that the net benefit is at least moderate. Grade C actions are to be considered on an individual patient basis, and Grade D actions are not recommended. Grade I means there is insufficient evidence to assess the balance of benefits and harms of the service. The evidence may be lacking, of poor quality, or conflicting (USPSTF, 2008). The Guide to Community Preventive Services uses a three-tier system: recommended, recommended against, and insufficient evidence. Because evidence exists on a continuum, practitioners seek to use the best available information, which can be derived through information about the outcomes, the context, and professional insight, in their decision-making.

Experience and Context

In addition to information about outcomes, professional experiences and community factors are important sources of evidence to consider in the decision-making process (Brownson et al., 2009; Puddy & Wilkins, 2011). **Experiential evidence** comes from the prior experiences, skills, and insights of professionals. **Contextual evidence** comes from information about the community and speaks to the feasibility and acceptability of a community's strategy. Experiential and contextual information is valuable when one is deciding if the program or strategy is right for a given situation. There may be information or prior experiences from within a community that suggest particular strategies are unlikely to be successful in a specific situation, even though they are supported by research. Contextual conditions for an intervention are important to consider when selecting interventions.

Designing and implementing practical, feasible, theory-based programs can be labor, skill, and time intensive. Using existing programs also allows communities to capitalize on the knowledge and learning experiences of others to increase the likelihood of success. Fortunately, repositories of evidence-based programs exist and are continuing to grow. Practitioners

are encouraged to research existing evidence-based programs. Table 10-3 includes some starting places.

Rarely do programs developed for a particular situation get fully adopted in their original state by others. The need to adapt evidence-based programs is common. People may change names, alter handouts, give local examples, and alter media channels in an attempt to tailor materials to their audience. Furthermore, teachers and practitioners tend to implement select strategies, omit others, and add strategies or content. Program adaptations may be due to time, available resources, staff expertise, or other contextual factors.

In adapting evidence-based health promotion programs, practitioners must be careful not to omit critical elements of change from the evidence-based program. The more pieces of a program that are changed, the less likely the program is to be based on evidence. When programs are adapted, project staff should revisit the theoretical framework and ensure that strategies addressing the influential factors of the behavior remain intact. Organizations try to help others develop programs by identifying the critical strategies of the program and labeling elements as core, essential, or critical. When programs have been altered, process and outcome evaluations of core elements are needed (National Cancer Institute, 2006).

Creating A Local Program

Despite the benefits and efficiencies associated with the use of evidence-based health promotion programs, local programs may need to be developed. This section discusses general considerations for developing a program plan and detailed action plans. While at times it may seem like the program is starting from scratch, that should not be the case. All practice should be based on evidence. Minimally, program development builds on theoretical understandings about the behavior, prior evidence of efficacy about the types of interventions, and information about particular types of strategies.

Developing a health promotion program plan is an extension of the previous work of creating a theoretical behavior model. The behavioral model illustrates the behavioral antecedents, behavioral building blocks (the really important antecedents), and the relationship between the antecedents. Theoretical modeling becomes "real-world" or applied to practice when programs are created to bring about change in the behavioral factors illustrated in the behavioral model. Aligning program strategies to specific high-priority predisposing, enabling,

TABLE 10-3 Evidence-Based Health Promotion Strategies and Programs

Resource	Description	Topic Areas	Source
Research-Tested Intervention Programs (RTIPS)	RTIPS offers programs developed from scientifically based studies that have been shown to be effective. The database is organized to make it easy to find and compare various intervention programs that address the main areas of interest, be they a particular cancer site, a demographic, a delivery setting, or another intervention component. Program materials can be downloaded or ordered.	• Breast cancer screening • Cervical cancer screening • Colorectal screening • Diet and nutrition • Obesity • Physical activity • Public health genomics • Sun safety • Survivorship • Tobacco control	National Cancer Institute
Guide to Clinical Preventive Services	The U.S. Preventive Services Task Force is an independent group of national experts in prevention and evidence-based medicine that works to improve the health of all Americans by making evidence-based recommendations about clinical preventive services such as screenings, counseling services, and preventive medications.	• Cancer screenings • Heart, vascular, and respiratory disease screenings • Infectious diseases • Injury and violence • Mental health and substance abuse • Metabolic, nutritional, and endocrine conditions • Musculoskeletal conditions • Obstetric and gynecologic conditions • Vision disorders • Children and adolescent screenings	Agency for Healthcare Research and Quality; U.S. Preventive Services Task Force
Guide to Community Preventive Services (The Community Guide)	The Community Guide is a resource for evidence-based recommendations and findings about what works to improve public health. A task force or independent researchers make practice recommendations based on systematic scientific reviews of published literature.	• Adolescent health • Alcohol • Asthma • Birth defects • Cancer • Cardiovascular disease • Diabetes • Emergency preparedness • Health communication • Health equity • HIV/AIDS, STIs and pregnancy • Mental health • Motor vehicle injury • Nutrition • Obesity • Oral health	Centers for Disease Control and Prevention

continues

TABLE 10-3 *continued*

Resource	Description	Topic Areas	Source
		• Physical activity • Social environment • Tobacco use • Vaccines • Violence • Worksite	
Substance Abuse and Mental Health Services Administration (SAMHSA) National Registry of Evidence-Based Programs and Practices (NREPP)	NREPP is a searchable online registry of interventions and supporting mental health promotion, substance abuse prevention, and mental health and substance abuse treatments. Members of the public are connected to intervention developers so that they can learn how to implement these approaches in their communities.	• Alcohol • Crime/delinquency • Drugs • Employment • Family • Homelessness • Mental health • Suicide • Tobacco • Trauma/injuries	Substance Abuse and Mental Health Services Administration (SAMHSA)
University of North Carolina (UNC) Center for Health Promotion and Disease Prevention	A CDC Prevention Research Center, the UNC Center for Health Promotion and Disease Prevention (HPDP) works to bring public health research findings to the daily lives of individuals and communities, with a special focus on North Carolina and populations vulnerable to disease.	• Cancer, cardiovascular disease, and stroke prevention • Healthy aging • HIV/AIDS and STI prevention • Obesity prevention and control • Research translation and dissemination • Social and economic determinants of health • Sustainable food system *Note:* The CDC funds other prevention institutes that specialize in other topic areas	University of North Carolina
HIV/AIDS Prevention Research Synthesis Project (PRS)	The goal of PRS is to translate scientific evidence from the research literature into practical information that can be used by prevention providers as well as state and local health departments throughout the United States. PRS identifies evidence-based behavioral interventions (EBIs) related to HIV and also engages in other activities.	• Behavioral interventions to reduce the outcomes associated with HIV/AIDS *Note:* Other CDC Centers also have evidence-based programs	Centers for Disease Control and Prevention

and reinforcing (PER) factors is the absolute most fundamental aspect of designing theory-based interventions (Green & Kreuter, 2005). The importance of intervention specificity cannot be overstated. Without designing strategies to change the influential behavioral factors and related antecedents, programs are atheoretical, and behavior is less likely to change. As discussed in the previous chapter, the program plan and evaluation gets represented in an outcome logic model.

Pooling Strategies and Patching Gaps

In their popular book on health promotion planning, Green and Kreuter (2005) describe the process of creating and tailoring programs from other interventions through a process of pooling and patching. Pooling occurs when practitioners gather information about other strategies and programs and blend evidence-based strategies to create a program base. Patching is the process of filling gaps in the program framework (Green & Kreuter, 2005). Gaps can occur for a variety of reasons, including a lack of available strategies or evidence and due to specific needs of the audience.

Organizing strategies into activity blocks that target specific antecedents can be one of the more difficult steps in the process of building an outcome logic model. The 20 or so behavioral antecedents listed on a PER worksheet need to be grouped by some type of commonality. It is logical to place similar types of antecedents into a block and then create common activities to address them. For example, information and awareness antecedents (e.g., knowledge, beliefs and reminders) could be placed in one block. A second block may include the environment and product resources, with a third block containing skill and social support–type antecedents. This creates a structure to sort and order antecedents; the boxes are not exclusive, and individual antecedents may be moved between blocks until the best fit for the antecedents has been achieved. This sorting and grouping of antecedents began with the development of the theoretical behavioral model. It is revisited and refined in the activity building phase.

A second method for structuring activity blocks is to organize antecedents and strategies by the target audience. Blocks of strategies are organized around a target audience or environments from which the mediator resides. In Figure 10-8, the Smarter Lunchrooms Statewide Dissemination Model is organized around activities and resources for two important audiences: (1) university and extension agent partners

and (2) school food service teams. Partners provide training, implementation, and evaluation support to area school districts. Food service teams implement the cafeteria-based strategies in their local school buildings (Orlowski, Narayan, & Spears, 2014b). Smarter lunchrooms initiatives are emerging programs with emerging evidence (see the Behavioral Science in Action feature). Therefore, programs are built on gathering information about evidence-based strategies and developing local strategies to fill gaps in the program model. Also, school district populations vary widely across any state; a program framework model that allows for the experience and contextual evidence is important. The Smarter Lunchrooms Statewide Dissemination Model is used as the model for understanding in the upcoming section.

Pooling Intervention Strategies

Pooling intervention strategies involves gathering information about other programs and strategies and reviewing the application to the objectives and context at hand. Unless a program is truly groundbreaking, information on strategies and corresponding outcomes likely exist. Minimally, programmers should address, in earnest, the behavioral buildings blocks of the theoretical model. Researchers and program planners note that "three" is an important number in this initial program planning. Effective multi-component programs tend to address at least three major determinants (theoretical constructs) of change (Green & Kreuter, 2005; McKenzie, Neiger, & Thackeray, 2009). Pooling information on strategies to address the behavior building blocks is an excellent starting point.

Activity boxes begin with one or two main programming ideas to address the multiple behavioral antecedents. Again, starting with three activity boxes organized around the three or more primary behavioral mediators is one method of starting. As the program plans grow, additional activities often are identified. In the Smarter Lunchroom Outcome Logic Model (Figure 10-8), the partnership activity box started as a means for evaluating the dissemination project. Faculty and students would collect observational and plate waste data in school cafeterias. As the plan developed and during the early stages of implementation, the need for standardized processes and a common storage area was identified as a related activity. In this manner, activities can be initially anchored in evidence-based practice and provide structure to where other strategies can be added.

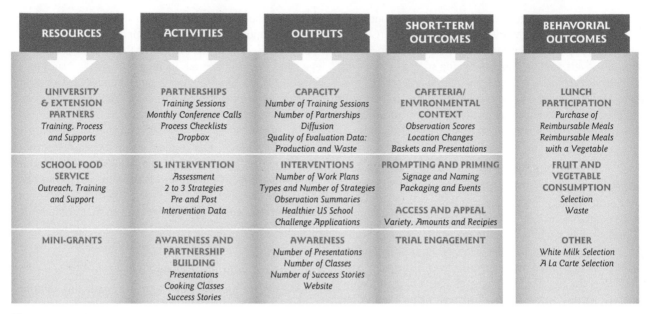

Figure 10-8 Statewide Dissemination Program Model

Source: Adapted from Orlowski, Narayan, & Spears (2014b)

The original sorting of the antecedents and strategies may be refined as activity categories become flushed out. One or more of the antecedents originally placed in one thematic box may be moved elsewhere to be addressed through the strategies of another box. Activity boxes may be assigned descriptive names at this point, too. The names are simple phrases or words that communicate the unique focus of that program component. Names can be based on the target audience, main programming components, or behavioral buildings blocks. In Figure 10-8, activity blocks describe the behavioral building block: (a) Partnerships, (b) Cafeteria Interventions, and (c) Awareness Building.

Finally, synergistic opportunities are another means of building efficient and multicomponent programs. Synergistic opportunities are situations in which two or more people and/or programs can work together to achieve similar goals. In health promotion, collaborative efforts can achieve resource and expertise sharing and message reinforcement. Synergistic opportunities can come from current community programs, existing media campaigns, or individuals with a common interest. Within a school environment, numerous

departments or services work to improve the health and well-being of students and staff. Specific entities identified in the Coordinated School Health Model include nutrition services, classroom instruction, physical education, counseling services, staff wellness programs, school nursing staff, family and community partners, and facilities staff. Coordinated efforts can improve the outcome of most school initiatives (USDHHS, n.d.b.). Synergistic opportunities can also be identified with a program. Strategies in one block or activity can be linked to subsequent activities and learning.

Patching Gaps

Once the activity boxes are sorted and labeled, the next step involves filling gaps in the program framework. Gaps are areas where there is no strategy for a given behavioral antecedent. The outcome logic model process can visually highlight gaps, that is, places in the model where activities that target specific factors or outcomes are missing in the plan. Patching is the process of filling gaps in the program (Green & Kreuter, 2005). The process of patching is much like that described in pooling. Teams will want to research and brainstorm different ways to address the antecedents and be mindful of the types of strategies (health education, communication, policy, engineering, or community mobilization) that work best with select antecedents. In the Smarter Lunchrooms model, minigrant resources were added later to address schools' needs for intervention items such as signage, coolers, and baskets. Schools could apply for funding to purchase items identified in their action plans. Similarly, as the program grew and community members provided input, the list of specific types of awareness activities grew to include cooking classes and onsite presentations.

Building Action Plans

After the program framework is complete (theoretical framework, activity boxes with targeted strategies), action plans develop and outline a content progression within the strategies. Action plans are similar to lesson plans in a classroom. A curriculum is typically shown in a block plan, but lessons plans contain the smaller details of a daily plan. It is the plan from which a teacher or facilitator can implement the strategy. Action plans are much more detailed than the blocks identified in outcome logic models. Action plans are organized as a handful of short-term objectives. They include the materials and procedures for reaching those objectives. Well thought out and clearly written action plans are an essential part of the program planning process.

Creating local health promotion programs is the topic of many textbooks and courses. The purpose of the previous section was to introduce the topic and demonstrate how planning health promotion activities is based on theoretical frameworks and is carried out through a systematic process that is illustrated in an outcome logic model. Additional programming planning resources are available. The next chapter is a community case study on infant mortality. It illustrates the process of assessing community need and adopting and modifying evidence-based programs that align to clear behavioral objectives.

SUMMARY

Individuals must be motivated to act, be able to act, and be reinforced and reminded to act. To address the various factors related to motivation, abilities, and reinforcements, multicomponent programs are needed. Multicomponent programs consist of a combination of strategies from across five categories of health promotion interventions: health education, health communication, health engineering, health policy, and community mobilization. Programs should be based on evidence, meaning that there is documentation of effectiveness. Interventions that address socioeconomic factors and contextual factors have a wider impact on population health.

BEHAVIORAL SCIENCE IN ACTION

Engineering Choice in the School Cafeteria

New school meal guidelines described in the opening section of this chapter changed the types of foods offered via the National School Lunch Program. Policy alone, though, is unlikely to change children's eating behaviors. Using environmental strategies and paying attention to how and where foods are positioned in the cafeteria work synergistically with the policy changes to alter student consumption of targeted food items. Research has documented that the impact of environmental nudging can be significant. In one study, moving a food item to the front of the entree line increased purchases by 11% (Wansink & Just, 2011). Renaming vegetables using descriptive terms increased selection of the vegetable by 16%, and relocating healthy beverage options to eye level changed a quarter of the beverage sales (Thorndike et al., 2012; Wansink et al., 2012).

Choice engineering maintains personal choice but "nudges" individuals to make healthy choices. The power of environmental strategies is that they are simple, sustainable, and nonintrusive to the individual. The environment is altered, and thus intervention effort is not required daily. A labeling system is adopted, a display area is reconfigured, or a price is adjusted. Furthermore, the strategies reach the *population* served, which is a greater reach than through education or counseling-type interventions. Choice architecture in a cafeteria tends to fall into two broad categories: setup and food presentation.

Setup

The manner in which a cafeteria and food service line is set up is functional, but the method in which items are placed and offered also influences food selection. Location, convenience, and the type of choices can alter which foods students select.

Location: Moving an entree to the front of a service area and placing low-fat (1%) milk in the front of a cooler or at eye level increase consumption of that food. Conversely, moving sugar-sweetened beverages and snacks to less convenient locations, such as top shelves or behind a counter, can decrease consumption of the higher-calorie choices. The ideal placement of food for influencing choice appears to be first or at the front of the line. Moving items into the path of the line also dramatically increased selection. For example, moving a salad bar into the main flow of the line has doubled and tripled selection and consumption of vegetables off the salad bar. In two separate case studies, a salad bar was moved just 2 feet, and use increased by greater than 250% (Smith, Just, & Wansink, 2010) and 650% (Orlowski, Narayan, & Spears, 2014a).

Default choice: Default options are what the chooser will receive if he or she does nothing. The default option is the option that requires the least effort (Thaler & Sunstein, 2008). Common defaults are

French fries with a children's meal and an automated magazine renewal. In a cafeteria setting, food selections remain the same, but the default item is chosen and consumed at much higher frequencies. Adding a healthier food option as the default increases consumption of the healthier option. For example, placing low-fat salad dressing in the dispensers on the salad bar increases use of those salad dressings and decreases calorie consumption. Selections of salad dressing remain the same, but what is offered as the default is chosen and consumed at much higher frequencies. Individuals still may choose the regular salad dressing, but that option is provided in packets found at a different location.

Convenience: The more convenient an item is, the more likely it is to be chosen. Location and default choices increase convenience. Additional convenience strategies include quick service lines for healthy options, placing fruit in multiple locations, and providing preorder/prepay options (Just et al., 2008). Placing fruit in multiple serving locations in the cafeteria doubles fruit sales (Wansink, 2011).

Presentation

Presenting a food involves appealing to all senses and enhancing taste expectations. How a food looks, smells, and is described establishes a taste expectation. The expectation then influences the actual experience. Enhancing taste expectations for fruits, vegetables, and unfamiliar foods is particularly important for altering school lunch food choice.

Packaging: How a food is packaged and the service tray that it is presented in are part of the visual "taste" of the food. A clear, interesting-shaped container, a shiny fruit bowl, a colored service tray, lighting of the item, and use of stickers all are part of the visual presentation of the food item.

Naming: The use of appealing names draws attention to the food item and raises taste expectations. Super-charged carrots or Spiderman spinach salad are names associated with increased food consumption (Thapa & Lyford, 2014).

Labeling: Easy to understand labeling systems have also been associated with changes in food choice. Two popular labeling systems, Red/Yellow/Green and Slow/Whoa/Go, make healthier choice easier to identify (Levy et al., 2012; Thorndike et al., 2012; Thorndike, Sonnenberg & Levy, 2014). Red items are high in calories and fat and should be chosen infrequently. Green items are low in calories and fat and should be chosen more frequently. Yellow items are less nutritious than green items and can be chosen occasionally. In a worksite cafeteria after a labeling system started, the sale of green items increased by from 41% to 46% of sales, and red item sales decreased from 24% to 20% (Thorndike et al., 2014).

Suggestive selling: The use of prompts and encouragement increases the likelihood of a person trying a food. Prompts can be endorsements such as a teacher saying, "I tried it earlier, and it was so crunchy!" or a food service worker smiling and saying, "Would you like to try it? I made it myself."

Smarter Lunchrooms is a national school-based initiative that aims to improve the consumption of healthier school lunch items through the use of subtle, easy to sustain environmental changes. The smarter lunchrooms movement was initiated at the Cornell Center for Behavioral Economics for Child Nutrition Programs at Cornell University. Visit www.smarterlunchrooms.org to watch a video of smarter environmental strategies in action.

IN THE CLASSROOM ACTIVITIES

1) Nutrition and healthy eating are content areas. Create a list of five specific forms of nutrition-type health behaviors. Discuss how strategies could vary across the categories of interventions by the specific form of the behavior.

2) Go to the Become an EX website. Review the materials in the three activity blocks: relearn habit, relearn addiction, and relearn support. Match intervention strategies to specific antecedent targets. List the targets by categories on the PER worksheet.

3) Go to the Community Guide website and review the evidence-based strategies for one topic area.

Share and compare the strategies with another student.

4) Practices described in this chapter's Behavioral Science in Action feature are used regularly in the retail food industry. Study the produce section of a local grocery store and create a list of environmental cues and product nudges.

5) Brainstorm how health communication and community mobilization strategies could be used to support food selection in school cafeterias. What types of antecedents could be targeted by each strategy?

WEB LINKS

Act against AIDS: http://www.cdc.gov/actagainstaids/

Become an EX Smoking Cessation Program: http://www.becomeanEx.org

The Community Guide: http://www.thecommunityguide.org

U.S. Department of Agriculture, National School Lunch Program: http://www.fns.usda.gov/nslp/national-school-lunch-program-nslp

REFERENCES

American Legacy Foundation. (2012). *EX: Re-learn life without cigarettes.* Retrieved from http://www.becomeanex.org

Andreasen, A. R. (1995). *Marketing social change: Changing behavior to promote health, social development, and the environment.* San Francisco: Jossey-Bass.

Association of State and Territorial Directors of Health Promotion and Public Health Education & Centers for Disease Control and Prevention (CDC). (2001). Policy and environmental change: New directions for public health. Atlanta: Centers for Disease Control and Prevention.

Biener, L., Hamilton, W. L., Siegel, M., & Sullivan, E. M. (2010). Individual, social-normative, and policy predictors of smoking cessation: A multilevel longitudinal analysis. *American Journal of Public Health, 100*(3), 547–554.

Brownson, R. C., Fielding, J. E., & Maylahn, C. M. (2009). Evidence-based public health: A fundamental concept for public health practice. *Annual Review of Public Health, 30,* 175–201.

Centers for Disease Control and Prevention (CDC). (n.d.a.). *Community health worker training materials for cholera prevention and control.* Retrieved from http://www.cdc.gov/cholera/materials.html

Centers for Disease Control and Prevention (CDC). (n.d.b.). *Components of coordinated school health.* Retrieved from http://www.cdc.gov/healthyyouth/cshp/components.htm

Centers for Disease Control and Prevention (CDC). (n.d.c.). *Gateway to health communication & social marketing practice.* Retrieved from http://www.cdc.gov/healthcommunication/index.html

Centers for Disease Control and Prevention (CDC), Division of Adolescent and School Health (DASH). (2011). *Characteristics of effective health education.* Retrieved from http://www.cdc.gov/HealthyYouth/SHER/characteristics/index.htm

Cheng, H., Kotler, P., & Lee, N. R. (2011). *Social marketing in public health: Global trends and success stories.* Sudbury, MA: Jones and Bartlett.

Community Preventive Services Task Force. (2005). Tobacco. In S. Zaza, P. A. Briss, & K. W. Harris (Eds.), *The guide to community preventive services: What works to promote health?* (pp. 3–79) New York: Oxford University Press.

Community Preventive Services Task Force. (2012). Updated recommendations for client- and provider-oriented interventions to increase breast, cervical, and colorectal cancer screening. *American Journal of Preventive Medicine, 43*(1), 760–764.

Emmons, K. M., & Rollnick, S. (2001). Motivational interviewing in health care settings: Opportunities and limitations. *American Journal of Preventive Medicine, 20*(1), 68–74.

Fernandez, M. E., Gonzales, A., Tortolero-Luna, G., Williams, J., Saavedra-Embesi, M., Chan, W., & Vernon, S. W. (2009). Effectiveness of *Cultivando la salud*: A breast and cervical cancer screening promotion program for low-income Hispanic women. *American Journal of Public Health, 99*(5), 936–943.

Frieden, T. R. (2010). A framework for public health action: The health impact pyramid. *American Journal of Public Health, 100*(4), 590–595.

Gilbert, G. G., Sawyer, R. G., & McNeil, E. B. (2011). *Health education: Creating strategies for school & community health.* Sudbury, MA: Jones and Bartlett.

Global Health Workforce Alliance, World Health Organization (WHO). (2010). *Global experience of community health workers for delivery of health related millennium development goals: A systematic review, country case studies, and recommendations for integration into national health systems.* Geneva, Switzerland: World Health Organization.

Green, L.W., & Kreuter, M. W. (2005). *Health promotion planning: An educational and ecological approach* (4th ed.). Boston: McGraw Hill.

Heckman, C. J., Egleston, B. L., & Hofmann, M. T. (2010). Efficacy of motivational interviewing for smoking cessation: A systematic review and meta-analysis. *Tobacco Control, 19*(5), 410–416.

Hinman, A. R., Orenstein, W. A., & Schuchat, A. (2011). Vaccine-preventable diseases, immunizations, and *MMWR, 1961–2011. Morbidity and Mortality Weekly, 60*(Suppl.), 49–57.

Joint Committee on Health Education and Promotion Terminology. (2001). Report of the 2000 Joint Committee on Health Education and Promotion Terminology. *American Journal of Health Education, 32*(2), 89–103.

Joint Committee on National Health Education Standards. (2007). *National health education standards: Achieving excellence* (2nd ed.). Atlanta: American Cancer Society.

Just, D. R., Wansink, B., Mancino, L., & Guthrie, J. (2008). *Behavioral economic concepts to encourage healthy eating in school cafeterias* (Economic Research Report, No. ERR-68). Washington, DC: U.S. Department of Agriculture, Economic Research Service.

Kash, B., May, M. L., & Tai-Seale, M. (2007). Community health workers training and certification programs in United States: Findings from a national survey. *Health Policy, 80*(1), 32–42.

Kerr, N. A., Yore, M. M., Ham, S. A., & Dietz, W. H. (2004). Increasing stair use in a worksite through environmental changes. *American Journal of Health Promotion, 18*(4), 312–315.

Lai, D. T., Cahill, K., Qin, Y., & Tang, J. L. (2010). Motivational interviewing for smoking cessation. Cochrane Collaboration. Retrieved from http://www.thecochranelibrary.com

Levy, D. E., Riis, J., Sonnenberg, L. M., Barraclough, S. J., & Thorndike, A. N. (2012). Food choices of minority and low-income employees: A cafeteria intervention. *American Journal of Preventive Medicine, 43*(3), 240–248.

McKenzie, J. F., Neiger, B. L., & Thackeray, R. (2009). *Planning, implementing, and evaluating health promotion programs: A primer* (5th ed.). San Francisco: Pearson.

Meissner, H. I., Breen, N., Taubman, M. I., Vernon, S. W., & Graubard, B. I. (2006). Which women aren't getting mammograms and why? (United States). *Cancer Causes Control, 18*, 61–70.

Merzel, C., & D'Afflitti, J. (2003). Reconsidering community-based health promotion: Promise, performance and potential. *American Journal of Public Health, 93*(4), 557–574.

National Cancer Institute (NCI). (2001). *Five A Day For Better Health program: Monograph.* Bethesda, MD: National Institutes of Health, National Cancer Institute.

National Cancer Institute. (2006). *Using what works: Adapting evidence-based programs to fit your needs.* Bethesda, MD: U.S. Department of Health and Human Services, National Institutes of Health, National Cancer Institute.

National Cancer Institute (NCI). (2007). *Designing print materials: A communications guide for breast cancer screening.* Bethesda, MD: U.S. Department of Health and Human Services, National Institutes of Health, National Cancer Institute.

National Cancer Institute (NCI). (2008). *Pink book: Making health communication work* (2nd ed.). Bethesda, MD: U.S. Department of Health and Human Services, National Institutes of Health, National Cancer Institute. Retrieved from http://www.cancer.gov/pinkbook/

National Committee on Health Education Standards. (2007). *National health education standards: Achieving excellence* (2nd ed.) Atlanta: American Cancer Society.

National Conference of State Legislatures. (2011). *Immunizations policy issues overview*. Retrieved from http://www.ncsl.org/issues-research/health/immunizations-policy-issues-overview.aspx

National Institute of Alcohol Abuse and Alcoholism (NIAAA). (2005). *Alcohol alert: Brief interventions* (No. 66). Bethesda, MD: U.S. Department of Health and Human Services, National Institutes of Health. Retrieved from http://www.niaaa.nih.gov

Norris, S. L., Chowdhury, F. M., Van Le, K., Horsley, T., Brownstein, J. N., Zhang, X., . . . Satterfield, D. W. (2006). Effectiveness of community health workers in care of persons with diabetes. *Diabetic Medicine, 23*(5), 544–556.

Orlowski, M., Narayan, R., & Spears, B. (2014a). *Salad bar relocation increases vegetable consumption: Smarter Lunchrooms; Ohio success story* (program report). Columbus: Ohio Department of Education.

Orlowski, M., Narayan, R., & Spears, B. (2014b). *Smarter Lunchrooms: Ohio project evaluation, 2012–2014* (program report). Columbus: Ohio Department of Education.

Pedestrian and Bicycle Information Center. (2007). *Safe Routes to School guide*. Retrieved from http://saferoutesinfo.org/

Puddy, R. W., & Wilkins, N. (2011). Understanding evidence, part 1: Best available research evidence. In *A Guide to the Continuum of Evidence of Effectiveness*. Atlanta: Centers for Disease Control and Prevention.

Randolph, W., & Viswanath, K. (2004). Lessons learned from public health mass media campaigns: Marketing health in a crowded media world. *Annual Review of Public Health, 25*, 419–437.

Ranney, L., Melvin, C., Lux, L., McClain, E., Morgan, L., & Lohr, K. (2006). *Tobacco use: prevention, cessation, and control* (Evidence Report/Technology Assessment No. 140, AHRQ Publication No. 06–E015). Rockville, MD: Agency for Healthcare Research and Quality.

Robert Wood Johnson Foundation (RWJF). (2011). *Vulnerability 2030*. Retrieved from http://www.rwjf.org

Rollnick, S, Miller, W. R., & Butler, C. C. (2007). *Motivational interviewing in health care: Helping patients change behavior*. New York: Guildford.

Rubak, S., Sandbaek, A., Lauritzen, T., & Christensen, B. (2005). Motivational interviewing: A systematic review and meta-analysis. *British Journal of General Practice, 55*(513), 305–312.

Sabatino, S. A., Lawrence, B., Elder, R., Mercer, S. L., Wilson, K. M., DeVinney, B., . . . Glanz, K. (2012). Effectiveness of interventions to increase screening for breast, cervical, and colorectal cancers: Nine updated systematic reviews for the Guide to Community Preventive Services. *American Journal of Preventive Medicine, 43*(1), 765–786.

Shults, R. A., Elder, R. W., Nichols, J. L., Sleet, D. A., Compton, R., & Chattopadhyay, S. K. (2009). Effectiveness of multicomponent programs with community mobilization for reducing alcohol-impaired driving. *American Journal of Preventive Medicine, 37*(4), 360–371.

Smith, L. E., Just, D. R., & Wansink, B. (2010). Convenience drives choice in school lunch rooms: A salad bar success story. Paper presented at the Experimental Biology 2010 Annual Meeting, Anaheim, California. Abstract retrieved from http://www.fasebj.org

Story, M., Kaphingst, K. M., Robinson-O'Brien, R., & Glanz, K. (2008). Creating healthy food and eating environments: Policy and environmental approaches. *Annual Review of Public Health, 29,* 253–272.

Thaler, R., & Sunstein, C. (2008). *Nudge: Improving decisions about health, wealth and happiness.* New Haven, CT: Yale University Press.

Thapa, J. R., & Lyford, C. P. (2014). Behavioral economics in the school lunchroom: Can it affect food supplier decisions? A systematic review. *International Food and Agribusiness Management Review, 17*(A), 187–208.

Thorndike, A. N., Sonnenberg, L. M, Riis, J., Barraclough, S., & Levy, D. E. (2012). A 2-phase labeling and choice architecture intervention to improve healthy food and beverage choices. *American Journal of Public Health, 102*(3), 527–533.

Thorndike, A. N., Sonnenberg, L., & Levy, D. E. (2014). Traffic-light labels and choice architecture: Promoting healthy food choices. *American Journal of Preventive Medicine, 46*(2), 143–149.

U.S. Department of Agriculture (USDA). (2011). *Choose MyPlate.* Retrieved from http://www.choosemyplate.gov

U.S. Department of Agriculture (USDA), U.S. Department of Health and Human Services (USDHHS). (2010). *Dietary guidelines for Americans, 2010* (7th ed.). Washington, DC: U.S. Government Printing Office.

U.S. Department of Health and Human Services (USDHHS). (2000). *Reducing tobacco use: A report of the surgeon general.* Atlanta: U.S. Department of Health and Human Services, Centers for Disease Control and Prevention, National Center for Chronic Disease Prevention and Health Promotion, Office on Smoking and Health.

U.S. Department of Health and Human Services (USDHHS), Health Resources and Services Administration, Bureau of Health Professions. (2007). *Community Health Workers National Workforce Study.* U.S. Department of Health and Human Services. Retrieved from http://bhpr.hrsa.gov/healthworkforce/reports/chwstudy2007.pdf

U.S. Department of Health and Human Services (USDHHS), Centers for Disease Control and Prevention (CDC). (2011). *Childcare and school vaccination requirements.* Retrieved from http://www2a.cdc.gov/nip/schoolsurv/schImmRqmt.asp

U.S. Department of Health and Human Services (USDHHS), Centers for Disease Control and Prevention (CDC). (2012). *Act against AIDS: Second year-end report, April 2010–March 2011.* Retrieved from http://www.cdc.gov/actagainstaids/

U.S. Preventive Services Task Force (USPSTF). (2008). *Grade definitions.* Retrieved from http://www.uspreventiveservicestaskforce.org/uspstf/grades.htm

Victor, R. G., Ravenell, J. E., Freeman, A., Leonard, D., Bhat, D. G., Shafig, M., . . . Haley, R. W. (2010). Effectiveness of a barber-based intervention for improving hypertension control in black men. *Archives of Internal Medicine, 171*(4), 342–350.

Villanti, A. C., McKay, H. S., Abrams, D. B., Holtgrave, D. R., & Bowie, J. V. (2010). Smoking cessation interventions for U.S. young adults: A systematic review. *American Journal of Preventive Medicine, 39*(6), 564–574.

Viswanathan, M., Kraschnewski, J., Nishikawa, B., Morgan, L. C., Thieda, P., Honeycutt, A., . . . Jonas, D. (2009). *Outcomes of community health worker interventions* (Evidence Report/Technology Assessment No. 181). Retrieved from http://www.ahrq.gov/downloads/pub/evidence/pdf/comhealthwork/comhwork.pdf

Wansink, B. (2011). Move the fruit: Putting fruit in new bowls and new places doubles lunchroom sales. *Journal of Nutrition Education & Behavior, 43*(4 Supple 1), 1.

Wansink, B., & Just, D. R. (2011). Healthy foods first: Students take the first lunchroom food 11% more often than the third. *Journal of Nutrition Education & Behavior, 43*(4 Supple 1), 8.

Wansink, B., Just, D. R., Payne, C. R., & Klinger, M. Z. (2012). Attractive names sustain increased vegetable intake in schools. *Preventive Medicine, 55*, 330–332.

World Health Organization (WHO). (January 2007). *Community health workers: What do we know about them? The state of evidence of programmes, activities, costs and impact on health outcomes of using community health workers* (Policy Brief). Geneva, Switzerland: Author.

CHAPTER 11

Infant Mortality in Montgomery County, Ohio: A Case Study

KEY TERMS

allostasis	infant mortality	preterm birth
allostatic load	life course perspective	progesterone
CenteringPregnancy®	life expectancy	sudden infant death syndrome (SIDS)

LEARNING OBJECTIVES

1. List five established causes of infant mortality.
2. Discuss behaviors that significantly impact population-level infant mortality.
3. Identify traits and conditions of the social environment associated with birth outcomes.
4. Locate local infant mortality rates and sources of behavioral, social, and geographical factors of influence.
5. Discuss aspects of a life course perspective to improving birth outcomes and how this may differ from traditional health promotion programs.
6. Classify infant death, birth outcomes, and influential factors into correct levels of the disease prevention model.
7. Explain the behavioral assumptions, aligned activities, and anticipated outcomes in an established health promotion program.

Introduction

Life expectancy and infant mortality are the two most commonly used community health status indicators. Both indicators are used as a proxy measure for the overall health of the population being measured. **Infant mortality** (IM) is the death of a child less than 1 year of age. Infant mortality is an important indicator for a community because it measures the health and well-being of both children and mothers, as well as the overall health of the community. High infant mortality rates are associated with social determinants of health and biological causes. Some social determinants of health that impact infant mortality include high rates of poverty; substandard housing; illiteracy; and exposure to alcohol, illicit drugs, or pollutants such as cigarette smoke, paint, lead, and asbestos. Biological causes include congenital malformations, preterm birth, sudden infant death syndrome (SIDS), maternal complications, maternal substance abuse, and maternal age. IM also reflects the accessibility and quality of primary health care and the availability of supportive services in the community.

Like life expectancy, infant mortality indicators are used to make community comparisons at the international, country, regional, and local levels. The United States and other countries use infant mortality rates to compare the health of their country to peer countries. Similarly, states, counties, and cities compare their infant mortality rates to those of their peers. Businesses that are relocating or starting up will often use infant mortality and life expectancy to gauge the health of the community in which they are thinking of locating. A high infant mortality rate could indicate higher health insurance costs for a community.

This chapter discusses how one public health community assessed and designed evidence-based behavioral strategies to improve high rates of infant deaths.

Infant Mortality

Infant mortality is measured by the infant mortality rate (IMR), defined as the number of deaths in children less than 1 year of age per 1000 live births in the same year (Blaxter, 1981) (Figure 11-1). The IMR can be useful for comparing the health status of a population over time or different populations at a single point in time. Figure 11-2 is a good example of infant mortality data that initiated action for a population.

$$\text{Infant Mortality Rate} = \frac{\text{\# of deaths of children} < 1 \text{year of age in a specific year}}{\text{\# of live births in the same year}}$$

Figure 11-1 Infant Mortality Rate Calculation

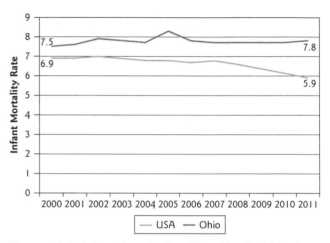

Figure 11-2 Infant Mortality Rate Trend for the United States and Ohio

This figure depicts the IMRs from 2000 to 2011 for the United States and Ohio. One can see from the figure that while the United States and Ohio had similar IMRs in 2000 (Ohio was approximately 9% worse), the U.S. IMR had improved by 2011, while Ohio's IMR was slightly worse. Ohio's 2011 IMR went from 9% worse to 32% worse than the United States' rate. These data initiated discussion about what was happening, or not happening, in Ohio that was causing the state's IMR to stagnate while the rest of the country was improving. The Ohio Infant Mortality Task Force was initiated based on the lack of improvements in IMR.

Disparity

Infant mortality rates also vary by population subgroups. In the United States, black infant mortality rates are more than twice as high as non-Hispanic white rates (see Table 11-1). Racial disparity in infant deaths cannot be explained by differences in socioeconomic status. For example, black mothers with college degrees or higher face similar risk of infant mortality as white women who have not finished high school (Loggins & Andrade, 2014). Biological differences and

TABLE 11-1 Infant Mortality Rates by Race: United States, 2010

Race	Infant Mortality Rate
Non-Hispanic White	5.1
Black or African American	11.6
American Indian	7.6
Asian or Pacific Islander	3.6
Hispanic or Latino	5.5
Total	6.1

Source: Centers for Disease Control and Prevention, National Center for Health Statistics.

genetics also do not account for the observed racial and ethnic differences in infant mortality. Researchers who have reviewed epidemiological patterns in infant mortality do not find support for the idea of biology or genetics as the driving force in observed differences. Instead, the patterns of racial disparity in mortality, and changing prematurity rates for infants from African immigrant populations, point to social explanations (David & Collins, 2007).

Actual Causes of Infant Death

For every 1000 babies that are born in the United States, approximately six die during their first year of life. Over half of these babies (57%) die due to one of five major causes (Hoyert & Xu, 2012). The top cause of infant deaths (21%) is congenital malformations, commonly known as birth defects (Figure 11-3). There are many types of birth defects, which vary greatly in severity. An example of a less severe birth defect is polydactyly, which occurs when a baby is born with additional fingers or toes that can be removed surgically. An example of a severe birth defect is Down syndrome, which is a genetic mutation of chromosome 21. Some birth defects can be prevented, while others cannot. Spina bifida, a major birth defect of the spine, is an example of a preventable birth defect. If a woman has enough folic acid (a B vitamin) in her body at least 1 month *before* and also *during* pregnancy, it can help prevent the disorder (CDC, 2004). Birth defects that are not preventable include genetic birth defects such as heart defects, Down syndrome, and blood disorders.

The second leading cause of infant deaths (17%) is preterm birth (Hoyert & Xu, 2012). **Preterm birth** is defined as a birth less than 37 weeks gestation. U.S. infants' chances of surviving through the first year of life are closely associated with preterm birth rates. Full-term birth is considered to occur

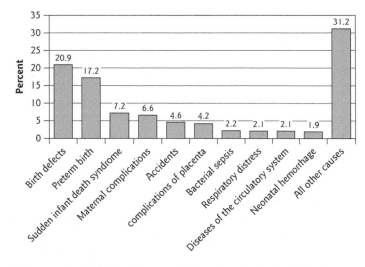

Figure 11-3 Leading Causes of Infant Deaths in the United States, 2011

from 37 to 41 weeks, though there has been more recently an emphasis on 39 weeks as a minimum full term. For population changes in infant mortality to occur, decreases in the number of premature births must also occur. Preterm birth is a key reason the U.S. infant mortality rate is so much higher than other industrialized countries. Maternal and child health researchers examined infant mortality data from industrialized nations and adjusted the data to take into account differences in the way infant mortality is defined. When the United States is compared to other industrialized nations' adjusted data, premature birth stands out as a key factor in the U.S. lag to improve infant mortality (MacDorman & Mathews, 2009; Williams, 2013).

Sudden infant death syndrome (SIDS) is the third leading cause of death (7.2%). SIDS is defined as the sudden death of an infant less than 1 year of age that cannot be explained after a thorough investigation is conducted, including a complete autopsy, examination of the death scene, and review of the clinical history. The good news is that the overall rate of SIDS in the United States has declined by more than 50% since 1990 (Shapiro-Mendoza et al., 2006). However, disparities in SIDS remain disproportionately high for non-Hispanic black and American Indian/Alaska Native infants (MacDorman & Matthews, 2011). Reducing infant deaths due to SIDS remains an important public health priority.

The fourth leading cause of infant deaths is maternal complications of pregnancy (6.6%). Complications of pregnancy are health problems that occur during pregnancy. These may include the mother's health, the baby's health, or both. Some women have health problems that begin during pregnancy, and other women have health problems before they become pregnant that could lead to problems during pregnancy. Thus, it is vital for women to receive health care both before and during pregnancy in order to decrease the risk of complications during pregnancy.

Accidents are the fifth leading cause of infant death (4.6%). Accidental deaths are often predictable and preventable. The top five causes of accidental infant deaths are suffocation (77%), motor vehicle crashes (8%), drowning (4%), fire/burns (2%), and poisoning (2%) (Murphy, Xu, & Kochanek, 2013). Suffocation accounts for more than three-quarters of all accidental infant deaths, and the majority of these suffocations happen while the infants are in unsafe sleeping environments. Unsafe bedding, furniture, a toy, or the body of another sleeper can lead to suffocation.

Infant Mortality Risk and Protective Factors

Risk factors and protective factors for infant mortality can be varied in origin. Risks associated with preterm birth are often a special focus due to the opportunities for prevention of prematurity as a leading cause of infant mortality. When examining the risks associated with preterm birth, the three main risk categories are medical, behavioral, and social (see Figure 11-4).

Medical and Biological Risk Factors

Medical risk factors impacting preterm birth include infections during pregnancy, having a previous preterm birth, being pregnant with more than one baby, and having high blood pressure or diabetes. In addition to impacting preterm birth, some overall infant mortality risk factors also have to do with biological factors. These factors include serious birth defects such as congenital malformations, deformations, and chromosomal abnormalities.

Behavioral Risk Factors

Behavioral factors, including lifestyle and health care, can impact preterm birth and infant mortality. One of the most important behavioral factors related to infant mortality is a woman's overall health status. Good preconception health care means living a safe, healthy lifestyle and managing any current health conditions before getting pregnant. Smoking tobacco, both during pregnancy and after childbirth, is a risk factor. Smoking during pregnancy increases the risk of a baby being born too early. Smoking during pregnancy also contributes to low birth weight. Both of these are serious risk factors for infant death. Smoking during and after pregnancy is a risk factor for SIDS. Alcohol use during pregnancy contributes to certain birth defects and fetal alcohol spectrum disorders. Receiving late prenatal care (starting after the second trimester) or no prenatal care contributes to the risk of having a baby with health problems. Receiving no prenatal care also increases the risk of low birth weight and infant mortality (USDHHS, n.d.).

Women of childbearing age can lower their risk of poor birth outcomes by adopting recommended healthy behaviors. Taking folic acid supplements before and during pregnancy helps to prevent major defects in the baby's spine and brain. Maintaining a healthy weight is important, as women who are overweight or obese are at higher risk for complications during pregnancy. Engaging in regular physical activity is another

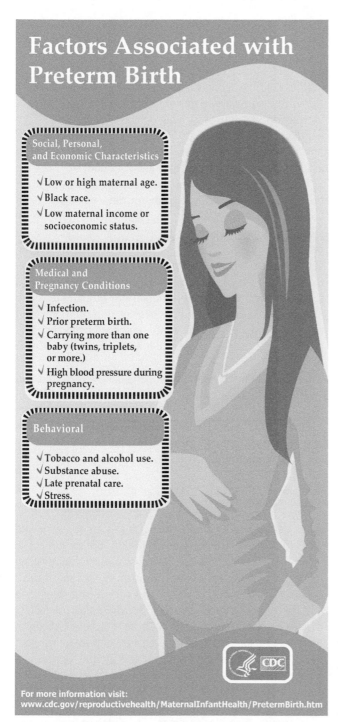

Factors Associated with Preterm Birth

Social, Personal, and Economic Characteristics

√ Low or high maternal age.
√ Black race.
√ Low maternal income or socioeconomic status.

Medical and Pregnancy Conditions

√ Infection.
√ Prior preterm birth.
√ Carrying more than one baby (twins, triplets, or more.)
√ High blood pressure during pregnancy.

Behavioral

√ Tobacco and alcohol use.
√ Substance abuse.
√ Late prenatal care.
√ Stress.

CDC

For more information visit:
www.cdc.gov/reproductivehealth/MaternalInfantHealth/PretermBirth.htm

Figure 11-4 Preterm Birth Risk Factors

Source: Courtesy of Centers for Disease Control and Prevention.

healthy pregnancy behavior. Activities that are of moderate intensity, such as brisk walking, support heart and lung health during pregnancy.

After birth, breastfeeding is an important part of keeping babies healthy. Manufactured infant formula does not contain the immune system protective factors that human milk does. Feeding infant formula, rather than breastfeeding, contributes to increased infant mortality (Chen & Rogan, 2004). Injury prevention is also important for keeping babies safe and healthy during their first year of life. Protective measures include considering the safety of the home environment and the general safety of babies when not at home (e.g., car seats, seat belts, smoke alarms, taking CPR classes, safe sleeping, day care setting safety) (CDC, 2013).

Environmental Risk Factors

Though environmental exposure plays a part in health outcomes, including infant mortality, there are few well-understood environmental contributors to infant mortality at this time. More research is needed in this area (CDC, 2012).

Social Risk Factors

Pregnancy-related health outcomes are influenced by factors such as race, ethnicity, age, and income. Even when studies take into account well-established risk factors for preterm birth and infant mortality, there are still unexplained differences in infant mortality between different populations. For example, women receiving Medicaid are more likely to have a preterm birth. The same is true for women in lower income groups. Black women are more likely to have a preterm birth than white women. Blacks also experience a much higher rate of infant mortality than whites. This racial disparity holds true regardless of socioeconomic status. Social factors, sometimes referred to as the social environment, play an important part in infant mortality. The social factors most often associated with preterm birth include poverty and black race (CDC, 2012). When considering the impact of the larger social environment on infant mortality, the life course perspective, adopted by leading maternal and child health researchers, offers a particularly useful framework.

Life Course Perspective

The **life course perspective** describes a newer way of looking at maternal and child health, as an integrated continuum and not as disconnected stages unrelated to each other. This view is based on work in public health and the social sciences highlighting the influence that each stage of life has on the next stage. Emphasis is placed on the ways in which social, economic, and physical environments interact to strongly impact the health of individuals and the community (Fine & Kotelchuck, 2010; Lu & Halfon, 2003).

Instead of focusing on differences in health patterns for one disease or condition at a time, the life course perspective examines larger social, economic, and environmental factors as underlying causes of persistent inequalities in health for a wide range of diseases and conditions across population groups. The life course perspective focuses on populations versus individuals. Its foundation is in the social determinants and social equity models of health (Fine & Kotelchuck, 2010).

Key life course perspective concepts include time line, timing, environment, and equity. Time line refers to the idea that today's life experiences influence tomorrow's health. Timing is the idea that one's health can be affected differently during critical periods of life. Environment refers to a larger community environment, including biological, physical, and social aspects. The community environment has a strong impact on a person's ability to be healthy. Equity addresses health differences between groups with an approach that acknowledges that health inequality is about more than genetic makeup and personal choices (Fine & Kotelchuck, 2010).

When applied to infant mortality, the life course perspective expands the view farther than simply getting mothers good health care during pregnancy. So much focus has been on what happens during the 9 months of pregnancy that we overlook the many influences outside that time period that can influence birth outcomes. The life course perspective takes into account the pregnant woman's larger life experience, her full life course, and its impact on her health. Many factors over a woman's entire life course impact the ability to successfully carry a pregnancy through a full 40 weeks. These include overall health, chronic stress, access to safe housing, food or financial insecurity, and many other quality of life considerations. These are things that prenatal care cannot be expected to fix, and they need to be addressed much earlier than when a woman is already pregnant. The two key aspects of the life course view of infant mortality are early (or fetal) programming and cumulative pathways (Fine & Kotelchuck, 2010; Lu & Halfon, 2003).

Early programming relates to the concept that exposures and development very early in life, even when in one's mother's uterus, can impact the functioning of body systems in adulthood. This can result in a different health status, including the ability to successfully carry a pregnancy to full term. Cumulative pathways relates to understanding the difference between short-term stress, which our bodies are designed to handle, and chronic stress, which wears on our body systems over time. When presented with a major stressor, such as a surprise grizzly bear appearance, your body activates the fight-or-flight response. This produces high levels of stress hormones to help you fight harder or run away faster. After you get away from the bear, your body calms down, with stress hormones, heart rate, breathing, and blood pressure returning to normal. This self-regulation is called **allostasis**, and it allows our bodies to maintain stability through change. Conversely, if the grizzly bear never leaves, and you are always in danger, your body loses the ability to properly regulate. Stress response is activated but does not shut off. High levels of stress hormones maintained for prolonged periods of time produce what is called **allostatic load**, or weathering. Unlike being briefly stressed out, living with chronic stress wears on the body's ability to function properly. For women, this can lead to poor birth outcomes, including preterm birth. Types of chronic stress than can impact women's health include unsafe neighborhoods, violence in relationships, chronic under- or unemployment, homelessness, food insecurity, and poverty. For black women, the added impact of institutionalized racism as a part of daily life can explain racial differences in birth outcomes (Lu & Halfon, 2003; Lu et al., 2010).

Figure 11-5, from the work of Lu and Halfon (2003), illustrates lifetime reproductive potential separately for white and for black women. The arrows pushing upward are protective factors that raise reproductive potential. These include higher income, higher educational opportunity, optimal health behaviors, low maternal stress, and access to a safe living environment. The arrows pushing downward are risk factors that lower reproductive potential. These include lack of education, poverty, food insecurity, adverse childhood events, poor overall health, and chronic stress. The reproductive potential for whites reaches and maintains a higher level over the life course than that of blacks. White women have more protective factors (upward arrows) and fewer risk factors (downward arrows) than black women. The different levels of risk factors and protective factors illustrated over the life course

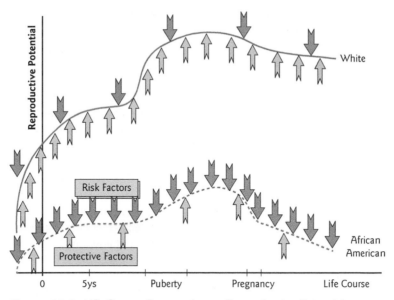

Figure II-5 Life Course Perspective on Reproductive Potential

Source: Springer and the original publisher / Maternal and Child Health Journal, Issue 1, volume 7, 2003 by Michael C. Lu, Figure 1. Lifecourse Perspective is given to the publication in which the material was originally published by adding with kind permission from Springer Science and Business Media.

contribute to racial disparities in birth outcomes. In the life course perspective, black women's lower reproductive potential, compared to that of white women, can be explained as a result of exposure to more risk factors and fewer protective factors across the life course. One of those risk factors particular to black women is institutionalized racism (Jones, 2000; Lu & Halfon, 2003; Lu et al., 2010). Interventions planned over the life course, such as risk reduction and health promotion strategies, might help close the black–white difference in reproductive potential.

> **Check for Understanding** Draw the disease prevention model for infant mortality. Fill in level one and level two of the model.

Infant Mortality in Montgomery County, Ohio

While the rest of the country has been celebrating a decrease in infant mortality, Ohio's IMR has not improved (MacDorman, Hoyert, & Mathews, 2013), and in some communities, including Montgomery County, the IMR has become even

worse over the past few years. The state of Ohio ranked 47th in infant mortality in 2010 and 49th in black infant mortality (Mathews & MacDorman, 2013; Murphy et al., 2013). Only the states of Mississippi (9.62), Alabama (8.73), and Tennessee (7.87) had a worse overall IMR than Ohio (7.73). For black infant mortality, only Indiana had a worse IMR at 14.96 versus 14.78 for Ohio. By contrast, Alaska had the best overall IMR of 3.57, and Minnesota had the best black IMR of 6.35; both have an IMR over 50% lower than the overall and black IMR of Ohio (Mathews & MacDorman, 2013).

Montgomery County is located in the mid-to-southwest region of Ohio, and it encompasses 464 square miles of rural, suburban, and mostly urban areas, with the city of Dayton located in the center. The population is 75% white and 21% black. In addition, 16.8% of the population is living in poverty (U.S. Census Bureau, 2014). This geographic area has a significant need for assistance due to a variety of economic, social, and institutional problems. These issues contribute to the increasing IMR in the community, particularly in the black community, where the IMR was 2.3 times higher for black babies versus white babies in 2012 (Ohio Department of Health, Office of Vital Statistics, 2012) (see Figure 11-6).

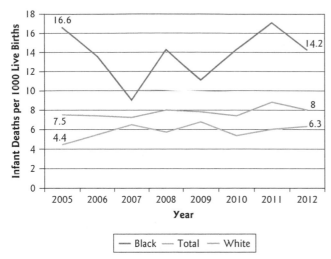

Figure 11-6 Infant Mortality by Race in Montgomery County, 2005–2012

Community Assessment

In April 2012, the Infant Mortality Coalition (IMC) was formed in Montgomery County. The community-wide coalition was spearheaded by representatives from Public Health–Dayton & Montgomery County (PHDMC) and the Greater Dayton Area Hospital Association. This combined effort is significant, as recent literature emphasizes the need for public health and medicine to work together in order to have the biggest impact on the community's health issues (IOM, 2012). Because infant mortality is a multifaceted issue, cooperative relationships throughout the community are needed to work together to decrease infant mortality. The initial IMC had 31 members from more than 25 agencies (see Table 11-2). Membership continued to grow throughout the first 2 years of the coalition. The organizations that are represented include state-mandated agencies, nonprofit organizations, faith-based organizations, community and parent representatives, volunteer leaders, representatives from funding sources, and experts in various fields that impact infant mortality (i.e., experts in infant mortality medical interventions and experts in specific topics, including breastfeeding and outcome evaluations).

For the first several months after the IMC was formed, the group worked diligently to conduct a thorough needs assessment, with the objective of using a data-driven process to select an evidence-based infant mortality reduction initiative. Because there are many factors that can impact IM, it was necessary to determine which populations are disproportionately affected. These populations could be defined by race, location, socioeconomic status, or specific risk factors. A variety of analytical tools were used for the needs assessment, including Geographical Information Services (GIS) mapping, vital statistics analysis, U.S. Census Bureau data, analysis of the Behavioral Risk Factor and Surveillance System (BRFSS) data, a Perinatal Periods of Risk (PPOR) analysis of Montgomery County, analysis of a local low birth weight registry, and an environmental scan. In addition to the needs assessment, a review of existing evidence-based infant mortality initiatives was conducted and discussed at IMC meetings.

> **Check for Understanding** List 10 agencies from your community that might be valuable participants in an infant mortality coalition.

Risk Factors and Birth Outcomes

Table 11-3 illustrates some of the analysis conducted with the birth certificate data from 2012. The analysis indicates that 14% of births in Montgomery County were preterm, with over 20% of black babies being born preterm. In addition, almost a quarter of all women had late or no prenatal care, and almost a third of black women had late or no prenatal care. Thirteen percent of pregnant women smoked throughout their pregnancy, and about 70% of women were breastfeeding at discharge from the hospital.

Behavioral Risk Factor Surveillance System data was analyzed to determine overall health and risk factors of the population. Table 11-4 provides a summary of a portion of the analysis. The analysis highlighted numerous disparities. Almost a quarter of the black population indicated they had fair or poor health, versus 16% of the white population. Rates of diabetes, high blood pressure, and the percent eating less than one fruit and vegetable serving per day were also higher for the black population. Also concerning is that about two-thirds of the population was overweight or obese, and over a quarter of the population reported not participating in any leisure time physical activity or exercise.

TABLE 11-2 Montgomery County Infant Mortality Coalition Membership

Agency	Representative	Roles and Responsibilities on the Team
1. Help Me Grow Brighter Futures	Director of Evidence-Based Birth Outcome program	Expertise in home care services
2. Health Ministry Program of Good Samaritan Hospital	Health Ministries program coordinator	Represents faith-based programs
3. Good Samaritan Hospital	United against Violence of Greater Dayton Initiative	Expertise on violence in the community
4. Five Rivers Women's Health Center	Nurse coordinator	Federally qualified health center expertise
5. Ohio Pediatrics	Pediatrician	Expertise in children with disabilities
6. Montgomery County Department of Job and Family Services	Director of Department of Job and Family Services	Administers Federal, State, and local Employment, Public Assistance, Medical Assistance, service & day care, and Support Enforcement programs
7. Public Health	Epidemiologist	Conducts data analysis
8. Wright State University	Research instructor, epidemiologist, and demographer	Breastfeeding expertise, data analyst
9. Community Health Centers of Greater Dayton	Practice manager at Victor Cassano Health Center	Federally qualified health care expertise
10. Haines Children's Center	Family Advocacy Intervention and Review coordinator	Advocacy expertise
11. Board of Developmental Disabilities	Parent and Child Enrichment (PACE) program nurse	Disability expertise
12. Public Health	Health Commissioner	Co-chair of IMC, environmental health expertise, policy maker
13. Public Health	Assistant to the health commissioner	Assists with running of IMC, policy maker
14. Public Health	Public health nurse supervisor, community outreach	Home health care expertise, nurse
15. CityMatCH	Public health project coordinator	National representative for CityMatCH
16. Greater Dayton Area Hospital Association	Director, Health Initiatives	Co-chair of IMC, hospital administration

continues

TABLE 11-2 **Montgomery County Infant Mortality Coalition Membership** *continued*

Agency	Representative	Roles and Responsibilities on the Team
17. Haines Children's Center	Adolescent Services supervisor	Adolescence expertise
18. Public Health	Ohio Infant Mortality Reduction Initiative director	Expertise in health inequities and minority health
19. Miami Valley Hospital	Obstetrics department chair	High-risk obstetrician
20. Parent representative	Has had an infant death in the family	Community perspective
21. Family and Children First Council	Program coordinator at Montgomery County Family and Children First Council	Safe sleep expertise
22. Alcohol, Drug Addiction, and Mental Health Services (ADAMHS) Board	Community Initiatives Division	Substance abuse expertise
23. Dayton Council on Health Equity	Community coordinator for Health Equity	Health inequities expertise
24. Public Health	Administrative secretary	Coordinates meetings, records minutes, distributes information among the group
25. Care Source	Vice president of Clinical Operations	Health care expertise
26. Bright Future Lactation Resource Center Ltd.	Breastfeeding consultant for the World Health Organization (WHO)	Breastfeeding expertise
27. University of Dayton	Family and Children First Council Research administrator	Policy expertise
28. Dayton Children's Medical Center	Neonatal nurse practitioner	Ohio Perinatal Quality Collaborative representative
29. Miami Valley Hospital	Perinatal clinical nurse specialist	Women's health expertise
30. Women, Infants, and Children (WIC)	Supervisor of WIC program	Nutrition, fetal alcohol spectrum disorders, and breastfeeding expertise
31. Parity, Inc.	Executive director	Expertise in health inequities in minority populations

TABLE 11-3 Birth Outcomes and Risk Factors of Pregnant Women in Montgomery County, 2012

	Total	White	Black
Preterm birth[a]	14.0%	11.5%	21.1%
Smoking during pregnancy[b]	13.1%	15.1%	10.1%
Late or no prenatal care[c]	24.2%	21.4%	32.1%
Breastfeeding at discharge[d]	72.5%	75.6%	61.2.%

[a]Less than 37 weeks gestation
[b]A woman who reported smoking any cigarettes during her third trimester was counted as smoking during her pregnancy
[c]Late or no prenatal care is defined as a woman receiving her first prenatal visit after the first trimester of pregnancy
[d]Breastfeeding at discharge is the percentage of women who are breastfeeding when they leave the hospital after giving birth
Data Source: Ohio Department of Health, Center for Public Health Statistics and Informatics
Data Analysis: Public Health–Dayton & Montgomery County, Office of Epidemiology

TABLE 11-4 Behavioral Risk Factor Surveillance System: Montgomery County, Ohio, 2011–2013

Risk Factor	White	Black
Fair or poor health status	16.4%	22.2%
Less than 1 fruit & vegetable serving per day[a]	40.1%	46.1%
No physical activity[a]	26.5%	32.2%
Obese or overweight	65.4%	70.8%
High blood pressure[a]	34.4%	44.9%
Ever diagnosed with diabetes	11.6%	13.9%

a) 2011 and 2013 data combined

Mapping

Mapping is an important community assessment tool used to identify places within a community that show disparities in outcomes. Several maps of Montgomery County were generated to identify infant mortality disparities in the community. The map of Montgomery County shown in Figure 11-7 identifies the infant mortality rates by zip codes for the combined years 2009–2011. IMR varies greatly depending on the zip code of residence. The IMR ranges from 0 in zip codes 45325, 45418, 45429, and 45440 to as high as 22.5 per 1000 live births in zip code 45426. The zip codes with the highest IMRs also had a high percentage of poverty and black population.

Additional maps on low birth weight, very low birth weight, preterm birth, race, smoking during pregnancy, prenatal care, poverty, and household income were created to assess where specific risk factors and outcomes were located within the county. Analysis of the additional maps revealed that the zip codes with the highest IMRs were also associated with high proportions of black population and poverty. This information was useful in identifying the areas in Montgomery County

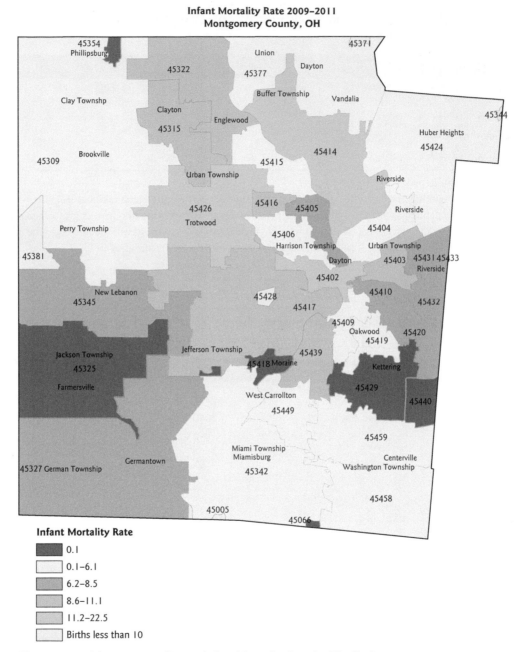

Figure 11-7 Montgomery County Infant Mortality Rate by Zip Code

to target with interventions, and additionally where the IMC needed to provide education to promote these interventions.

Target Population and Behavioral Focus

Based on Public Health–Dayton & Montgomery County's data analysis, it was clear that preterm births and the risk factors associated with them had the greatest impact on Montgomery County infant mortality (Tables 11-3 and 11-4). This meant that factors including the very poor health of the population (diabetes, obesity, and high blood pressure) and risk factors (e.g., smoking, not breastfeeding, no physical activity, and late prenatal care) were contributing to unhealthy pregnancies, preterm births, and thus a high IMR (Table 11-3). These risk factors and outcomes were especially poor within the black population. The IMC took these data into consideration to determine the area that would be targeted for infant mortality interventions.

After considering the data about infant mortality and preterm birth, the final step in the needs assessment was to identify the appropriate target population for interventions. The needs assessment clearly indicated that black babies were having worse outcomes for both infant mortality and preterm birth. Because many of the preterm birth issues were due to maternal health, black women of childbearing age were therefore chosen to be the focus of the selected interventions. With the focus on black mothers and infants, the maps that had been generated allowed the IMC to identify zip codes with higher IMR, preterm births, and a higher proportion of black population. After consideration of these three main maps, the target area became the zip codes in Montgomery County that had an IMR greater than 7.5 per 1000 live births (the average) and that had more than 100 black births for the years analyzed (see Figure 11-8).

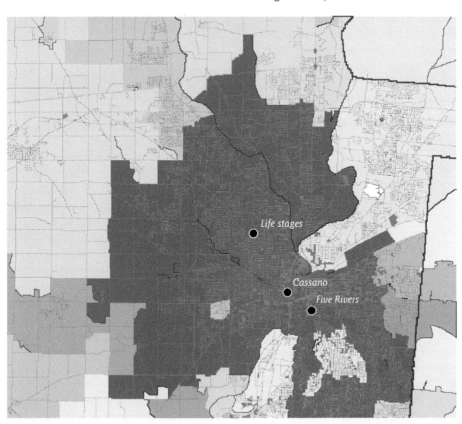

Figure 11-8 Montgomery County Infant Mortality Initiative Target Area, Clinical Partners Highlighted

Interventions to Improve Preterm Birth

In addition to conducting a needs assessment, the coalition applied to become a member of the new national Institute for Equity in Birth Outcomes (IEBO) that was formed by CityMatCH, a national maternal and child health organization focused on urban communities. The IEBO's focus was to decrease disparities in birth outcomes in urban areas. The IEBO accepted four teams from across the nation for their first cohort, and Montgomery County was one of those teams. The IEBO provided training and guidance in selecting appropriate evidence-based strategies and systems that would best address the community issues that were contributing to infant mortality. The IEBO also provided technical and evaluation support, which included designing evaluation plans that captured overall outcomes, such as preterm birth and infant mortality rates, as well as social and behavioral targets such as adherence to interventions, attending prenatal care, and stress. The IEBO also facilitated the connection of the coalition with other professionals to assist with interventions. These resources were often people who had already successfully implemented relevant interventions in their community. Finally, the IEBO provided momentum to the IMC to begin an infant mortality strategy in Montgomery County.

Table 11-5 shows types of evidence-based programs that were discussed at the first IEBO training. In addition to discussing what these strategies are, the estimated impact of implementing these initiatives in the community was given based on local community data. Team members were given time to discuss each intervention and how it might be implemented in the community.

After discussing the evidence-based strategies, a review of the systems in which evidence-based strategies worked the best was presented (see Table 11-6). Systems are the vehicle for implementing a program. For example, implementing universal progesterone to eligible pregnant women is a great evidence-based strategy to decrease preterm birth. However, to implement this program, communities need to have a system that can effectively implement this strategy. The facilitating system includes that of health care providers (particularly an obstetrics and gynecology care provider), public clinic support, reimbursement policy for the progesterone, and pregnant women seeking prenatal care. Another program from the list in Table 11-5 may require an entirely different system.

TABLE 11-5 Evidence-Based Programs to Improve Infant Mortality

Behavioral or Social Factor Target
Vaginal and oral progesterone universal screening
Safe sleep
Family planning
Maternal stress prevention and management
High-risk pregnancy and delivery management
Tobacco, alcohol, and other drug cessation
Breastfeeding and kangaroo mother care
Social factors of health equity
Policy and system change

Source: Adapted from Gilbert & Kasehagen, 2013a.

Dayton and Montgomery County Infant Mortality Reduction Initiatives

The Montgomery County Infant Mortality Coalition chose reduction of preterm birth as its primary focus. In part because it is a leading cause of infant mortality, preterm birth was also chosen due to the existing ability to improve it, as well as the racial inequity in preterm birth in the community. The Montgomery County goal is to reduce preterm births by 10%. One requirement of membership in the IEBO was the implementation of at least one downstream intervention to address infant mortality. Downstream factors addressing preterm birth impact women who are already pregnant and at risk for preterm birth. Risk factors include having had a prior preterm birth and being diagnosed with a short cervix during ultrasound. Although it was not required by the IEBO, Montgomery County added an upstream intervention as well in order to reach more pregnant women in the target area beyond those already at risk for preterm birth due to prior experience or diagnosis. The downstream and upstream interventions were chosen based on the community assessment data, community readiness for selected behavioral targets and strategies, and available evidence-based interventions.

TABLE 11-6 Systems for Moving Infant Mortality Programs to Practice

System	Brief Description
1. Medical home	A team-based health care delivery model led by a physician, physician's assistant, or nurse practitioner that provides comprehensive and continuous medical care to patients with the goal of obtaining maximized health outcomes.
2. Providers	An individual or an institution that provides preventive, curative, promotional, or rehabilitative health care services in a systematic way to individuals, families, or communities.
3. Hospitals/Baby-Friendly hospitals and birthing clinics	A health care institution providing patient treatment with specialized staff and equipment. Hospitals become designated as Baby-Friendly by implementing the Ten Steps to Successful Breastfeeding.
4. Title X/family planning clinics	A federal grant program that is completely devoted to providing comprehensive family planning and other related preventive health services to individuals. It is designed to prioritize the needs of individuals from low-income families and/or uninsured people who might not otherwise have access to these health care services.
5. CenteringPregnancy®	A model of group prenatal care that promotes individual health empowerment and community building.
6. Home visitation	Home visiting programs offer a variety of family-focused services to expectant parents and families with new babies and young children. They address issues such as maternal and child health, positive parenting practices, safe home environments, and access to services.
7. Case management	Maternity case management includes nurses, social workers, and other professionals trained to help pregnant women who have situations in their lives that could lead to problems with their pregnancies or childbirth.
8. Doula care	Trained and experienced professionals provide continuous physical, emotional, and informational support to mothers before, during, and just after birth
9. WIC	The Special Supplemental Nutrition Program for Women, Infants, and Children (WIC) is a federal assistance program for health care and nutrition of low-income pregnant women, breastfeeding women, and infants and children under the age of 5.

Source: Adapted from Gilbert & Kasehagen, 2013b.

The focus of the infant mortality interventions was to increase the number of deliveries that reach greater than 37 weeks. After this long-term objective was agreed upon, information about the available interventions (see Table 11-5) was shared with the coalition as a means to foster communication about community readiness and resources. Coalition members shared information about which interventions they supported and could provide resources for implementation. Selecting programs and behavioral targets that the community at large supported and felt confident in implementing was an important part of the project's planning phase. Imbedded in the intervention selection was also the identification of centralized locations for the program. Three prenatal clinic partners were identified (1) Community Health Centers of Greater Dayton (CHCGD): Victor Cassano Health Center; (2) Samaritan Centers for Women: Life Stages; and (3) Five Rivers Health Centers: Center for Women's Health.

Progesterone Therapy

Progesterone therapy was selected as the downstream intervention. **Progesterone** is a hormone that plays an important role in maintaining pregnancy. When given to appropriately screened pregnant women, progesterone therapy reduces the rate of recurrent preterm deliveries in women with a prior preterm birth. Progesterone therapy also reduces the rate of preterm births in women diagnosed with a short cervix at ultrasound (Likis et al., 2012). The behavioral target of the progesterone therapy intervention was to increase the percentage of pregnant women who adhere to the prescribed progesterone therapy. Once identified as eligible, treatment adherence involved weekly injections for the women with prior preterm birth or daily vaginal suppositories for women with a diagnosis of short cervix (see the Intermediate Outcomes in Figure 11-9).

Primary activities of the progesterone therapy intervention included screening and identifying at-risk pregnant women, prescribing and filling progesterone prescriptions, encouraging adherence with the treatment, and following up with the patient. Screening for progesterone eligibility was done via a standardized clinical algorithm. First, prior to 16 weeks of pregnancy, women were screened for having had a prior preterm birth. Next, around 20 weeks of pregnancy, women were screened during their ultrasound for a short cervix. Initiation of the treatment was an important behavioral milestone; the target behavior, though, was continuation and completion (adherence) of the therapy through the pregnancy. Factors associated with successful progesterone therapy implementation and maintenance included ease of prescription access; insurance coverage and other payment options, including Medicaid; keeping weekly appointments for injections; and maintaining scheduled home administration of vaginal suppositories.

Key outputs for the progesterone initiative included patient education and outreach materials that were finalized and distributed for recruitment, the number of participating health centers, the number of women who enrolled in prenatal care, and the number of pregnant women identified as candidates for treatment. The short-term outcomes measured the antecedents that influence motivation, ability, and support for adhering to progesterone therapy. The indicators that were deemed important and measurable included the number of eligible pregnant women initiating treatment, the number of ultrasounds performed, and levels of care management at the health care sites.

CenteringPregnancy®

The Dayton and Montgomery County upstream infant mortality intervention was CenteringPregnancy. **CenteringPregnancy** is a model of prenatal care that integrates the three care components of health assessment, education, and support within a group setting. Eight to 12 women with similar due dates meet regularly to learn care skills, participate in facilitated discussion, and develop a support network. CenteringPregnancy care starts around the beginning of the second trimester. Centering® groups meet 10 times throughout pregnancy and soon after delivery. Each group has a facilitator and a health practitioner. The practitioner, within the group space, completes standard prenatal physical health assessments.

CenteringPregnancy groups provide a richer setting in which women can learn, share, and support one another. This model differs from the exchanges in standard one-on-one prenatal care appointments. When group members share similar concerns and experiences with each other, the peer support can make the whole process of pregnancy feel more normal. Groups provide support to the women and increase individual motivation to learn and make positive change. CenteringPregnancy group discussions address infant mortality risk factors such as smoking, maternal stress, safe sleep, and breastfeeding. Through Centering, women are empowered and socially supported to choose health-promoting behaviors. The specific behavioral targets of a Centering program include the percentage of women who complete the prenatal care and the percentage of women who improve risk and protective behaviors (see intermediate outcomes in Figure 11-10). Health outcomes of this prenatal care model include decreased preterm birth, increased birth weight, and increased gestational age at

Montgomery County, Ohio – Progesterone Therapy for Preventing Preterm Birth in Vulnerable Populations

Goals:

1. To reduce preterm birth through the prescribed administration of progesterone to women who are candidates for treatment.
2. To reduce inequalities in preterm birth and infant mortality.

Inputs/Resources	Activities	Outputs	Outcomes
<u>Pregnant women</u> • Pregnant women — Medicaid — Uninsured <u>Health care providers</u> • Participating health centers — Providers — Care managers — Administrative staff • "Change agents" • Social support service providers • Referring healthcare and social service providers • Medicaid insurance providers • Medical records • Reimbursement for treatment <u>Implementation and evaluation Supports</u> • CityMatCH resources • Evidence-based interventions for vulnerable populations • Treatment algorithms • Epidemiologist • Foundations • Hospitals/birthing centers	• Identify, recruit, train, & task improved birth outcome "change agents" • Outreach to women of childbearing age by change agents • Health center outreach and site recruitment • Partnerships with Centers developed • Provider, care manager, and staff education • Patient education • Screening for progesterone therapy eligibility • Care management to patients (which includes: Medication administration, Patient follow up, and Adherence monitoring) <u>Communication</u> • Assessment of appropriate targets & message • Develop messages to be delivered • Develop database of partners	• # of change agents recruited • # of participating health centers • # training sessions completed & # and type of participants • # and type of patient education & outreach materials finalized & distributed • # of women initiating prenatal care • # of pregnant women identified as candidates for treatment • # of standardized progesterone treatment algorithms developed and initiated • # and type of care management instances provided <u>Communication</u> • # and type of communications delivered • # of community champions	<u>Short Term</u> • % pregnant women enrolled into prenatal care who are aware of importance of progesterone therapy • % pregnant women who initiate progesterone therapy • % of health care staff who have knowledge of the role of 17P and transvaginal progesterone in preventing preterm birth • % of women who receive ultrasounds between 16–24 weeks to measure cervix length • # and % of pregnant women recommended for progesterone therapy receiving shots weekly from diagnosis to delivery • Number of providers and sites in which progesterone therapy and care management are available (treatment capacity) <u>Intermediate</u> • Adherence score for pregnant women receiving progesterone therapy • Mean adherence score for pregnant women receiving therapy by participating health center • Percentage of women eligible for progesterone therapy who complete the therapy

Figure 11-9 Progesterone Therapy Logic Model

continues

Montgomery County, Ohio – Progesterone Therapy for Preventing Preterm Birth in Vulnerable Populations

Inputs/Resources	Activities	Outputs	Outcomes
	• Create communication products • Disseminate media products Infrastructure supports • Program adherence monitoring • Data collection • Evaluation • Identifying potential funding sources/ revenue streams	Infrastructure support • Written reports • Data (patient and aggregate) regarding performance • Information usable for quality improvement • Distilled best practices/ lessons learned • Grant applications	Long term • % of deliveries ≥ 37 weeks of gestational age among women by race/ethnicity • % of deliveries ≥ 32 weeks of gestational age among women by race/ethnicity • % of newborns born weighing ≥ 1500 grams (VLBW) among women by race/ ethnicity • % of newborns born weighing ≥ 2500 grams (LBW) among women by race/ ethnicity

Assumptions

1. External funds and well-placed change agents can facilitate behavior change
2. Awareness, normative and facility barriers to participating in prenatal care
3. Pregnant women are able and willing to initiate and then sustain treatment
4. Health centers and providers are amenable to changing practice
5. Support services are accessible and utilized by patients

Contextual Factors

1. Social norms and personal experiences of the target population
2. Politics
3. Service and pharmacy reimbursement
4. Availability of medication

Figure 11-9 (continued)

delivery (Centering Healthcare Institute, 2014; Tanner-Smith, Steinka-Fry, & Lipsey, 2013).

Thirteen essential elements (see Table 11-7) define the Centering model of care. These elements highlight the important social network aspects of this model of care delivery. Centering is more than meeting in a group—it involves how the group is facilitated. Group meetings are conducted in a circle with ample opportunities for socializing and establishing strong social ties. Information about self-care and infant care is discussed, not lectured or taught. Members own the group, and the leader is there as a facilitator and resource guide.

Primary activities of the CenteringPregnancy intervention involve recruiting and training clinical staff, reaching out to women of childbearing age in the community, and establishing Centering group care meetings (see Figure 11-10). Factors associated with successful CenteringPregnancy

---

TABLE 11-7 Centering Healthcare's 13 Essential Elements

1. Health assessment occurs within the group space.

2. Participants are involved in self-care activities.

3. A facilitative leadership style is used.

4. The group is conducted in a circle.

5. Each session has an overall plan.

6. Attention is given to the core content, although emphasis may vary.

7. There is stability of group leadership.

8. Group conduct honors the contribution of each member.

9. The composition of the group is stable, not rigid.

10. Group size is optimal to promote the process.

11. Involvement of support people is optional.

12. Opportunity for socializing with the group is provided.

13. There is ongoing evaluation of outcomes.

Source: Centering Healthcare Institute.

---

implementation include acceptance of the group care model, ease of keeping longer Centering group meeting appointments, and possibly transportation and child care issues. Key outputs of the activities include number of pregnant women beginning Centering care, number of Centering group sessions conducted, and number of participants per session.

Short-term outcomes measure the antecedents that influence motivation, ability, and support for completing a Centering program. The indicators to be measured include knowledge among pregnant women of the importance of prenatal care, improved patient satisfaction, and the creation of a network of social support for the pregnant women. The Centering model establishes a supportive social environment for self and infant care. A secondary behavioral outcome of the program is change in maternal risk and protective factors. Specifically, changes in maternal stress and coping, substance use, nutrition, tobacco, and breastfeeding are of interest. The third behavioral measure of great interest is attendance at a postpartum visit. After the baby is born, mothers attend another group session that transitions maternal and infant care into an important part of the continuum of care and outcomes. Through the supportive environment previously established, new mothers share information and seek information and resources related to motherhood and infant care.

The logic models for both (see Figures 11-9 and 11-10) interventions were developed through a planning process. The coalition began with resources from the IEBO and then created models for the local initiative. System supports and evaluation were an important grouping or story line on each model. Epidemiologists and program evaluators from a local university, health department, and state health department are responsible for the process and impact monitoring of the project. As one of four nationally selected community projects, this work aimed not only to improve birth outcomes in Montgomery County but also to add to the evidence base for other communities to follow. The models also served as a communication tool within the coalition and the outside groups. The logic models clearly described the behavioral targets and the activities, inputs, and behavioral assumption on which the program was grounded.

Policy and Systems Change

Policy, systems, and environmental changes have the most widespread impact on a population health issue, and infant

Montgomery County, Ohio - Centering Pregnancy® (CP) for Preventing Preterm Birth

Goals:
1. To reduce preterm birth
2. To reduce inequalities in preterm birth
3. To expand the use of the CenteringPregnancy® group prenatal care model in Montgomery County (system change)

Inputs/Resources	Activities	Outputs	Outcomes
Pregnant nulliparous women • Medicaid • Uninsured • Childcare • Transportation Health care providers • Participating health centers — CP® coordinator — CP® facilitator — Providers — Administrative Staff • "Change agents" • Social support service providers • Referring healthcare & social service providers System supports and evaluation • Insurance companies • CP® expert/consultant • CP® training • Meeting space, supplies, & food • Reimbursement for services • Medical records	CenteringPregnancy® • Identify, recruit, train and task improved birth outcome "change agents" • Identify, recruit, and train health center staff • Outreach to women of childbearing age by "change agents" & screening at health centers • Implement Centering group sessions — Health assessment — Self-care activities — Education — Sharing/Socialization • Facilitate partnerships among prenatal providers • Develop referral network Communication • Assessment of appropriate targets & message • Develop messages to be delivered • Develop database of partners	CenteringPregnancy® • # of change agents recruited • # of participating health centers • # of training sessions completed and # and type of participants • # of pregnant women screened at health centers • # of pregnant women referred to CP • # of pregnant women beginning CP • Average gestational age of pregnant women enrolled in CP • # of CP groups started (and size) • # and type of CP sessions conducted • # of participants per session Communication • # and type of communications delivered • # of community champions	Short Term • % of pregnant women enrolled in CP who are aware of importance of early entry and maintenance of prenatal care • # and % of women enrolled in CP satisfied with their experience in the program • Average # of sessions attended by women enrolled in CP • % of pregnant women enrolled in CP who report a support network for delivery and post-partum care. • % of women who initiate a trial health promotion behavior Intermediate • % of pregnant women who complete CP • % of pregnant women enrolled in CP who improve health behaviors: alcohol and other substance use, tobacco, nutrition, stress/coping, and breastfeeding • % of women enrolled in CP completing a postpartum visit Long Term • % of deliveries ≥ 37 weeks of gestational age among women by race/ethnicity • % of deliveries ≥ 32 weeks of gestational age among women by race/ethnicity

Figure 11-10 CenteringPregnancy® Logic Model

continues

Inputs/Resources	Activities	Outputs	Outcomes
• CityMatCH resources • Epidemiologist • Funding for start-up & other expenses • HCP education materials	• Create communication products • Disseminate media products Infrastructure support • Data collection & evaluation • Written reports/ reporting • Quality improvement • Identifying potential funding sources/ revenue streams to ensure sustainability • Advocacy for CP adoption	Infrastructure support • Written reports • Data (pt. & aggregate) regarding performance • Information usable for quality improvement • Distilled best practices/ lessons learned • Grant applications	• % of newborns born weighing ≥ 1500 grams (VLBW) among women by race/ ethnicity • % of newborns born weighing ≥ 2500 grams (LBW) among women by race/ ethnicity • % change in disparity in pre-term birth, VLBW, and LBW by race/ethnicity

Assumptions

1. Pregnant women are receptive to participating in CenteringPregnancy®.
2. Healthcare clinics and staff are committed to implementing & sustaining the CenteringPregnancy® model.
3. Support services are accessible and utilized by patients.
4. Change agents can facilitate & nurture behavior change.
5. Social support from peers and the establishment of a social network facilitate prenatal care and other behavior change.
6. Trial of healthy behaviors and cessation of other behaviors can be prompted and supported by peers.

Contextual Factors

1. Social norms & personal experiences of the target population
2. CenteringPregnancy® services are billable

Figure 11-10 (continued)

mortality is no exception. The infant mortality reduction interventions chosen by the IMC, progesterone therapy and CenteringPregnancy, included both policy and system changes. Policy and system supports provide the context from which the interventions were implemented and maintained. Neither of these interventions would have worked in the long term without system supports and policy interventions.

The progesterone therapy intervention was driven by policy change. This was seen mainly in the adoption of a standardized clinical screening algorithm for providers to use with all newly pregnant women. After the new screening process was made official clinical policy, the new way in which pregnant women were screened improved diagnosis of risk factors for preterm birth. Since adoption of the process, all women, instead of some, have been screened specifically for a history of a previous preterm birth and for short cervix length to see if they are eligible for progesterone therapy. Changing the policy to universal screening identified more women who were eligible for progesterone therapy, and if providers continue to adhere to it, it will have a broader impact on preterm birth and infant mortality than previous policy.

The CenteringPregnancy intervention is a total system change for prenatal care delivery. The Centering Healthcare Institute prides itself on transforming health care through disruptive system design (Rising, Kennedy, & Klima, 2004). The way appointments are planned, scheduled, timed—as well as their content—is a complete change from traditional prenatal care. Methods of staff scheduling, space needs and allocation, and other details need to be worked out before CenteringPregnancy can be implemented. This can be a challenging process for providers to engage in after being used to another method. In the long run, however, a successful system change to CenteringPregnancy can improve many outcomes for patients and increase satisfaction of both the patients and providers.

Current Project Status

The progesterone therapy and CenteringPregnancy intervention activities started in earnest in May 2014. The clinic partners started actively widening coverage of progesterone treatment and investigating broader payment coverage options. Progesterone in Montgomery County became part of a statewide initiative that has received Medicaid funding. CenteringPregnancy training for clinic partners was completed

over the summer of 2014, and new Centering groups started in late 2014. The Infant Mortality Coalition hosted site visits from CityMatCH in both June and October 2014. The first site visit involved a working meeting regarding the next steps and evaluation planning. A community forum was scheduled in the intervention target community area to share information about the infant mortality situation and ask for community input regarding the best ways to engage community members. The second site visit was a community training related to issues of institutionalized racism and the part it plays in community health improvement efforts.

Lessons Learned

Embarking on a community-wide intervention is often challenging. The rewards in community health, however, make this type of endeavor worth pursuing. From the experience of developing an infant mortality initiative, as well as other health initiatives in Montgomery County, many lessons have been learned. A few of the key lessons are discussed here.

Earn the Trust of Your Community

According to PHDMC Commissioner Jim Gross, earning the trust of the community is the first and most important step to building a public health system. Without trust, the leading organization will be unable to create the relationships necessary to foster meaningful collaborations. This requisite trust requires the leading organization to establish an understandable vision for the creation of a healthier community. The organization and community members must work every day with integrity and in an unbiased manner, focusing entirely on serving the citizens efficiently and effectively. Once trust has been established, an organization's ability to create partnerships and lead population-based health improvements is achievable. Without the respect of the community, fewer people will participate, and they will be less engaged with the initiative's efforts (J. Gross, personal communication, April 22, 2014).

Use Data to Make Decisions

Thorough analysis of high-quality data forms a solid foundation for any public health initiative. Data provide the basis for what health problems should be addressed in the community, as well as the who, what, when, and where of the problem. When beginning any coalition or task force, it is a good idea to begin the first few meetings with a detailed data analysis of the health issue in the community. The data analysis could identify health disparities within the community, specific areas in the community where there is an excess of the health problem being addressed, and risk factors associated with the health problem. Review of data also ensures that the coalition is fully aware of the health issue in the community and that all are on the same level of understanding. Data will thus help address the health problem in the community more effectively and gain buy-in from coalition members who might not be as aware of the health issue. When the IMC began meeting monthly, approximately half of each of the first six meetings was spent reviewing data. This included overall infant mortality data for the community, state, and nation, followed by more specific analyses related to risk factors, mapping, and disparities.

A Champion for the Health Issue

Community-wide campaigns need a champion or multiple champions. Champions are credible community members—whether appointed or assumed leaders—who can be counted upon to speak enthusiastically in support of the cause. They often become the face and messenger of the cause. They may be appointed leaders such as elected officials, a fire chief, executive directors, or school superintendents. Alternatively, they may be assumed leaders such as a mail carrier, a teacher, or a physician who knows everyone in the community and has the confidence of the community. Champions can help the cause in several ways by:

- Recruiting new members or volunteers
- Raising resources
- Increasing public awareness of the cause
- Making formal and informal presentations
- Serving as board or advisory council members
- Increasing support for the organization
- Initiating new relationships to help the cause

To be most effective in a community, the person or people leading the coalition should be champions of the cause. It is also good to have champions as other members of the coalition. The heads of the IMC in Montgomery County were the health commissioner and the director of health initiatives at the area hospital association. Both had decision-making capabilities for organizations that were pivotal in the efforts to reduce infant mortality, and both were well known and respected in the community.

Leaders for the Intervention Efforts

Once goals have been developed and interventions selected, there is a need for people with expertise in specific interventions to head up implementation. This could be an individual or a team. Montgomery County has an implementation team that includes eight members. The team meets more frequently than the IMC, and, in addition to leading the intervention efforts, they also attend CityMatCH trainings, webinars, and conference calls as part of the IEBO. This team includes experts in the medical field, epidemiology, health care program management, and policy implementation.

Additionally, if there is a content expert on the subject of the intervention, having him or her as part of the effort will increase the capacity to proceed and will likely speed up the process. These experts provide valuable knowledge on the many details that will come up as the intervention is implemented, and their experience will help avoid pitfalls as well as provide connections to other experts who can provide additional expertise. In Montgomery County, two content experts are part of the coalition: a physician expert in implementing progesterone therapy and a nurse midwife currently running a CenteringPregnancy program at a local obstetrics and gynecology practice.

Patience

Community-wide health improvement projects require patience. System change and changes in upstream factors take time and most often occur in incremental steps. The work of one agency may move more quickly than others; however, that quicker agency is unlikely to achieve population-level changes in health status on its own. The involvement of representative groups can increase the time needed for accomplishing tasks. Calling meetings, sharing information across and within organizations, building consensus, and gathering resources will likely require more time when more partners are involved. The trade-off for time and patience, though, can be the achievement of a sustainable change.

Perseverance is needed. There are often lag periods when it does not seem that much is happening toward improving outcomes. During these times, it is good to look at incremental progress that is being made. For example, it could take several months to have a few key meetings between organizations that result in an agreement being reached that will allow the initiative to take the next important step.

It is unreasonable to expect to see population health impacted in the first years of a community initiative. Implementing a community-wide initiative takes significant time. Find ways to keep the coalition and community engaged in the effort. Celebrate smaller goals that take less time to achieve in order to demonstrate that progress has been made toward the overarching goal. For example, the first goal that the Montgomery County IMC achieved was selection into the national IEBO. Next was identification of the appropriate infant mortality reduction initiatives to be used in the community, which was followed by the development of clinical partnerships for the initiatives. The next milestones to be celebrated were the completion of CenteringPregnancy training and startup of new Centering groups.

SUMMARY

Infant mortality is one of the two primary measures of population health. The community of Montgomery County targeted initiatives toward decreasing pre-term birth in order to accomplish the overall goals of decreasing overall infant mortality and the racial disparities that exist in infant mortality rates. Implementing community-wide interventions presents considerable challenges and requires perseverance of effort. To positively transform the health and well-being of the community, women's health must be improved, and inequities must be decreased. While Montgomery County has made some significant strides toward addressing the infant mortality situation, much more needs to be done. Underlying all of the infant mortality reduction efforts is the ultimate benefit for the community—reducing the number of babies that die before their first birthday. With approximately 60 babies dying per year in Montgomery County, that is about three kindergarten classes that will not start in the next 5 years. The costs to the community are immeasurable when children never get to start school, learn, and grow up as productive, contributing citizens.

IN THE CLASSROOM ACTIVITIES

1) Visit the County Health Rankings website. Go to Measures and locate infant mortality data (in Additional Measures then Health Outcomes) for your county and state. How do the rates vary across the state, and how does your state's data compare to other states? Locate low birth weight data (Health Outcomes then Quality Of Life). What are the trends in birth weight?

2) Visit your state health department's website and locate infant mortality data. What are the actual causes of death? Are there similar trends in disparities?

3) List the behavioral risk factors for infant death. How might social factors alter a person's ability to cease unhealthy behaviors and/or initiate a healthy behavior?

4) Visit the Unnatural Causes: Is Inequality Making Us Sick? California Newsreel documentary site. Watch the episode *When the Bough Breaks* that explores the impact of racism on infant mortality. Download the discussion guides and share your thoughts about the comprehension questions.

5) Visit the CityMatCH website and watch or read *A Gardener's Tale*, Dr. Camara Jones' presentation about the impacts of racism on the nation's health and well-being. (http://www.citymatch.org/special-reports/gardeners-tale-dr-camara-jones)

6) In teams of five, play the Life Course game, which is available for download through CityMatCH (Life Course Toolbox, http://www.citymatch.org:8080/lifecoursetoolbox/index.php). After completing the game, discuss the following questions: What events in the game reminded you of something from your own life? What aspects of the game caught your attention? What issues or concepts does the game help illustrate?

7) Use the outcome logic models in this chapter (Figures 11-9 and 11-10) to check your understanding. Link the assumptions and contextual factors to theoretical constructs and categories within the PER worksheet. What activities align to the theoretical constructs? How do the behavioral targets differ in the two models?

WEB LINKS

Child Trends: http://www.childtrends.org

CityMatCH: http://www.citymatch.org

County Health Rankings & Roadmaps Project at the University of Wisconsin Population Health Institute: www.countyhealthrankings.org

Federal Interagency Forum on Child and Family Statistics: http://childstats.gov

Public Health, Dayton & Montgomery County: http://www.phdmc.org

Public Health, Dayton & Montgomery County health reports: http://www.phdmc.org/health-reports

Unnatural Causes... is inequality making us sick? Documentaries: www.unnaturalcauses.org

REFERENCES

Blaxter, M. (1981). The health of children: *A review of research on the place of health in cycles of disadvantage.* London: Heinemann Educational, 1981.

California Newsreel. (2008). *When the bough breaks, Unnatural causes: Is inequality making us sick?* Available from www.unnaturalcauses.org

Centering Healthcare Institute. (2014). *Centering: Model overview.* Retrieved from http://www.centeringhealthcare.org.

Centers for Disease Control and Prevention (CDC). (2004). Spina bifida and anencephaly before and after folic acid mandate: United States, 1995–1996 and 1999–2000. *Morbidity and Mortality Weekly, 53*(17), 362–365.

Centers for Disease Control and Prevention (CDC). (2009). National Center for Health Statistics CDC Wonder On-line Database, compiled from Compressed Mortality File 1999–2006 (Series 20 No. 2L, 2009) http://wonder.cdc.gov/cmf-icd10-archive2006.html

Centers for Disease Control and Prevention (CDC). (2010). *Behavioral Risk Factor Surveillance System.* Retrieved from http://www.cdc.gov/brfss/

Centers for Disease Control and Prevention (CDC). (2012). *Infant and perinatal mortality and the environment.* National Center for Environmental Health, Environmental Health Tracking Branch. Retrieved from http://ephtracking.cdc.gov/showRbInfantMortalityEnv.action

Centers for Disease Control and Prevention (CDC). (2013). *Reproductive health.* Retrieved from http://www.cdc.gov/reproductivehealth

Centers for Disease Control and Prevention (CDC). (2014). Web-Based Injury Statistics Query and Reporting System (WISQARS). Retrieved from http://www.cdc.gov/injury/wisqars/index.html

Chen, A., & Rogan, W. J. (2004). Breastfeeding and the risk of postneonatal death in the United States. *Pediatrics, 113*(5), e435–e439.

David, R., & Collins, J. (2007). Disparities in infant mortality: What's genetics got to do with it? *American Journal of Public Health, 97*(7), 1191–1197.

Fine, A., & Kotelchuck, M. (2010). *Rethinking MCH: The life course model as an organizing framework.* U.S. Department of Health and Human Services, Health Resources and Services Administration. Retrieved from http://mchb.hrsa.gov/lifecourse/rethinkingmchlifecourse.pdf

Gilbert, C., & Kasehagen, L. (2013a). *Strategies for improving birth outcome inequities.* CityMatCH Institute for Equity in Birth Outcomes, Training #1, Omaha, NE, April 29–May 2. Retrieved from http://www.citymatch.org/projects/iebo/institute-training

Gilbert, C., & Kasehagen, L. (2013b). *Frameworks for improving birth outcome inequities.* CityMatCH Institute for Equity in Birth Outcomes, Training #1, Omaha, NE, April 29–May 2. Retrieved from http://www.citymatch.org/projects/iebo/institute-training

Hoyert, D. L., & Xu, J. Q. (2012). Deaths: Preliminary data for 2011. *National Vital Statistics Reports, 61*(6).

Institute of Medicine (IOM). (2012). *Primary care and public health: Exploring integration to improve population health.* Washington, DC: National Academies Press.

Jones, C. P. (2000). Levels of racism: A theoretic framework and a gardener's tale. *American Journal of Public Health, 90*(8), 1212–1215.

Likis, F. E., Andrews, J. C., Woodworth, A. L., Velez Edwards, D. R., Jerome, R. N., Fonnesbeck, C. J., …Hartmann, K. E. (2012). Progestogens for prevention of preterm birth. *Comparative Effectiveness Review, 74* (AHRQ Publication No. 12-EHC105-EF). Rockville, MD: Agency for Healthcare Research and Quality. Retrieved from www.effectivehealthcare.ahrq.gov/reports/final.cfm

Loggins, S., & Andrade, F. C. (2014). Despite an overall decline in U.S. infant mortality rates, the black/white disparity persists: Recent trends and future projections. *Journal of Community Health, 39*(1), 118–123.

Lu, M. C., & Halfon, N. (2003). Racial and ethnic disparities in birth outcomes: A life-course perspective. *Maternal Child Health Journal, 7*, 13–30.

Lu, M. C., Kotelchuck, M., Hogan, V., Jones, L., Wright, K., & Halfon, N. (2010). Closing the black–white gap in birth outcomes: A life-course approach. *Ethnicity & Disease, 20*(S2), 62–76.

MacDorman, M. F., Hoyert, D. L., & Mathews, T. J. (2013). *Recent declines in infant mortality in the United States, 2005–2011* (NCHS data brief, No. 120). Hyattsville, MD: National Center for Health Statistics.

MacDorman, M. F., & Mathews, T. J. (2009). The challenge of infant mortality: Have we reached a plateau? *Public Health Reports, 124*, 670–681.

MacDorman, M. F., & Mathews, T. J. (2011). Understanding racial and ethnic disparities in U.S. infant mortality rates (NCHS data brief, No. 74). Hyattsville, MD: National Center for Health Statistics.

Mathews, T. J., & MacDorman, M. F. (2013). Infant mortality statistics from the 2010 period linked birth/infant death data set. *National Vital Statistics Reports, 62*(8).

Murphy, S. L., Xu, J. Q., & Kochanek, K. D. (2013). Deaths: Final data for 2010. *National Vital Statistics Reports, 61*(4).

Ohio Department of Health, Office of Vital Statistics. (2012). *Neonatal, postneonatal, and infant mortality, Ohio and Selected counties, 2007–2012.* Retrieved from http://www.odh.ohio.gov/odhprograms/cfhs/octpim/latestoimd.aspx

Rising, S. S., Kennedy, H. P., & Klima, C. S. (2004). Redesigning prenatal care through CenteringPregnancy. *Journal of Midwifery & Women's Health, 49*(5), 398–404.

Shapiro-Mendoza, C. K., Tomashek, K. M., Anderson, R. N., & Wingo, J. (2006). Recent national trends in sudden, unexpected infant deaths: More evidence supporting a change in classification or reporting. *American Journal of Epidemiology, 163*(8), 762–769.

Tanner-Smith, E. E., Steinka-Fry, K. T., & Lipsey, M. W. (2013). The effects of CenteringPregnancy group prenatal care on gestational age, birth weight, and fetal demise. *Maternal & Child Health Journal, 18*, 801–809.

U.S. Census Bureau. (2014). *State & County QuickFacts: Montgomery County, Ohio.* Retrieved from http://quickfacts.census.gov/qfd/states/39/39113.html

U.S. Department of Health and Human Services (USDHHS). (n.d). *Prenatal services.* Maternal and Child Health Bureau, Health Resources and Services Administration. Retrieved from http://mchb.hrsa.gov/programs/womeninfants/prenatal.html

Williams, S. C. P. (2013). Gone too soon: What's behind the high U.S. infant mortality rate. *Stanford Medicine, 30*(3), 12. Retrieved from http://stanmed.stanford.edu/2013fall/documents/medmag_fall2013.pdf

GLOSSARY

A

ACE: Adverse childhood experiences that include childhood physical, emotional, or sexual abuse; witnessing domestic violence; and growing up with household substance abuse, mental illness, parental divorce, and/or an incarcerated household member.

Action: A stage of change in which a person is actively changing a health behavior. The behavior is performed at a risk-reducing level. This stage (action) follows the stage of preparation.

Activities: Planned actions to produce desirable changes in antecedents, the factors that influence health behaviors.

Activities of daily living: Basic self-care activities that include getting around inside the home, getting in and out of bed, bathing, dressing, eating, and toileting.

Actor: Term for a person in a social network.

Allostasis: Process by which the body responds to stressors in order to regain balance and stability.

Allostatic load: Wear and tear on the body that grows over time when an individual is exposed to repeated or chronic stress.

Antecedents: A range of factors that precede or influence risk and protective factors. Behavioral antecedents reflect knowledge, beliefs, demographic characteristics, skills, resources, reminders, reinforcements, and social support.

Appraisal support: Information from another that aids in self-evaluation.

Attitude: A feeling toward a person or thing. As a construct of the theory of planned behavior, attitude reflects the anticipated outcomes from the performance of a particular behavior.

Attributed: An outcome closely associated with a specific causative factor.

B

Baseline: Initial level or frequency of an indicator.

Behavioral building blocks: Antecedents or groupings of antecedents that are the foundation of the development of the logic model. Behavioral building blocks establish the initial framework from which other antecedents and relationships are displayed.

Behavioral capability: A person's ability to perform a given action, such as a skill.

Built environment: The part of the physical environment that is constructed by human activity. Elements of the built environment consist of the distribution of buildings (such as houses, schools, and businesses); the creation of spaces (such as parks, retail, open space, and aesthetic qualities); and transportation systems (including roads, public transportation, sidewalks, and bike paths).

C

CenteringPregnancy®: A group prenatal care model that empowers women to make healthier choices and provides strong social network support.

Centrality: Degree to which a person is centrally located in a network.

Chronic disease: A health condition that is slow in progression, is long on duration, is void of spontaneous resolution, and often limits the function, productivity, and quality of life of the individual who lives with it.

Cluster: A group of nodes. Each node is connected to at least one other node in the group.

Coalition: A group of people or agencies formed around a common purpose, often guided by large representative steering or advisory committees.

Cognitions: Activities of thinking, understanding, learning, and remembering.

Cohesion: The interconnectedness and solidarity of network actors; a function of the strength of ties, distance, and density.

Collective efficacy: A group's shared belief in its shared capabilities to organize and execute the courses of action required to produce given levels of attainment.

Community: A group of people with a common trait, experience, or interest.

Community assessment: Description of a community based on data from a broad range of sources. Included in the description are health-related factors and resources.

Community health workers: Members of a community who have been trained to assist in the implementation of a range of health promotion, screening, and basic medical care programs.

Community mobilization: A category of health promotion intervention in which members of the target audience assist in program implementation.

Community readiness: Degree to which a community is prepared to take action on a specific issue.

Concepts: Broad categories of elements within a theory.

Congenital malformations: Birth defects.

Constructs: Specific elements (antecedents) named within a theory.

Contemplation: A stage of change in which a person is thinking about changing a health behavior. This stage (contemplation) precedes the stage of preparation.

Contextual evidence: Information about the community. Contextual conditions for an intervention are important to consider when selecting interventions.

Cues to action: Simple actions or events that nudge or remind an individual to engage in a specific health behavior.

D

Decisional balance: Cognitive process of weighing the pros and cons of behavioral change.

Default: What the chooser will receive if he or she does nothing. The default option is the option that requires the least effort.

Density: The number of connections in the network as a proportion of those possible.

Determinant: The range of personal, social, and environmental factors that determine the health status of individuals or populations.

Diffusion: Process by which an innovation moves through channels of a social system.

Disability: A temporary or long-term reduction in a person's capacity to function. Persons with disabilities may experience limitations in hearing, vision, mobility, or cognition. They may also experience emotional or behavioral disorders.

Dissemination: Active process of using planned strategies to spread information to promote adoption of ideas and actions.

Distance: The number of steps connecting two people. Social distance is the number steps, or degrees of separation, between two people in a network. Geographic distance is the physical dispersion of members.

Downstream factor: Actions more closely linked to health outcomes. These actions are often seen as the "cause" of health conditions but may in fact be only symptoms.

Dynamic: Changing, not static.

E

Early adopters: Individuals who adopt innovations early in the process of diffusion, second only to innovators.

Early life: Childhood experiences; in a life course perspective of health, early experiences include developmental experiences as well as economic and social experiences.

Early majority: Individuals who adopt an innovation after early adopters and just before the average person.

Emotional support: The things that people do to make us feel loved and cared for and bolster a sense of self-worth.

Enabling factors: Environmental and skill-type antecedents that allow a person to accomplish a behavior.

Enactive attainment: Developing efficacy through one's own experiences.

Environment: Elements external to one's self consisting of physical surroundings as well as other people, cultural influences, and media.

Evidence: Some form of data for use in making judgments and decisions.

Evidence-based public health: The use of information related to health status, determinants of health, and interventions to make decisions about public health practice.

Experiential evidence: Evidence that comes from the prior experiences, skills, and insights of professionals.

Extrinsic: Factors external to a person.

F

Facilitation: The provision of resources, tools, or environmental change.

Fidelity: The degree to which a program was implemented as planned.

G

Geographic distance: Physical dispersion of members of a social network.

Geographic Information System (GIS): A tool to map various disease incidences and neighborhood properties such as connected streets, public transportation, and retail establishments.

Goals: Statements of desired outcomes to which people intend to commit action.

Gradient: A pattern of increase or decrease in a variable. In population health, a socioeconomic gradient in health refers to the pattern of health outcomes that corresponds to the socioeconomic position; generally as socioeconomic position improves, measured health improves in a stepwise fashion.

H

Habit: Established behavior pattern marked by increasing automaticity, decreasing awareness, and partial independence from reinforcement.

Health: A state of complete physical, mental, and social well-being; not merely the absence of disease or other infirmity.

Health behavior: An activity undertaken by an individual or group that promotes, protects, or maintains health.

Health communication: A category of health promotion intervention using communication strategies to inform and influence decisions that affect health.

Health disparity: A particular type of health difference that is closely linked with economic, social, or environmental disadvantage.

Health education: Any combination of planned learning experiences designed to facilitate voluntary changes in health behaviors.

Health engineering: A category of health promotion intervention in which a product or the environment is altered in a manner to meet a behavioral objective. Engineering strategies target access-type and reinforcement antecedents and enable persons to take and maintain action.

Health policy: A category of health promotion interventions in which laws, regulations, or formal and informal rules are established by the government or organizations. Policies alter access-type and reinforcement antecedents.

Homophily: The tendency for people to have relationships with others who have similar attributes.

I

Incentive motivation: The use of rewards and punishments to modify behavior.

Incidence: The number of newly diagnosed cases of disease during a specific time period.

Indicators: Measures that have been selected to represent a targeted variable, such as health status.

Induction: The spread of a behavior or trait from one person to another.

Infant mortality: The death of a child less than 1 year of age.

Influential factors: A component of outcome logic models that summarize key behavioral antecedents featured in a theoretical logical model. Activities are designed to change influential factors.

Informational support: Delivery of advice or information.

Injury: Intentional or unintentional damage or harm to the body resulting in impairment or a diminished level of health.

Innovation: Ideas, practices, or objects that are perceived as new by an individual or other unit of adoption.

Innovators: Initial users of an innovation.

Instrumental activities of daily living: Basic self-care activities associated with living independently. These include going outside the home, managing money, preparing meals, doing housework, taking prescription medications, and using the phone.

Instrumental support: Physical or tangible aid and services.

Intention: A construct of the theory of planned behavior. It signifies motivation and willingness to try or change.

Intermediate objectives: Statements of measurable change in risk or protective factors. Because of the target, these objectives may also be called behavioral objectives or outcome objectives.

Interpersonal: Characteristics of formal and informal relationships with others, including family, friends, co-workers, and peers.

Interventions: Categories of initiatives designed to improve health. Categories of health promotion interventions include health education, health communication, health engineering, health policy, and community mobilization.

Intrapersonal: Characteristics of an individual.

Intrinsic: Factors that originate from within a person.

Isolate: Person not connected to anyone in the network group.

K

Knowledge: The possession of information.

L

Laggards: The last individuals in a system to adopt an innovation.

Late majority: Individuals in a system who adopt an innovation after a majority of the members.

Life course perspective: A multidisciplinary approach to understanding the mental, physical, and social health of individuals. It incorporates both life span and life stage concepts that determine an individual's health trajectory.

Life expectancy: The expected (in the statistical sense) number of years of life remaining at a given age.

Lifestyle behaviors: Behaviors performed frequently and integrated into a way of living.

Lifestyle disease: A health condition in which behavioral factors represent a significant amount of the risk attributed to the condition.

Logic: A reasonable way of thinking or presenting information.

Logic model: A tool used to present a graphic depiction of how a program is supposed to work, including the relationships between inputs, activities, outputs, and outcomes.

Long-term objectives: Statements of measurable change in the expected outcome of the program. Long-term objectives clearly identify the health issue to be altered.

M

Maintenance: A stage of change that represents the integration of a health behavior into a person's lifestyle. This stage (maintenance) follows the stage of action.

Mass media: Radio, television, and/or print media with broad distribution channels.

Mastery: Improved confidence in a skill through the successful completion of the action in a number of situations and contexts.

Measurable: Able to be counted.

Mediate: Process through which variables facilitate change. Changes in a variable are associated with changes in an object of interest, such as a health behavior.

Mediating factor: Variable that explains the relationship between two other variables. Mediating variables act in the middle of the relationship.

Mental health: A state of well-being in which a person realizes his or her

potential, can cope with the normal stresses of life, can work productively and fruitfully, and is able to make a contribution to the community.

Milestone: An event marking a significant point in the process of change.

Mobility: Ability of individuals to move upward in a manner that improves conditions of living and social position.

Models: Graphic depictions of frameworks of large concepts, often from information across theories.

Moderating factor: Variable that influences the strength of a relationship between two other variables.

Modifying factors: Personal characteristics that influence perceived threat.

Morbidity: The number of disease cases during a specific time period.

Mortality: The number of deaths during a specific time period.

N

Node: A person who may or may not be connected to other objects in a network.

O

Objective: Measurable statements that communicate the target of intended change.

Observable: Possible to see or notice.

Observational learning: The process of watching the actions of others and the outcomes associated with the actions.

Operationalize: State in a measurable form.

Outcome evaluation: The collection of information to assess the impact of a program's activities. Outcome measures include indicators of short-term, intermediate (behavioral), and long-term (health) targets. Also called summative evaluations.

Outcome expectations: Beliefs about the likely consequences of a behavioral action.

Outcomes: Multilevel changes in someone or something that result from the program's activities.

Outputs: Direct measurable products of program activities. Outputs are indicators of program implementation, fidelity, and reach.

P

Perceived barriers: Obstacles an individual believes exist for engaging in the health behavior.

Perceived behavioral control: Difficulty a person associates with carrying out a health behavior; it is a reflection of confidence, ability, and opportunity.

Perceived benefits: Positive outcomes an individual believes will occur along with a behavioral action.

Perceived severity: Degree of seriousness an individual associates with experiencing a particular illness, disease, or injury. Severity includes physical as well as social outcomes.

Perceived social support: A person's anticipation of future potential aid.

Perceived susceptibility: Individual's belief about the personal likelihood of experiencing a particular illness or injury.

Perceived threat: Overall perception of the risk associated with a specific health issue or disease, developed as a combination of perceived susceptibility and perceived severity.

PER worksheet: A program planning and evaluation tool that combines constructs from the most popular health behavior theories into one framework and guides learners to organize facts across the different theories into general lay term prompts.

Photovoice: A data collection tool that uses photographs taken and summarized by members of the community.

Physiological arousal: A state of physiological alertness and readiness for action.

Policy: Local, state, and national laws, decisions, and plans that create built and social environments and systems.

Population health: The health outcomes of a group of individuals (a population), including the distribution of health outcomes within the group. Population health approaches seek also to understand the determinants of health and the interventions that impact health determinants.

Precontemplation: A stage of change in which a person is not thinking about or interested in changing a health behavior. This stage (precontemplation) precedes the stage of contemplation.

Predisposing factors: Cognitive, affective, and socio-demographic antecedents related to motivation or rationale for the target behavior.

Preparation: A stage of change that implies preparation for behavior change. This stage (preparation) precedes the stage of action.

Preterm birth: A birth before 37 weeks gestation.

Prevalence: The number of new and pre-existing (total) conditions or diseases in a population on a certain date.

Primary prevention: An approach that aims to prevent the incidence of disease, injury, and disability by promoting good health behaviors.

Prioritization: Interpreting information within the community health assessment and selecting priorities of action.

Procedural knowledge: Knowledge of how to do something.

Process evaluation: The collection of information (outputs) to assess how a program is implemented and the reach of the strategies. Also called formative or implementation evaluations.

Process measure: *See* outputs.

Progesterone: A hormone that is instrumental in sustaining pregnancy.

Program: A set of planned activities implemented over time to achieve specific objectives.

Protective factor: A behavior, trait, or environmental exposure that is associated with a lowered occurrence of a particular disease, injury, or other health condition.

R

Received social support: Support resources that have actually been received.

Reciprocal determinism: The bidirectional interactions of behavior, cognitions, and environmental influences in which factors operate interactively as determinants of each other.

Reciprocity: Degree to which social support and resources move both ways between actors in a network.

Reinforcements: Actions or consequences that occur after a behavior is performed.

Reinforcing factors: Actions from others or the environment related to the continuation or repetitiveness of the target behavior.

Relative risk: The measured association (relationship) between risk factors and a particular disease.

Resources: Financial, personnel, and in-kind resources from any source that are invested into a program.

Risk: The probability that an event will occur.

Risk factor: A behavior, trait, or environmental exposure that is associated with an increase in the occurrence of a particular disease, injury, or other health condition.

S

Secondary prevention: An approach that aims to identify and treat asymptomatic persons who have developed risk factors but in whom the health condition is not evident.

Self-efficacy: An individual's confidence in his or her ability to perform specific tasks or behaviors.

Self-regulation: The ability to set goals, track progress, and solve problems toward a behavioral target.

Sequence: A successive order of two or more items.

Shapeable: Alterable.

Short-term objectives: Statements of measurable change in activity targets, typically knowledge, beliefs, skills, resources, social support, and/or reinforcements.

Small media: Campaigns of small scope and distribution; mediums include patient education materials, fact sheets, newsletters, posters, displays, presentations, and promotional items such as pencils, magnets, and T-shirts.

Social capital: Social resources and benefits that emerge from strong social ties or social cohesion and facilitate collective action.

Social cohesion: Extent of connectedness and solidarity among members of the population.

Social determinant of health: The complex, integrated, and overlapping social structures and economic systems responsible for most health inequities. These social structures and economic systems include the social environment, physical environment, health services, and structural and societal factors. Social determinants of health are shaped by the distribution of money, power, and resources throughout local communities, nations, and the world.

Social engagement: Participation with other persons for companionship, activity, and completion of life tasks.

Social environment: People and relationship attributes of the environment.

Social influence: The normative guidance, from direct and indirect interactions, of a group.

Social integration: Participation in a broad range of relationships.

Social marketing: A particular form of health communication that applies commercial marketing techniques to campaigns designed to promote voluntary behavior change conducive to health.

Social networks: The structure, or the frame, of social relationships.

Social support: The various types of aid and assistance exchanged through social relationships. Emotional, instrumental, informational, and appraisal are specific types of social support.

Socioeconomic position: A composition of many individual concepts, the foundations being education, income, occupation and a prestige-based measure like rank or status in a social hierarchy.

Stages of change: A concept of the transtheoretical model stating that individuals go through a process of behavior change.

Strategy: General tactics within programs to achieve stated objectives and goals. Within programs, strategies can be grouped by type, such as media campaigns and policy advocacy.

Subjective norm: Pressure an individual perceives to perform or not perform a certain behavior. Subjective norm has been described as the perceived acceptability of a behavior within a specific community.

Sudden infant death syndrome (SIDS): The sudden death of an infant less than 1 year of age that cannot be explained after a thorough investigation is conducted, including a complete autopsy, examination of the death scene, and review of the clinical history.

System: A set of interconnected elements operating on multiple levels of influence and organized around a purpose or function.

T

Target: A desired amount.

Temptation: Challenge faced by an individual making a behavior change. It refers to the strength of the impulse to return to previous unhealthy behaviors when in a challenging or stressful situation.

Tertiary prevention: An approach that aims to minimize the negative effects of disease, prevent future complications/progressions, and restore function.

Theoretical logic model: A specific form of logic model that depicts a detailed explanation of the target behavior or environmental condition.

Theory: A set of interrelated concepts, definitions, and propositions that explain or predict events by specifying relationships among variables.

Ties: A social network term to represent relationships between people.

Toxic stress: Severe, chronic stress that becomes toxic to developing brains and biological systems.

Trajectories: Paths that are determined by one's previous experiences; current and future opportunities and resources available to a person on his or her path are based on prior experiences.

Trial use: To try out or experiment with a health behavior. Trial use is often a behavioral milestone in health behavior change.

Triangulation: Use of multiple sources of data for the same indicator.

U

Upstream factor: Issues or conditions located "up river," away from the person or object of interest. They may be out of immediate eyesight but can represent root causes of a health condition or circumstance.

V

Variable: A defined element that can vary in value. In relationship to health behavior theory, variables are content-specific versions of theoretical constructs.

Verbal persuasion: Information communicated via directions, encouragement, and feedback from another. Verbal persuasion, also called social persuasion, improves confidence, particularly when the action is within one's skill level.

Vicarious experiences: Watching, hearing about, or reading about someone else's experiences; can be a means for developing self-efficacy.

INDEX

Page numbers followed by "f" indicate figure; and those followed by "t" indicate table.